Orbit, Eyelids, and Lacrimal System

BASIC AND CLINICAL SCIENCE COURSE

Section 7

2012–2013

(Last major revision 2011–2012)

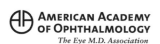
AMERICAN ACADEMY OF OPHTHALMOLOGY
The Eye M.D. Association

LEO

LIFELONG
EDUCATION FOR THE
OPHTHALMOLOGIST®

The Basic and Clinical Science Course (BCSC) is one component of the Lifelong Education for the Ophthalmologist (LEO) framework, which assists members in planning their continuing medical education. LEO includes an array of clinical education products that members may select to form individualized, self-directed learning plans for updating their clinical knowledge. Active members or fellows who use LEO components may accumulate sufficient CME credits to earn the LEO Award. Contact the Academy's Clinical Education Division for further information on LEO.

The American Academy of Ophthalmology is accredited by the Accreditation Council for Continuing Medical Education to provide continuing medical education for physicians.

The American Academy of Ophthalmology designates this enduring material for a maximum of 10 *AMA PRA Category 1 Credits*™. Physicians should claim only the credit commensurate with the extent of their participation in the activity.

The BCSC is designed to increase the physician's ophthalmic knowledge through study and review. Users of this activity are encouraged to read the text and then answer the study questions provided at the back of the book.

To claim *AMA PRA Category 1 Credits*™ upon completion of this activity, learners must demonstrate appropriate knowledge and participation in the activity by taking the post-test for Section 7 and achieving a score of 80% or higher. For further details, please see the instructions for requesting CME credit at the back of the book.

The Academy provides this material for educational purposes only. It is not intended to represent the only or best method or procedure in every case, nor to replace a physician's own judgment or give specific advice for case management. Including all indications, contraindications, side effects, and alternative agents for each drug or treatment is beyond the scope of this material. All information and recommendations should be verified, prior to use, with current information included in the manufacturers' package inserts or other independent sources, and considered in light of the patient's condition and history. Reference to certain drugs, instruments, and other products in this course is made for illustrative purposes only and is not intended to constitute an endorsement of such. Some material may include information on applications that are not considered community standard, that reflect indications not included in approved FDA labeling, or that are approved for use only in restricted research settings. **The FDA has stated that it is the responsibility of the physician to determine the FDA status of each drug or device he or she wishes to use, and to use them with appropriate, informed patient consent in compliance with applicable law.** The Academy specifically disclaims any and all liability for injury or other damages of any kind, from negligence or otherwise, for any and all claims that may arise from the use of any recommendations or other information contained herein.

Cover image courtesy of Timothy J. McCulley, MD.

Basic and Clinical Science Course

Gregory L. Skuta, MD, Oklahoma City, Oklahoma, *Senior Secretary for Clinical Education*

Louis B. Cantor, MD, Indianapolis, Indiana, *Secretary for Ophthalmic Knowledge*

Jayne S. Weiss, MD, New Orleans, Louisiana, *BCSC Course Chair*

Section 7

Faculty Responsible for This Edition

John Bryan Holds, MD, *Chair,* St Louis, Missouri

Warren J. Chang, MD, Bloomington, Indiana

Vikram D. Durairaj, MD, Denver, Colorado

Jill Annette Foster, MD, Columbus, Ohio

Roberta E. Gausas, MD, Philadelphia, Pennsylvania

Andrew R. Harrison, MD, Minneapolis, Minnesota

Morris E. Hartstein, MD, *Consultant,* Raanana, Israel

Robert G. Fante, MD, Denver, Colorado
   Practicing Ophthalmologists Advisory Committee for Education

Ron W. Pelton, MD, PhD, Colorado Springs, Colorado
   Practicing Ophthalmologists Advisory Committee for Education

The Academy wishes to acknowledge Robert Bernardino, MD, *Committee on Aging,* for his review of this edition.

The Academy also wishes to acknowledge the American Society of Ophthalmic Plastic and Reconstructive Surgery for recommending faculty members to the BCSC Section 7 committee.

Financial Disclosures

Academy staff members who contributed to the development of this product state that they have no significant financial interest or other relationship with the manufacturer of any commercial product discussed in this course or with the manufacturer of any competing commercial product.

The authors state the following financial relationships:

Dr Durairaj: Porex Surgical, lecturer/honoraria recipient; Stryker Corporation, lecturer/honoraria recipient

Dr Foster: Allergan, lecturer/honoraria recipient, consultant

Dr Harrison: Merz Pharmaceuticals, consultant

Dr Holds: QLT Phototherapeutics, consultant

Dr Pelton: Allergan, lecturer/honoraria recipient

The other authors state that they have no significant financial interest or other relationship with the manufacturer of any commercial product discussed in the chapters that they contributed to this course or with the manufacturer of any competing commercial product.

Recent Past Faculty

Roger A. Dailey, MD
Martin H. Devoto, MD
Michael Kazim, MD
Robert C. Kersten, MD
Timothy J. McCulley, MD

In addition, the Academy gratefully acknowledges the contributions of numerous past faculty and advisory committee members who have played an important role in the development of previous editions of the Basic and Clinical Science Course.

American Academy of Ophthalmology Staff

Richard A. Zorab, *Vice President, Ophthalmic Knowledge*
Hal Straus, *Director, Publications Department*
Christine Arturo, *Acquisitions Manager*
Stephanie Tanaka, *Publications Manager*
D. Jean Ray, *Production Manager*
Ann McGuire, *Medical Editor*
Steve Huebner, *Administrative Coordinator*

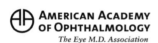

**AMERICAN ACADEMY
OF OPHTHALMOLOGY**
The Eye M.D. Association

655 Beach Street
Box 7424
San Francisco, CA 94120-7424

Contents

11 Periocular Malpositions and Involutional Changes 189

13 Abnormalities of the Lacrimal Secretory and Drainage Systems 249

These references are intended to be selective rather than exhaustive, chosen by the BCSC faculty as being important, current, and readily available to residents and practitioners.

Related Academy educational materials are also listed in the appropriate sections. They include books, online and audiovisual materials, self-assessment programs, clinical modules, and interactive programs.

Study Questions and CME Credit

Each volume of the BCSC is designed as an independent study activity for ophthalmology residents and practitioners. The learning objectives for this volume are given on page 1. The text, illustrations, and references provide the information necessary to achieve the objectives; the study questions allow readers to test their understanding of the material and their mastery of the objectives. Physicians who wish to claim CME credit for this educational activity may do so by following the instructions given at the end of the book.

Conclusion

The Basic and Clinical Science Course has expanded greatly over the years, with the addition of much new text and numerous illustrations. Recent editions have sought to place a greater emphasis on clinical applicability while maintaining a solid foundation in basic science. As with any educational program, it reflects the experience of its authors. As its faculties change and as medicine progresses, new viewpoints are always emerging on controversial subjects and techniques. Not all alternate approaches can be included in this series; as with any educational endeavor, the learner should seek additional sources, including such carefully balanced opinions as the Academy's Preferred Practice Patterns.

The BCSC faculty and staff are continuously striving to improve the educational usefulness of the course; you, the reader, can contribute to this ongoing process. If you have any suggestions or questions about the series, please do not hesitate to contact the faculty or the editors.

The authors, editors, and reviewers hope that your study of the BCSC will be of lasting value and that each Section will serve as a practical resource for quality patient care.

Objectives

Upon completion of BCSC Section 7, *Orbit, Eyelids, and Lacrimal System,* the reader should be able to

- describe the normal anatomy and function of orbital and periocular tissues

- identify general and specific pathophysiological processes (including congenital, infectious, inflammatory, traumatic, neoplastic, and involutional) that affect the structure and function of these tissues

- choose appropriate examination techniques and protocols for diagnosing disorders of the orbit, eyelids, and lacrimal system

- select from among the various imaging and ancillary studies available those that are most useful for the particular patient

- describe appropriate differential diagnoses for disorders of the orbital and periocular tissues

- state the indications for enucleation, evisceration, and exenteration

- describe functional and cosmetic indications in the surgical management of eyelid and periorbital conditions

- state the principles of medical and surgical management of conditions affecting the orbit, eyelids, and lacrimal system

- identify the major postoperative complications of orbital, eyelid, and lacrimal system surgery

PART I

Orbit

CHAPTER 1

Orbital Anatomy

Dimensions

The orbits are the bony cavities that contain the globes, extraocular muscles, nerves, fat, and blood vessels. Each bony orbit is pear shaped, tapering posteriorly to the apex and the optic canal. The medial orbital walls are approximately parallel and are separated by 25 mm in the average adult. The widest dimension of the orbit is approximately 1 cm behind the anterior orbital rim. Approximate measurements of the adult orbit are shown in Table 1-1. The orbital segment of the optic nerve is slightly curved and moves with the eye. This curve allows the eye to move forward with proptosis without damaging the nerve.

Topographic Relationships

The orbital septum arises from the orbital rims anteriorly. The paranasal sinuses are either rudimentary or very small at birth, and they increase in size through adolescence. They lie adjacent to the floor, medial wall, and anterior portion of the orbital roof. The orbital walls are composed of 7 bones: ethmoid, frontal, lacrimal, maxillary, palatine, sphenoid, and zygomatic. The composition of each of the 4 walls and the location in relation to adjacent extraorbital structures are shown in Figures 1-1, 1-2, and 1-3 and summarized in the following sections.

Roof of the Orbit
- composed of the frontal bone and the lesser wing of the sphenoid
- important landmarks: the *lacrimal gland fossa,* which contains the orbital lobe of the lacrimal gland; the *fossa for the trochlea of the superior oblique tendon,* located

Table 1-1 Adult Orbital Dimensions

Volume	30 cm³
Entrance height	35 mm
Entrance width	40 mm
Medial wall length	45 mm
Distance from posterior globe to optic foramen	18 mm
Length of orbital segment of optic nerve	25–30 mm

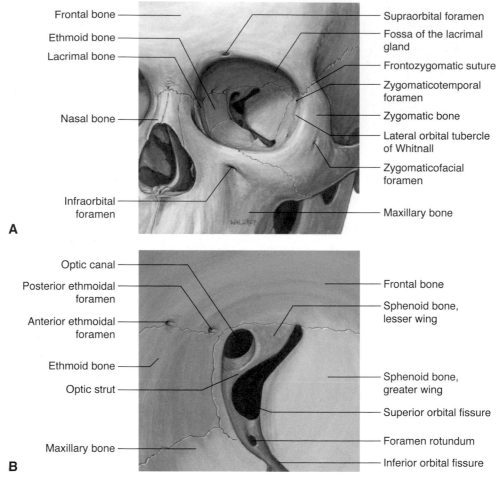

Frontal bone

Ethmoid bone

Lacrimal bone

Nasal bone

Infraorbital foramen

A

Supraorbital foramen

Fossa of the lacrimal gland

Frontozygomatic suture

Zygomaticotemporal foramen

Zygomatic bone

Lateral orbital tubercle of Whitnall

Zygomaticofacial foramen

Maxillary bone

Optic canal

Posterior ethmoidal foramen

Anterior ethmoidal foramen

Ethmoid bone

Optic strut

Maxillary bone

B

Frontal bone

Sphenoid bone, lesser wing

Sphenoid bone, greater wing

Superior orbital fissure

Foramen rotundum

Inferior orbital fissure

Figure 1-1 **A,** Orbital bones, frontal view. **B,** Orbital bones, apex. *(Reproduced with permission from Dutton JJ. Atlas of Clinical and Surgical Orbital Anatomy. Philadelphia: Saunders; 1994:8.)*

5 mm behind the superior nasal orbital rim; and the *supraorbital notch,* or *foramen,* which transmits the supraorbital vessels and branch of the frontal nerve
- located adjacent to anterior cranial fossa and frontal sinus

Lateral Wall of the Orbit

- composed of the zygomatic bone and the greater wing of the sphenoid; separated from the lesser wing portion of the orbital roof by the superior orbital fissure
- important landmarks: the *lateral orbital tubercle of Whitnall,* with multiple attachments, including the lateral canthal tendon, the lateral horn of the levator aponeurosis, the check ligament of the lateral rectus, the Lockwood ligament (the suspensory ligament of the globe), and the Whitnall ligament; and the *frontozygomatic suture,* located 1 cm above the tubercle

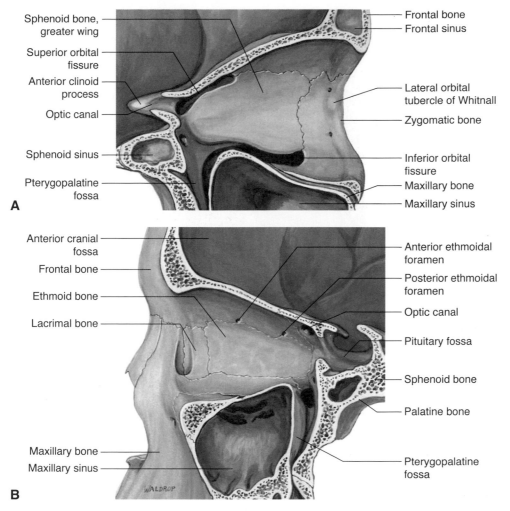

Sphenoid bone, greater wing
Superior orbital fissure
Anterior clinoid process
Optic canal
Sphenoid sinus
Pterygopalatine fossa

Frontal bone
Frontal sinus
Lateral orbital tubercle of Whitnall
Zygomatic bone
Inferior orbital fissure
Maxillary bone
Maxillary sinus

A

Anterior cranial fossa
Frontal bone
Ethmoid bone
Lacrimal bone

Anterior ethmoidal foramen
Posterior ethmoidal foramen
Optic canal
Pituitary fossa
Sphenoid bone
Palatine bone

Maxillary bone
Maxillary sinus

Pterygopalatine fossa

B

WALDROP

Figure 1-2   A, Orbital bones, lateral wall, internal view. **B,** Orbital bones, medial wall, internal view. *(Reproduced with permission from Dutton JJ. Atlas of Clinical and Surgical Orbital Anatomy. Philadelphia: Saunders; 1994:9–10.)*

- located adjacent to the middle cranial fossa and the temporal fossa
- commonly extends anteriorly to the equator of the globe, helping to protect the posterior half of the eye while still allowing wide peripheral vision
- is the thickest and strongest of the orbital walls

Medial Wall of the Orbit

- composed of the ethmoid, lacrimal, maxillary, and sphenoid bones
- important landmark: the *frontoethmoidal suture,* marking the approximate level of the cribriform plate, the roof of the ethmoids, the floor of the anterior cranial fossa, and the entry of the anterior and posterior ethmoidal arteries into the orbit

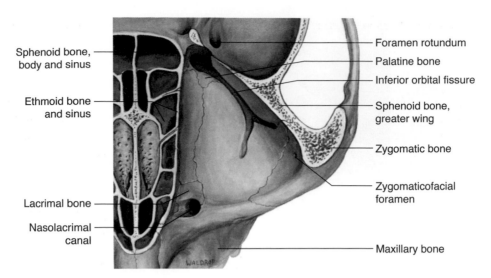

Figure 1-3 Orbital bones, inferior wall, internal view. *(Reproduced with permission from Dutton JJ.* Atlas of Clinical and Surgical Orbital Anatomy. *Philadelphia: Saunders; 1994:11.)*

- located adjacent to the ethmoid and sphenoid sinuses and nasal cavity
- medial wall of the optic canal forms the lateral wall of the sphenoid sinus

The thinnest walls of the orbit are the *lamina papyracea,* which covers the ethmoid sinuses along the medial wall, and the *maxillary bone,* particularly in its posteromedial portion. These are the bones most frequently fractured as a result of indirect, or blowout, fractures (see Chapter 6). Infections of the ethmoid sinuses may extend through the lamina papyracea to cause orbital cellulitis and proptosis.

Floor of the Orbit

- composed of the maxillary, palatine, and zygomatic bones
- forms the roof of the maxillary sinus; does not extend to the orbital apex but instead ends at the pterygopalatine fossa; hence, it is the shortest of the orbital walls
- important landmarks: the *infraorbital groove* and *infraorbital canal,* which transmit the infraorbital artery and the maxillary division of the trigeminal nerve

Apertures

The orbital walls are perforated by several important apertures (see Figs 1-1 through 1-3).

Ethmoidal Foramina

The anterior and posterior ethmoidal arteries pass through the corresponding ethmoidal foramina in the medial orbital wall along the frontoethmoidal suture. These foramina provide a potential route of entry into the orbit for infections and neoplasms from the sinuses.

Superior Orbital Fissure

The superior orbital fissure separates the greater and lesser wings of the sphenoid and transmits cranial nerves III, IV, and VI; the first (ophthalmic) division of cranial nerve (CN) V; and sympathetic nerve fibers. Most of the venous drainage from the orbit passes through this fissure by way of the superior ophthalmic vein to the cavernous sinus.

Inferior Orbital Fissure

The inferior orbital fissure is bounded by the sphenoid, maxillary, and palatine bones and lies between the lateral orbital wall and the orbital floor. It transmits the second (maxillary) division of CN V, including the zygomatic nerve, and branches of the inferior ophthalmic vein leading to the pterygoid plexus. The infraorbital nerve, which is a branch of the maxillary nerve, leaves the skull through the foramen rotundum and travels through the pterygopalatine fossa to enter the orbit at the infraorbital groove. This fossa extends laterally to become the infratemporal fossa. The nerve travels anteriorly in the floor of the orbit through the infraorbital canal, emerging on the face of the maxilla 1 cm below the inferior orbital rim. The infraorbital nerve carries sensation from the lower eyelid, cheek, upper lip, upper teeth, and gingiva. Numbness in this distribution often accompanies blowout fractures of the orbital floor and typically improves with time.

Zygomaticofacial and Zygomaticotemporal Canals

The zygomaticofacial canal and zygomaticotemporal canal transmit vessels and branches of the zygomatic nerve through the lateral orbital wall to the cheek and the temporal fossa, respectively.

Nasolacrimal Canal

The nasolacrimal canal extends from the lacrimal sac fossa to the inferior meatus beneath the inferior turbinate in the nose. Through this canal passes the nasolacrimal duct, which is continuous from the lacrimal sac to the nasal mucosa (see Part III, Lacrimal System).

Optic Canal

The optic canal is 8–10 mm long and is located within the lesser wing of the sphenoid. This canal is separated from the superior orbital fissure by the bony optic strut. The optic nerve, ophthalmic artery, and sympathetic nerves pass through this canal. The orbital end of the canal is the optic foramen, which normally measures less than 6.5 mm in diameter in adults. Optic canal enlargement accompanies the expansion of the nerve, as seen with optic nerve gliomas. Blunt trauma may cause an optic canal fracture, hematoma at the orbital apex, or shearing of the nerve at the foramen, resulting in optic nerve damage.

Soft Tissues

Periorbita

The periorbita is the periosteal covering of the orbital bones. At the orbital apex, it fuses with the dura mater covering the optic nerve. Anteriorly, the periorbita is continuous with the orbital septum and the periosteum of the facial bones. The line of fusion of these layers at the orbital rim is called the *arcus marginalis*. The periorbita adheres loosely to the bone except at the orbital margin, sutures, fissures, foramina, and canals. In an exenteration, the periorbita can be easily separated except where these firm attachments are present. Subperiosteal fluid, such as pus or blood, is usually loculated within these boundaries. The periorbita is quite sensitive, being innervated by the sensory nerves of the orbit.

Intraorbital Optic Nerve

The intraorbital portion of the optic nerve is approximately 30 mm long. The nerve is somewhat longer than the orbit, making an S-shaped curve to allow for movement with the eye. The optic nerve is 4 mm in diameter and surrounded by the pia mater, arachnoid, and dura mater, which are continuous with the same layers covering the brain. The dura mater covering the posterior portion of the intraorbital optic nerve fuses with the annulus of Zinn at the orbital apex and is continuous with the periosteum of the optic canal.

Extraocular Muscles and Orbital Fat

The extraocular muscles are responsible for the movement of the eye and for synchronous movements of the eyelids. All of the extraocular muscles, except the inferior oblique muscle, originate in the orbital apex and travel anteriorly to insert onto the eye or eyelid. The 4 rectus muscles (superior, medial, lateral, and inferior recti) originate in the annulus of Zinn. The levator muscle arises above the annulus on the lesser wing of the sphenoid. The superior oblique muscle originates slightly medial to the levator muscle and travels anteriorly through the trochlea on the superomedial orbital rim, where it turns posterolaterally toward the eye. The inferior oblique muscle originates in the anterior orbital floor lateral to the lacrimal sac and travels posterolaterally within the lower eyelid retractors to insert inferolateral to the macula.

In the anterior portion of the orbit, the rectus muscles are connected by a membrane known as the *intermuscular septum*. When viewed in the coronal plane, this membrane forms a ring that divides the orbital fat into the *intraconal fat (central surgical space)* and the *extraconal fat (peripheral surgical space)*. These anatomical designations on a magnetic resonance (MR) or computed tomographic (CT) scan are helpful for describing the location of a mass. A knowledge of these spaces helps direct the surgical dissection to the mass.

The orbit is further divided by many fine fibrous septa that unite and support the globe, optic nerve, and extraocular muscles (Fig 1-4). Accidental or surgical orbital trauma can disrupt this supporting system and contribute to globe displacement and restriction. In many cases of diplopia after fracture, restriction of eye movement is caused by the entrapment of the orbital connective tissue rather than by the muscles themselves.

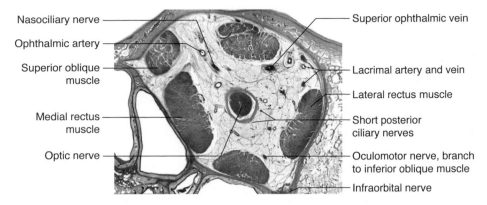

Nasociliary nerve

Ophthalmic artery

Superior oblique muscle

Medial rectus muscle

Optic nerve

Superior ophthalmic vein

Lacrimal artery and vein

Lateral rectus muscle

Short posterior ciliary nerves

Oculomotor nerve, branch to inferior oblique muscle

Infraorbital nerve

Figure 1-4 Mid-orbit at the widest extent of the extraocular muscles. *(Modified from Dutton JJ.* Atlas of Clinical and Surgical Orbital Anatomy. *Philadelphia: Saunders; 1994:151. Used with permission.)*

The motor innervation of the extraocular muscles arises from cranial nerves III, IV, and VI. The superior rectus and levator muscles are supplied by the superior division of CN III (oculomotor nerve). The inferior rectus, medial rectus, and inferior oblique muscles are supplied by the inferior division of CN III. The lateral rectus is supplied by CN VI (abducens nerve). The cranial nerves to the rectus muscles enter the orbit posteriorly through the superior orbital fissure and travel through the intraconal fat to enter the muscles' intraconal surface at the junction of the posterior third and anterior two-thirds. Cranial nerve IV (trochlear nerve) crosses over the levator muscle and innervates the superior oblique on the superior surface at its posterior third. The nerve to the inferior oblique muscle travels anteriorly on the lateral aspect of the inferior rectus to enter the muscle on its posterior surface.

Annulus of Zinn

The annulus of Zinn is the fibrous ring formed by the common origin of the 4 rectus muscles (Fig 1-5). The ring encircles the optic foramen and the central portion of the superior orbital fissure. The superior origin of the lateral rectus muscle separates the superior orbital fissure into 2 compartments. The portion of the orbital apex enclosed by the annulus is called the *oculomotor foramen.* This opening transmits CN III (upper and lower divisions), CN VI, and the nasociliary branch of the ophthalmic division of CN V (trigeminal). The superior and lateral aspect of the superior orbital fissure external to the muscle cone transmits CN IV as well as the frontal and lacrimal branches of the ophthalmic division of CN V. Cranial nerve IV is the only nerve that innervates an extraocular muscle and does not pass directly into the muscle cone when entering the orbit. Cranial nerves III and VI pass directly into the muscle cone through the oculomotor foramen. The superior ophthalmic vein passes through the superior and lateral portion of the superior orbital fissure outside the oculomotor foramen.

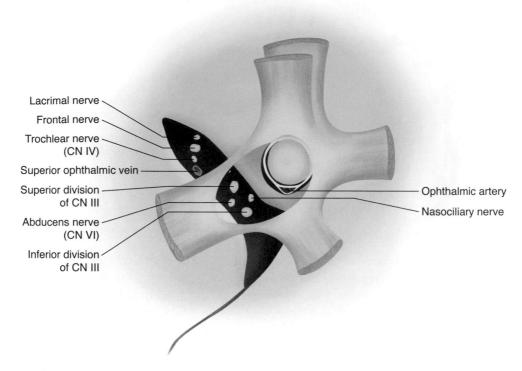

Lacrimal nerve
Frontal nerve
Trochlear nerve
(CN IV)
Superior ophthalmic vein
Superior division
of CN III
Abducens nerve
(CN VI)
Inferior division
of CN III

Ophthalmic artery
Nasociliary nerve

Figure 1-5 View of orbital apex, right orbit. The ophthalmic artery enters the orbit through the optic canal, whereas the superior and inferior divisions of cranial nerve III, cranial nerve VI, and the nasociliary nerve enter the muscle cone through the oculomotor foramen. Cranial nerve IV, the frontal and lacrimal nerves, and the ophthalmic vein enter through the superior orbital fissure and thus lie within the periorbita but outside of the muscle cone. Note that the presence of many nerves and arteries along the lateral side of the optic nerve mandates a superonasal surgical approach to the optic nerve in the orbital apex. *(Modified from Housepian EM. Intraorbital tumors. In: Schmidek HH, Sweet WH, eds.* Current Techniques in Operative Neurosurgery. *Orlando, FL: Grune & Stratton; 1976:148. Used with permission. Illustration by Cyndie C. H. Wooley.)*

Vasculature of the Orbit

The blood supply to the orbit arises primarily from the ophthalmic artery, which is a branch of the internal carotid artery. Smaller contributions come from the external carotid artery by way of the internal maxillary and facial arteries. The ophthalmic artery travels underneath the intracranial optic nerve through the dura mater along the optic canal to enter the orbit. The major branches of the ophthalmic artery are the

- branches to the extraocular muscles
- central retinal artery (to the optic nerve and retina)
- posterior ciliary arteries (long to the anterior segment and short to the choroid)

Terminal branches of the ophthalmic artery travel anteriorly and form rich anastomoses with branches of the external carotid in the face and periorbital region (Fig 1-6).

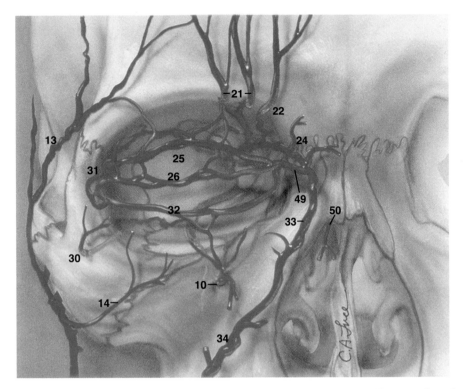

Figure 1-6 Anterior view of the arterial supply to the eyelids and orbit. The arteries shown are *10*, infraorbital; *13*, superficial temporal; *14*, transverse facial; *21*, supraorbital; *22*, supratrochlear; *24*, infratrochlear; *25*, superior peripheral arcade; *26*, superior marginal arcade; *30*, zygomaticofacial; *31*, lateral palpebral; *32*, inferior marginal arcade; *33*, angular; *34*, facial; *49*, medial palpebral; *50*, dorsal nasal. *(Reproduced with permission from Zide BM, Jelks GW, eds.* Surgical Anatomy of the Orbit. *New York: Raven; 1985:11.)*

The superior ophthalmic vein provides the main venous drainage of the orbit. This vein originates in the superonasal quadrant of the orbit and extends posteriorly through the superior orbital fissure into the cavernous sinus. Frequently, the superior ophthalmic vein appears on axial orbital CT scans as the only structure coursing diagonally through the superior orbit. Many anastomoses occur anteriorly with the veins of the face as well as posteriorly with the pterygoid plexus (Figs 1-7, 1-8).

Nerves

Sensory innervation to the periorbital area is provided by the ophthalmic and maxillary divisions of CN V (Fig 1-9). The ophthalmic division of CN V travels anteriorly from the ganglion in the lateral wall of the cavernous sinus, where it divides into 3 main branches: frontal, lacrimal, and nasociliary. The frontal and lacrimal nerves enter the orbit through the superior orbital fissure above the annulus of Zinn (see Fig 1-5) and travel anteriorly in the extraconal fat to innervate the medial canthus (supratrochlear branch), upper eyelid (lacrimal and supratrochlear branches), and forehead (supraorbital branch). The

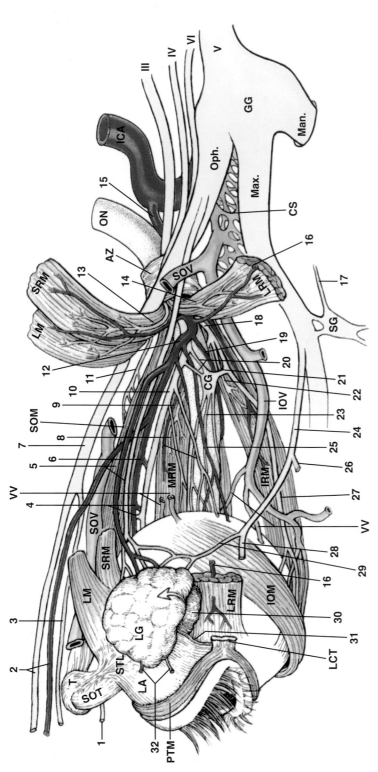

Figure 1-7 Side view of left orbit. *AZ*, annulus of Zinn; *CG*, ciliary ganglion; *CS*, cavernous sinus; *GG*, Gasserian ganglion; *ICA*, internal carotid artery; *IOM*, inferior oblique muscle; *IOV*, inferior ophthalmic vein; *IRM*, inferior rectus muscle; *LA*, levator aponeurosis; *LCT*, lateral canthal tendon; *LG*, lacrimal gland; *LM*, levator muscle; *LRM*, lateral rectus muscle; *Man.*, mandibular nerve; *Max.*, maxillary nerve; *MRM*, medial rectus muscle; *ON*, optic nerve; *Oph.*, ophthalmic nerve; *PTM*, pretarsal muscle; *SG*, sphenopalatine ganglion; *SOM*, superior oblique muscle; *SOT*, superior oblique tendon; *SOV*, superior ophthalmic vein; *SRM*, superior rectus muscle; *STL*, superior transverse ligament; *T*, trochlea; *VV*, vortex veins; *1*, infratrochlear nerve; *2*, supraorbital nerve and artery; *3*, supratrochlear nerve; *4*, anterior ethmoid nerve and artery; *5*, lacrimal nerve and artery; *6*, posterior ethmoid artery; *7*, frontal nerve; *8*, long ciliary nerves; *9*, branch of cranial nerve III to medial rectus muscle; *10*, nasociliary nerve; *11*, cranial nerve IV; *12*, ophthalmic (orbital) artery; *13*, superior ramus of cranial nerve III; *14*, cranial nerve VI; *15*, ophthalmic artery, origin; *16*, anterior ciliary artery; *17*, vidian nerve; *18*, inferior ramus of cranial nerve III; *19*, central retinal artery; *20*, sensory branches from ciliary ganglion to nasociliary nerve; *21*, motor (parasympathetic) nerve to ciliary ganglion from nerve to inferior oblique muscle; *22*, branch of cranial nerve III to inferior rectus muscle; *23*, short ciliary nerves; *24*, zygomatic nerve; *25*, posterior ciliary arteries; *26*, zygomaticofacial nerve; *27*, nerve to inferior oblique muscle; *28*, zygomaticotemporal nerve; *29*, lacrimal secretory nerve; *30*, lacrimal gland–palpebral lobe; *31*, lateral horn of levator aponeurosis; *32*, lacrimal artery and nerve terminal branches. *(Reproduced from Stewart WB, ed. Ophthalmic Plastic and Reconstructive Surgery. 4th ed. San Francisco: American Academy of Ophthalmology Manuals Program; 1984.)*

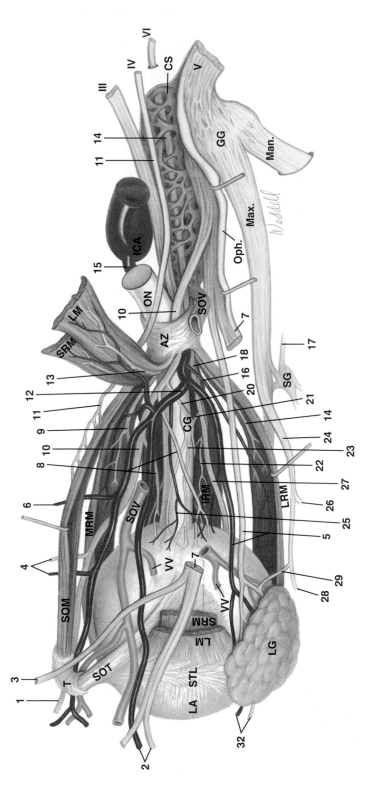

Figure 1-8 Top view of left orbit. *AZ,* annulus of Zinn; *CG,* ciliary ganglion; *CS,* cavernous sinus; *GG,* Gasserian ganglion; *ICA,* internal carotid artery; *IRM,* inferior rectus muscle; *LA,* levator aponeurosis; *LG,* lacrimal gland; *LM,* levator muscle; *LRM,* lateral rectus muscle; *Man.,* mandibular nerve; *Max.,* maxillary nerve; *MRM,* medial rectus muscle; *ON,* optic nerve; *Oph.,* ophthalmic nerve; *SG,* sphenopalatine ganglion; *SOM,* superior oblique muscle; *SOT,* superior oblique tendon; *SOV,* superior ophthalmic vein; *SRM,* superior rectus muscle; *STL,* superior transverse ligament; *T,* trochlea; *VV,* vortex veins; *1,* infratrochlear nerve; *2,* supraorbital nerve and artery; *3,* supratrochlear nerve; *4,* anterior ethmoid nerve and artery; *5,* lacrimal nerve and artery; *6,* posterior ethmoid artery; *7,* frontal nerve; *8,* long ciliary nerves; *9,* branch of cranial nerve III to medial rectus muscle; *10,* nasociliary nerve; *11,* cranial nerve IV; *12,* ophthalmic (orbital) artery; *13,* superior ramus of cranial nerve III; *14,* cranial nerve VI; *15,* ophthalmic artery, origin; *16,* anterior ciliary artery; *17,* vidian nerve; *18,* inferior ramus of cranial nerve III; *20,* sensory branches from ciliary ganglion to nasociliary nerve; *21,* motor (parasympathetic) nerve to ciliary ganglion from nerve to inferior oblique muscle; *22,* branch of cranial nerve III to inferior rectus muscle; *23,* short ciliary arteries; *24,* zygomatic nerve; *25,* posterior ciliary arteries; *26,* zygomaticofacial nerve; *27,* nerve to inferior oblique muscle; *28,* zygomaticotemporal nerve; *29,* lacrimal secretory nerve; *32,* lacrimal artery and nerve terminal branches. *(Reproduced from Stewart WB, ed. Ophthalmic Plastic and Reconstructive Surgery. 4th ed. San Francisco: American Academy of Ophthalmology Manuals Program; 1984.)*

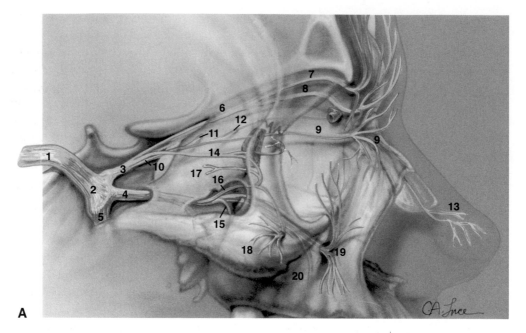

A

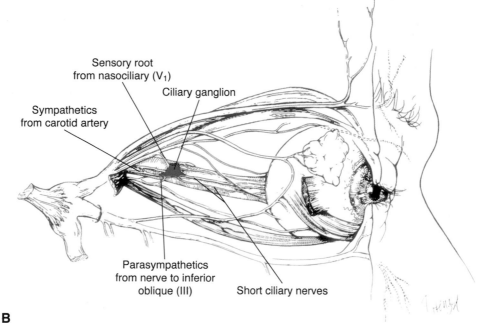

Sensory root
from nasociliary (V₁)

Ciliary ganglion

Sympathetics
from carotid artery

Parasympathetics
from nerve to inferior
oblique (III)

Short ciliary nerves

B

Figure 1-9 **A,** Sensory nerves. *1,* cranial nerve V; *2,* trigeminal ganglion; *3,* ophthalmic division of trigeminal nerve V_1; *4,* maxillary division of trigeminal nerve V_2; *5,* mandibular division of trigeminal nerve V_3; *6,* frontal nerve; *7,* supraorbital nerve; *8,* supratrochlear nerve (trochlea noted by *purple*); *9,* infratrochlear nerve; *10,* nasociliary nerve; *11,* posterior ethmoidal nerve; *12,* anterior ethmoidal nerve; *13,* external or dorsal nasal nerve; *14,* lacrimal nerve; *15,* posterior superior alveolar nerve; *16,* zygomatic nerve; *17,* zygomaticotemporal nerve; *18,* zygomaticofacial nerve; *19,* infraorbital nerve; *20,* anterior superior alveolar nerve. **B,** Contributions to the ciliary ganglion. *(Part A reproduced with permission from Zide BM, Jelks GW, eds.* Surgical Anatomy of the Orbit. *New York: Raven; 1985:12. Part B reproduced with permission from Doxanas MT, Anderson RL.* Clinical Orbital Anatomy. *Baltimore: Williams & Wilkins; 1984.)*

nasociliary branch enters the orbit through the superior orbital fissure within the annulus of Zinn, entering the intraconal space and traveling anteriorly to innervate the eye via the ciliary branches. The short ciliary nerves penetrate the sclera after passing through the ciliary ganglion without synapse. The long ciliary nerves pass by the ciliary ganglion and enter the sclera, where they extend anteriorly to supply the iris, cornea, and ciliary muscle.

The muscles of facial expression, including the orbicularis oculi, procerus, corrugator superciliaris, and frontalis muscles, receive their motor supply by way of branches of CN VII (the facial nerve) that penetrate the undersurface of each muscle.

The parasympathetic innervation, which controls accommodation, pupillary constriction, and lacrimal gland stimulation, follows a complicated course. Parasympathetic innervation enters the eye as the short posterior ciliary nerves after synapsing within the ciliary ganglion. Parasympathetic innervation to the lacrimal gland originates in the lacrimal nucleus of the pons and eventually joins the lacrimal nerve to enter the lacrimal gland.

The sympathetic innervation to the orbit provides for pupillary dilation, vasoconstriction, smooth muscle function of the eyelids and orbit, and hidrosis. The nerve fibers follow the arterial supply to the pupil, eyelids, and orbit and travel anteriorly in association with the long ciliary nerves. Interruption of this innervation results in the familiar signs of Horner syndrome: ptosis of the upper eyelid, elevation of the lower eyelid, miosis, anhidrosis, and vasodilation.

Lacrimal Gland

The lacrimal gland is composed of a larger orbital lobe and a smaller palpebral lobe. The gland is located within a fossa of the frontal bone in the superotemporal orbit. Ducts from both lobes pass through the palpebral lobe and empty into the upper conjunctival fornix temporally. Frequently, a portion of the palpebral lobe is visible on slit-lamp examination with the upper eyelid everted. Biopsy is generally not performed on the palpebral lobe or temporal conjunctival fornix because it can interfere with the lacrimal ductules draining the orbital lobe. With age, the orbital lobe of the lacrimal gland may prolapse inferiorly out of the fossa and present as a mass in the lateral upper eyelid.

Periorbital Structures

Nose and Paranasal Sinuses

The bones forming the medial, inferior, and superior orbital walls are close to the nasal cavity and are pneumatized by the paranasal sinuses, which arise from and drain into the nasal cavity. The sinuses may serve to decrease the weight of the skull, or they may function as resonators for the voice. The sinuses may also support the nasal passages in trapping irritants and in warming and humidifying the air. Pathophysiologic processes in these spaces that secondarily affect the orbit include sinonasal carcinomas, inverted papillomas, zygomycoses, Wegener granulomatosis, and mucoceles as well as sinusitis, which may cause orbital cellulitis or abscess.

The nasal cavity is divided into 2 nasal fossae by the nasal septum. The lateral wall of the nose has 3 bony projections: the superior, middle, and inferior conchae (turbinates). The conchae are covered by nasal mucosa, and they overhang the corresponding meatuses. Just cephalad to the superior concha is the sphenoethmoidal recess, into which the sphenoid sinus drains. The frontal sinus and the anterior and middle ethmoid air cells drain into the middle meatus. The nasolacrimal duct opens into the inferior meatus. The nasal cavity is lined by a pseudostratified, ciliated columnar epithelium with copious goblet cells. The mucous membrane overlying the lateral alar cartilage is hair bearing and therefore less suitable for use as a composite graft in eyelid reconstruction than the mucoperichondrium over the nasal septum, which is devoid of hair.

The frontal sinuses develop from evaginations of the frontal recess and cannot be seen radiographically until the sixth year of life. Pneumatization of the frontal bone continues through childhood and is complete by early adulthood (Fig 1-10). The sinuses can develop asymmetrically and vary greatly in size and shape. The frontal sinuses are almost always separated by the midline intersinus septum. Each sinus drains through separate frontonasal ducts and empties into the anterior portion of the middle meatus.

The ethmoid air cells are thin-walled cavities that lie between the medial orbital wall and the lateral wall of the nose. They are present at birth and expand as the child grows. Ethmoid air cells can extend into the frontal, lacrimal, and maxillary bones and may extend into the orbital roof (supraorbital ethmoids). The numerous small, thin-walled air cells of the ethmoid sinus are divided into anterior, middle, and posterior. The anterior and middle air cells drain into the middle meatus; the posterior air cells, into the superior

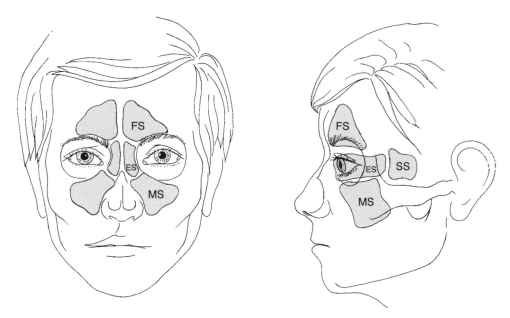

Figure 1-10 Relationship of the orbits to the paranasal sinuses: *FS,* frontal sinus; *ES,* ethmoid sinus; *MS,* maxillary sinus; *SS,* sphenoid sinus.

meatus. Orbital cellulitis develops most frequently from the spread of ethmoidal sinusitis through the lamina papyracea into the orbit.

The sphenoid sinus evaginates from the posterior nasal roof to pneumatize the sphenoid bone. It is rudimentary at birth and reaches full size after puberty. This sinus is divided into 2 cavities by a bony septum. Occasionally, pneumatization extends into the pterygoid and occipital bones. The sinus drains into the sphenoethmoidal recess of each nasal fossa. The optic canal is located immediately superolateral to the sinus wall. Visual loss and visual field abnormalities can be direct sequelae of pathologic processes involving the sphenoid sinus.

The maxillary sinuses are the largest of the paranasal sinuses. Together, the roofs of each maxillary sinus form the floor of the orbits. The maxillary sinuses extend posteriorly in the maxillary bone to the inferior orbital fissure. The infraorbital nerve and artery travel along the roof of the sinus from posterior to anterior. The bony nasolacrimal canal lies within the medial wall. The sinus drains into the middle meatus of the nose by way of the maxillary ostium. Orbital blowout fractures commonly disrupt the floor of the orbit medial to the infraorbital canal. The infraorbital nerve is often damaged, causing hypoesthesia of the cheek.

For further discussion and illustrations of ocular anatomy, see Chapter 1, Orbit and Ocular Adnexa, in BCSC Section 2, *Fundamentals and Principles of Ophthalmology.*

Dutton JJ. *Atlas of Clinical and Surgical Orbital Anatomy.* Philadelphia: Saunders; 1994.

Jordan DR, Anderson RA. *Surgical Anatomy of the Ocular Adnexa: A Clinical Approach.* Ophthalmology Monograph 9. San Francisco: American Academy of Ophthalmology; 1996.

CHAPTER **2**

Evaluation of Orbital Disorders

The evaluation of an orbital disorder should distinguish orbital from periorbital and intraocular lesions. This distinction provides a framework for development of a differential diagnosis. The evaluation begins with a detailed history to establish a probable diagnosis and guide the initial workup and therapy. Such a history should include

- onset, course, and duration of symptoms (pain, altered sensation, diplopia, changes in vision) and signs (erythema, palpable mass, globe displacement)
- prior disease (such as thyroid eye disease [TED] or sinus disease) and therapy
- injury (especially head or facial trauma)
- systemic disease (especially cancer)
- family history

Old photographs are frequently helpful for evaluating onset of globe displacement and establishing duration of the disease.

History

Pain

Pain may be a symptom of inflammatory and infectious lesions, orbital hemorrhage, malignant lacrimal gland tumors, invasion from adjacent nasopharyngeal carcinoma, or metastatic lesions.

Progression

The rate of progression can be a helpful diagnostic indicator. Disorders with onset occurring over days to weeks are usually caused by nonspecific orbital inflammation (NSOI), cellulitis, hemorrhage, thrombophlebitis, rhabdomyosarcoma, neuroblastoma, metastatic tumors, or granulocytic sarcoma. Conditions with onset occurring over months to years are usually caused by dermoid cyst, benign mixed tumor, neurogenic tumor, cavernous hemangioma, lymphoma, fibrous histiocytoma, fibrous dysplasia, or osteoma.

Periorbital Changes

Periorbital changes may provide clues indicative of the underlying disorders. Table 2-1 lists various signs and their common causes.

Table 2-1 Periorbital Changes Associated With Orbital Disease

Sign	Etiology
A salmon-colored mass in the cul-de-sac	Lymphoma (see Fig 5-14)
Eyelid retraction and eyelid lag	Thyroid eye disease
Vascular congestion over the insertions of the rectus muscles (particularly the lateral rectus)	Thyroid eye disease (see Fig 4-5A)
Corkscrew conjunctival vessels	Arteriovenous fistula (see Fig 4-5B)
Vascular anomaly of eyelid skin	Lymphangioma, varix, or capillary hemangioma
S-shaped eyelid	Plexiform neurofibroma or lacrimal gland mass (see Fig 5-7)
Eczematous lesions of the eyelids	Mycosis fungoides (T-cell lymphoma)
Ecchymoses of eyelid skin	Metastatic neuroblastoma, leukemia, or amyloidosis
Prominent temple	Sphenoid wing meningioma, metastatic neuroblastoma (see Fig 5-9A)
Edematous swelling of lower eyelid	Meningioma, inflammatory tumor, metastases
Optociliary shunt vessels on disc	Meningioma
Frozen globe	Metastases or zygomycosis
Black-crusted lesions in nasopharynx	Phycomycoses
Facial asymmetry	Fibrous dysplasia or neurofibromatosis (see Fig 5-12A)

Physical Examination

Special attention should be given to ocular motility, globe position, pupillary function, and ophthalmoscopy. Radiologic studies are often required in addition to the basic workup.

Inspection

Globe displacement is the most common clinical manifestation of an orbital abnormality. It usually results from a tumor, a vascular abnormality, an inflammatory process, or a traumatic event.

Several terms are used to describe the position of the eye and orbit. *Proptosis* denotes a forward displacement or bulging of a body part and is commonly used to refer to protrusion of the eye. *Exophthalmos* specifically means proptosis of the eye and is sometimes used to describe the bulging of the eye associated with TED. *Exorbitism* refers to an angle between the lateral orbital walls that is greater than 90°, which is usually associated with shallow orbital depth. This condition contrasts with *hypertelorism,* or *telorbitism,* which refers to a wider-than-normal separation between the medial orbital walls. Generally, exorbitism and hypertelorism refer to congenital abnormalities. *Telecanthus* refers to a wide intercanthal distance. The eye may also be displaced vertically *(hyperglobus* or *hypoglobus)* or horizontally by an orbital mass. Retrodisplacement of the eye into the orbit, called *enophthalmos,* may occur as a result of volume expansion of the orbit (fracture), in association with orbital varix, or secondary to sclerosing orbital tumors (eg, metastatic breast carcinoma).

Proptosis often indicates the location of a mass because the globe is usually displaced away from the site of the mass. *Axial displacement* is caused by retrobulbar lesions such as cavernous hemangioma, glioma, meningioma, metastases, arteriovenous malformations, and any other mass lesion within the muscle cone. *Nonaxial displacement* is caused by lesions with a prominent component outside the muscle cone. *Superior displacement* is produced by maxillary sinus tumors invading the orbital floor and pushing the globe upward. *Inferomedial displacement* can result from dermoid cysts and lacrimal gland tumors. *Inferolateral displacement* can result from frontoethmoidal mucoceles, abscesses, osteomas, and sinus carcinomas. *Bilateral proptosis* in adults is caused most often by TED; however, bilateral orbital involvement from lymphoma, vasculitis, NSOI, metastatic tumors, carotid cavernous fistulas, cavernous sinus thrombosis, or leukemic infiltrates can also produce bilateral proptosis. *Unilateral proptosis* in adults is also most frequently caused by TED. In children, bilateral proptosis may be caused by metastatic neuroblastoma, leukemic infiltrates, TED, or NSOI.

Exophthalmometry is a measurement of the anterior–posterior position of the globe, generally from the lateral orbital rim to the anterior corneal surface (Hertel exophthalmometry; Fig 2-1). On average, the globes are more prominent in men than in women and more prominent in black patients than in white patients. An asymmetry of greater than 2 mm between an individual patient's eyes suggests proptosis or enophthalmos. Proptosis may best be appreciated clinically when the examiner looks up from below with the patient's head tilted back (the so-called *worm's-eye view*; Fig 2-2).

Pseudoproptosis is either the simulation of abnormal prominence of the eye or a true asymmetry that is not the result of increased orbital contents. Diagnosis should be postponed until a mass lesion has been ruled out. Causes of pseudoproptosis are

- enlarged globe
- contralateral enophthalmos
- asymmetric orbital size
- asymmetric palpebral fissures (usually caused by ipsilateral eyelid retraction or facial nerve paralysis or contralateral ptosis)

Ocular movements may be limited in a specific direction of gaze by neoplasm or inflammation. In TED, the inferior rectus is the muscle most commonly affected, which restricts globe elevation and may cause hypotropia in primary gaze and restriction of

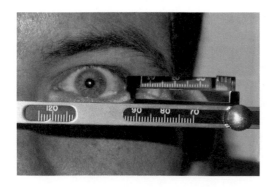

Figure 2-1 Hertel exophthalmometry device in use; reading 15.5, base 121. *(Courtesy of Jill Foster, MD.)*

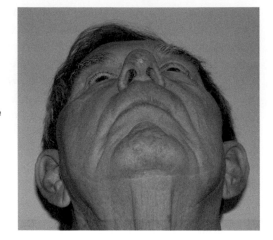

Figure 2-2 "Worm's-eye view" position. Note proptosis of left eye. *(Courtesy of Jill Foster, MD.)*

upgaze. A large or rapidly enlarging orbital mass can also impede ocular movements, even in the absence of direct muscle invasion.

Eyelid abnormalities are common in TED. The *von Graefe sign* refers to the delay in the upper eyelid's descent ("lid lag") during downgaze and is highly suggestive of a diagnosis of TED. In fact, such lid lag and the retraction of the upper and lower eyelids are the most common physical signs of TED.

Several eyelid signs of orbital pathology are seen in childhood disorders. Capillary hemangiomas in the orbit often involve the skin of the eyelids, producing strawberry birthmarks that usually grow during the first year of life and then regress spontaneously. Plexiform neurofibromas often involve the lateral upper eyelids as well as the orbits, producing a "bag of worms" appearance and texture beneath the skin and conjunctiva and sometimes causing an S-shaped curvature of the upper eyelids. Bilateral eyelid ecchymoses may occur in children with metastatic neuroblastoma.

Henderson JW, Campbell RJ, Farrow GM, et al. *Orbital Tumors.* 3rd ed. New York: Raven; 1994.

Rootman J, ed. *Diseases of the Orbit: A Multidisciplinary Approach.* 2nd ed. Philadelphia: Lippincott Williams & Wilkins; 2003.

Palpation

Palpation around the globe may disclose the presence of a mass in the anterior orbit, especially if the lacrimal gland is enlarged. Increased resistance to retrodisplacement of the globe is a nonspecific abnormality that may result either from a retrobulbar tumor or from diffuse inflammation such as TED. The physician should also palpate regional lymph nodes.

The differential diagnosis for a palpable mass in the superonasal quadrant may include mucocele, mucopyocele, encephalocele, neurofibroma, dermoid cyst, or lymphoma. A palpable mass in the superotemporal quadrant may be a prolapsed lacrimal gland, a dermoid cyst, a lacrimal gland tumor, lymphoma, or NSOI. A lesion behind the equator of the globe is usually not palpable.

Pulsations of the eye are caused by transmission of the vascular pulse through the orbit. This may result from either abnormal vascular flow or transmission of normal intracranial pulsations through a bony defect in the orbital walls. Abnormal vascular flow may be caused by arteriovenous communications, such as carotid cavernous or dural cavernous fistulas. Defects in the bony orbital walls may result from sinus mucoceles, surgical removal of bone, trauma, or developmental abnormalities, including encephalocele, meningocele, or sphenoid wing dysplasia (associated with neurofibromatosis).

Auscultation

Auscultation with a stethoscope over the globe or on the mastoid bone may detect bruits in cases of carotid cavernous fistula. The patient may also subjectively describe an audible bruit. Patients with such arteriovenous communications often have tortuous dilated epibulbar vessels (see Chapter 4, Fig 4-5B).

Primary Studies

Historically, plain-film radiography and tomography were used in evaluating patients with orbital disease. However, these techniques have been rendered largely obsolete by the widespread use of more current techniques, including computed tomography (CT) and magnetic resonance imaging (MRI). Ultrasonography may be helpful in some cases.

Computed Tomography

CT has revolutionized the management of orbital disorders. The tissues in a tomographic plane are assigned a density value proportional to their coefficient of absorption of x-rays. A 2-dimensional image is digitally constructed from these density measurements. CT is the most valuable technique for delineating the shape, location, extent, and character of lesions in the orbit (Fig 2-3). CT helps refine the differential diagnosis; moreover, when orbitotomy is indicated, CT guides the selection of the surgical approach by showing the relationship of the lesion to the surgical space or spaces of the orbit.

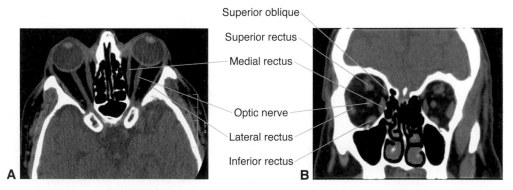

Superior oblique

Superior rectus

Medial rectus

Optic nerve

Lateral rectus

Inferior rectus

Figure 2-3 Axial **(A)** and coronal **(B)** CT views of the orbit demonstrating normal anatomy. *(Courtesy of Thomas Y. Hwang, MD, PhD, and Timothy J. McCulley, MD.)*

Orbital CT scans are usually obtained in 3-mm sections (as opposed to the thicker 5-mm sections usually utilized in head CT scans). "Fine cuts" of 1.5 mm may be requested for specific needs. Current CT scanners administer a dose of radiation of approximately 1–2 centigray (cGy) per scanning plane. By comparison, a posteroanterior and lateral chest radiograph administers a dose of radiation of approximately 5 milligray (mGy).

The visualization of tumors that are highly vascularized (eg, meningioma) or that have altered vascular permeability is improved by the use of intravenous contrast-enhancing agents. CT has resolution and tissue-contrast capabilities that allow imaging of soft tissues, bones, contrast-containing blood vessels, and foreign bodies.

Orbital images can be obtained in the axial plane, parallel to the course of the optic nerve; in the coronal plane, showing the eye, optic nerve, and extraocular muscles in cross section; or in the sagittal plane, parallel to the nasal septum. With older CT scanners, the patient's head has to be repositioned for direct imaging in each of the planes (coronal, sagittal, and axial) to obtain highly detailed images. Although these direct views provide the highest resolution, they require additional scanning time, increased radiation exposure, and sometimes difficult patient positioning. To avoid such difficulties, software on newer CT scanners can be used to reconstruct (reformat) any section in any direction (axial, coronal, or sagittal). Modern spiral (helical) CT scanners have multiple detector ports, and the scanner and the collecting tube move in a spiral fashion around the patient, generating a continuous data set. This results in rapid acquisition of a larger volume of data that, in combination with modern software, allows highly detailed reconstructions in all imaging planes.

Three-dimensional computed tomography allows reformatting of CT information into 3-dimensional projections of the bony orbital walls (Fig 2-4A, B). Because this type of imaging requires thin sections and additional computer time, 3-dimensional CT is typically reserved to assist in preparation for craniofacial surgery or repairs of complex orbital fractures.

Magnetic Resonance Imaging

Magnetic resonance imaging is a noninvasive imaging technique that does not employ ionizing radiation and has no known adverse biological effects (Fig 2-5). MRI is based on the interaction of 3 physical components: atomic nuclei possessing an electrical charge, radiofrequency (RF) waves, and a powerful magnetic field.

When a tissue containing hydrogen atoms is placed in the magnetic field, individual nuclei align themselves in the direction of the magnetic field. These aligned nuclei can be excited by an RF pulse emitted from a coil lying within the magnetic field. Excited nuclei align themselves against the static magnetic field; as the RF pulse is terminated, the nuclei flip back to their original magnetized position. The time it takes for this realignment to occur can be measured; it is called the *relaxation time.*

Each orbital tissue has specific magnetic resonance parameters that provide the information used to generate an image. These parameters include tissue proton density and relaxation times. *Proton density* is determined by the number of protons per unit volume of tissue. Fat has greater proton density per unit volume than bone and, therefore, has greater signal intensity. *T1,* or *longitudinal relaxation time,* is the time required for the net bulk

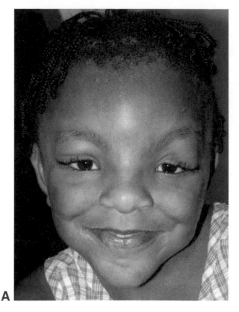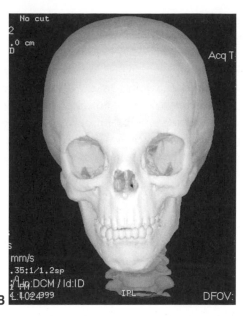

Figure 2-4   A, Patient with primary hypertelorism. **B,** Three-dimensional CT reconstruction of same patient. *(Courtesy of Jill Foster, MD.)*

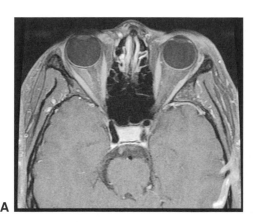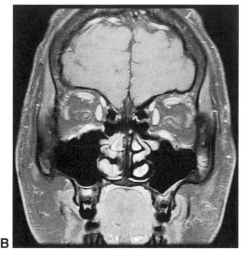

Figure 2-5   T1-weighted axial **(A)** and coronal **(B)** MR images of the orbit, with fat suppression. *(Courtesy of Thomas Y. Hwang, MD, PhD, and Timothy J. McCulley, MD.)*

magnetization to realign itself along the original axis. *T2, or transverse relaxation time,* is the mean relaxation time based on the interaction of hydrogen nuclei within a given tissue, an indirect measure of the effect the nuclei have on each other. Each tissue has different proton density and T1 and T2 characteristics, providing the image contrast necessary to differentiate tissues. Healthy tissues can have imaging characteristics different from those of diseased tissue, a good example being the bright signal associated with tissue edema seen on T2-weighted scans.

MRI is usually performed with images created from both T1 and T2 parameters. T1-weighted images generally offer the best anatomical detail of the orbit. T2-weighted images have the advantage of showing methemoglobin brighter than melanin, whereas these 2 substances have the same signal intensity on T1-weighted images. The difference in brightness seen on T2 images can be helpful in differentiating melanotic lesions from hemorrhagic processes. Gadolinium, a paramagnetic contrast agent given intravenously, allows enhancement of vascularized lesions so that they exhibit the same density as fat. It also demonstrates enhancement of lesions with abnormal vascular permeability. Special MR sequences have been developed to suppress the normal bright signal of fat on T1 images (fat suppression; see Fig 2-5) and the bright signal of cerebrospinal fluid on T2 images (fluid-attenuated inversion recovery, or FLAIR). Gradient echo sequences may reveal hemorrhage in vascular malformations that might be missed on T1- and T2-weighted images.

Comparison of CT and MRI

Although both CT and MRI are important modalities for the detection and characterization of orbital and ocular diseases, CT is currently the primary imaging technique. In general, CT provides better spatial resolution, allowing precise localization of a lesion. MRI generally provides better tissue contrast than CT; however, in most orbital conditions, the orbital fat provides sufficient natural tissue contrast to allow ready visualization of orbital tumors on CT. Each of the techniques has advantages in specific situations, some of which are discussed in the following text and in Table 2-2.

MRI offers advantages over CT in some situations. It allows the direct display of anatomical information in multiple planes (sagittal, axial, coronal, and any oblique plane).

Table 2-2 Comparison of CT and MRI in Orbital Disease

CT	MRI
Good technique for most orbital conditions, especially fractures and thyroid eye disease	Better technique for orbitocranial junction or intracranial imaging
Good view of bone and calcium	No view of bone or calcification
Poor definition of the orbital apex	Good view of orbital apex soft tissues unimpeded by bone
Better spatial resolution	More soft tissue detail
Reformatting or rescanning required to image in multiple planes	Simultaneous imaging of multiple planes
Improved imaging with contrast in many cases	Improved imaging with contrast in many cases
Less motion artifact because of shorter scanning time	More motion artifact because of longer scanning time
Less claustrophobic environment in scanner	Tighter confines in scanner
Good technique for patients with metallic foreign bodies	More contraindications (eg, patients with ferromagnetic metallic foreign bodies, aneurysm clips, and pacemakers)
Less expensive technique	More expensive technique

MRI provides better soft-tissue definition than does CT, a capability that is especially helpful in the evaluation of demyelination and in vascular and hemorrhagic lesions. As with CT, contrast agents are available to improve MRI detail.

Compared with CT, MRI also provides better tissue contrast of structures in the orbital apex, intracanalicular portion of the optic nerve, structures in periorbital spaces, and orbitocranial tumors, as there is no artifact from the skull base bones. Bone and calcification produce low signal on MRI. Bony structures may be evaluated by visualization of the signal void left by the bone. However, this is not possible when the bone is adjacent to structures that also create a signal void, such as air, rapidly flowing blood, calcification, and dura mater. Thus, *CT is superior to MRI for the evaluation of fractures, bone destruction, and tissue calcification.*

MRI is contraindicated in patients who have ferromagnetic metallic foreign bodies in the orbit or periorbital soft tissue, ferromagnetic vascular clips from previous surgery, magnetic intravascular filters, or electronic devices in the body such as cardiac pacemakers. If necessary, the presence of such foreign material can be ruled out with plain films or CT. Certain types of eye makeup can produce artifacts and should be removed prior to MRI. Dental amalgam is not a ferromagnetic substance and is not a contraindication to MRI, but this material does produce artifacts and degrades the images to some degree. Medical monitoring of a patient with serious health problems is easier in the environment of the CT room than in the MRI chamber. Because patients with acute head trauma are usually being evaluated for bone fractures, acute hemorrhagic problems, and possible foreign bodies, CT is usually the best choice in such cases, especially because it can be performed more rapidly. For subacute trauma, MRI may be preferable because it is better at differentiating between fresh and old hemorrhages (Fig 2-6).

Although CT and MRI yield different images, it is unusual for both techniques to be required in the evaluation of an orbital disorder. The choice between these modalities should be based on the specific patient's condition. In most cases, CT is the more effective and economical choice (see Table 2-2). When the orbitocranial junction or brain is involved, CT scanning and MRI may be complementary.

Ben Simon GJ, Annunziata CC, Fink J, Villablanca P, McCann JD, Goldberg RA. Rethinking orbital imaging: establishing guidelines for interpreting orbital imaging studies and evaluating their predictive value in patients with orbital tumors. *Ophthalmology.* 2005;112(12):2196–2207.

Buerger DE, Biesman BS. Orbital imaging: a comparison of computed tomography and magnetic resonance imaging. *Ophthalmol Clin North Am.* 1998;11(3):381–410.

Dutton JJ. *Radiology of the Orbit and Visual Pathways.* Philadelphia: Saunders Elsevier; 2010.

Wirtschafter JD, Berman EL, McDonald CS. *Magnetic Resonance Imaging and Computed Tomography.* Ophthalmology Monograph 6. San Francisco: American Academy of Ophthalmology; 1992.

Ultrasonography

Orbital ultrasonography may be used to examine patients with orbital disorders. The size, shape, and position of normal and abnormal orbital tissues can be determined by means of contemporary ultrasound techniques. Two-dimensional images of these tissues can be obtained with B-scan ultrasonography. Standardized A-scan ultrasonography provides

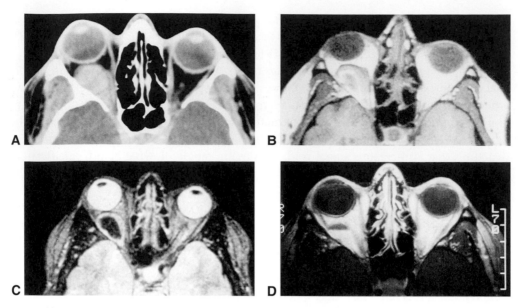

Figure 2-6 **A,** A CT scan of a patient with acute right exophthalmos resulting from a spontaneous orbital hemorrhage. The hematoma exhibits discrete margins, homogeneous consistency, and a radiodensity similar to that of blood vessels and muscle. **B,** A T1 MR scan obtained 4 days after the hemorrhage demonstrates the transient bull's-eye pattern characteristic of a hematoma beginning to undergo physical changes and biochemical hemoglobin degradation. **C,** A T2 MR scan obtained the same day as the T1 study shows a characteristic ring pattern. **D,** A T1 MR scan performed 3 months later shows that the hematoma has decreased in size. There is layering of the degraded blood components.

one-dimensional images of the orbital soft tissues characterized by a series of spikes of varying height and width that demonstrate the particular echogenic characteristics of each tissue. Areas of edema can sometimes be used to discern the degree of disease activity. Localization of foreign bodies is possible with ultrasonography. *Doppler ultrasonography* can provide specific information regarding blood flow (eg, the velocity and direction of blood flow in patients with occlusive vascular disease or vascular abnormalities associated with increased blood flow).

However, ultrasound analysis of orbital tissues and diseases requires specialized equipment and experienced personnel, and office-based equipment is generally not suitable for this purpose. Ultrasonography is of limited value in assessing lesions of the posterior orbit (because of sound attenuation) or the sinuses or intracranial space (because sound does not pass well through air or bone).

Aburn NS, Sergott RC. Orbital colour Doppler imaging. *Eye.* 1993;7(Pt 5):639–647.

Secondary Studies

Secondary studies that are performed for specific indications include venography and arteriography. These studies are rarely used but may be helpful in specific cases.

Venography

Before the era of CT and MRI, orbital venography was used in the diagnosis and management of orbital varices and in the study of the cavernous sinus. Contrast material is injected into the frontal or the angular vein to reveal a venous abnormality. Subtraction and magnification techniques have been used to increase the resolution of venography. Because moving blood generates a signal void during MR imaging, larger venous abnormalities and structures can be visualized well on MR venography. Some orbitocranial vascular malformations or fistulas are best accessed via the superior ophthalmic vein.

Arteriography

Arteriography is the gold standard for diagnosis of an arterial lesion such as an aneurysm or arteriovenous malformation. Retrograde catheterization of the cerebral vessels is accomplished through the femoral artery. However, since there is a small risk of serious neurological and vascular complications because the technique requires installation of the catheter and injection of radiopaque dye into the arterial system, the test is reserved for patients with a high probability of having a lesion.

Visualization can be maximized by the use of selective injection of the internal and external carotid arteries, magnification to allow viewing of the smaller caliber vessels, and subtraction techniques to radiographically eliminate bone.

CT and MR Angiography

The development of better hardware and software has made possible the precise CT and MR imaging of arteriovenous malformations, aneurysms, and arteriovenous fistulas without the expense, discomfort, and risks associated with intravascular catheterization and injection of contrast material. However, MR angiography is less sensitive than direct angiography for identifying carotid or dural cavernous sinus fistulas. When determining which test to use, the ophthalmologist may consult with a radiologist to discuss the suspected lesion and to ensure selection of the imaging modality best suited for the patient.

Pathology

The diagnosis of an orbital lesion usually requires analysis of tissue obtained through an orbitotomy. Appropriate handling of the tissue specimen is necessary to ensure an accurate diagnosis. The majority of tissue samples are placed in formalin for permanent-section analysis. Frozen-section analysis is generally not used for definitive diagnosis of an orbital tumor. However, when the area of proposed biopsy is not obvious, frozen sections are helpful to confirm that appropriate tissue has been obtained for permanent-section analysis. Frozen-section analysis is also used intraoperatively to determine tumor margins and ensure complete tumor removal. Tissue removed for frozen-section analysis should be placed in a dampened saline gauze and promptly sent to the frozen-section laboratory. If a lymphoproliferative lesion is suspected, some fresh tissue should be sent for analysis of flow cytometry.

Because of the vast array of possible unusual tumor types in the orbit, preoperative consultation with a pathologist familiar with orbital disease may be helpful to maximize the information gained from any orbital biopsy. In many cases, fresh tissue should be obtained and frozen for cell-surface marker studies. Cell-marker studies are required in the analysis of all orbital lymphoid lesions. These studies may permit differentiation of reactive lymphoid hyperplasia from lymphoma. Such studies may also indicate the presence of estrogen receptors in cases of metastatic prostate or breast carcinoma and thus provide useful information regarding sensitivity to hormonal therapy. Marker studies are also useful in the diagnosis of poorly differentiated tumors when light microscopy alone cannot yield a definitive diagnosis. Although cell-marker studies have largely replaced electron microscopy in the diagnosis of undifferentiated tumors, it may nevertheless be worthwhile in these cases to preserve fresh tissue in glutaraldehyde for possible electron microscopy. In noncohesive tumors (hematologic or lymphoid), a touch prep may permit a diagnosis.

All biopsy specimens must be treated delicately so that crush and cautery artifacts, which can confuse interpretation, are minimized. Permanent-section tissue biopsy specimens must be placed in fixatives immediately. If fine-needle aspiration biopsy is planned, a cytologist or trained technician must be available to handle the aspirate. In special cases, the biopsy can be performed under either ultrasonographic or CT control. Although a fine-bore needle occasionally yields a sufficient cell block, the specimen is usually limited to cytologic study. This technique may not permit as firm a diagnosis as is possible with larger biopsy specimens, in which light and electron microscopy can be used to evaluate the histologic pattern.

See BCSC Section 4, *Ophthalmic Pathology and Intraocular Tumors,* for more extensive discussion of pathology.

Laboratory Studies

Screening for abnormal thyroid function commonly includes T_3, T_4, and thyroid-stimulating hormone (TSH) tests. Results of these serum tests are abnormal in 90% of patients with TED. However, if thyroid disease is strongly suspected and these results are normal, additional endocrine studies, including studies of thyroid-stimulating immunoglobulins or TSH-receptor antibodies, can be considered.

Wegener granulomatosis (see Chapter 4) should be considered in patients with sclerokeratitis or coexisting sinus disease and orbital mass lesions. A useful test for this uncommon disease is the antineutrophil cytoplasmic antibody (ANCA) serum assay, which shows a cytoplasmic staining pattern (c-ANCA) in Wegener granulomatosis. The test results may be negative initially in localized disease. Biopsy of affected tissues classically shows vasculitis, granulomatous inflammation, and tissue necrosis, although necrotizing vasculitis is not always present in orbital biopsies.

Testing for serum angiotensin-converting enzyme and lysozyme may be helpful in the diagnosis of sarcoidosis. This multisystem granulomatous inflammatory condition may present with lacrimal gland enlargement, conjunctival granulomas, extraocular muscle or optic nerve infiltration, or solitary orbital granulomas. Diagnosis is confirmed through biopsy of 1 or more affected organs.

CHAPTER 3

Congenital Orbital Anomalies

Most congenital anomalies of the eye and orbit are apparent on ultrasound before birth. Developmental orbital defects can manifest at any time from conception until late in life. If an anomaly is caused by a slowing or cessation of a normal stage, the resulting deformity can be considered a pure arrest. An example is microphthalmia. However, a superimposed aberrant growth usually follows the original arrest, and the resulting deformity does not represent any previous normal stage of development. An example of this latter condition is formation of an orbital cyst following incomplete closure of the fetal fissure. As a rule, the more gross the abnormality, the earlier in development it occurred.

The examination of the child with an ocular or craniofacial malformation should focus on carefully defining the severity of the defect and ruling out associated changes. Some syndromes may have specific associated ocular changes or secondary ocular complications such as exposure keratitis or strabismus related to orbital malposition. For further discussion, including illustrations, see also Part II, Embryology, in BCSC Section 2, *Fundamentals and Principles of Ophthalmology;* and BCSC Section 6, *Pediatric Ophthalmology and Strabismus.*

Anophthalmia

True anophthalmia is defined by Duke-Elder as a total absence of tissues of the eye. Three types of anophthalmia have been described. *Primary anophthalmia* is rare and usually bilateral. It occurs when the primary optic vesicle fails to grow out from the cerebral vesicle at the 2-mm stage of embryonic development. *Secondary anophthalmia* is rare and lethal and results from a gross abnormality in the anterior neural tube. *Consecutive anophthalmia* presumably results from a secondary degeneration of the optic vesicle.

Because orbital development is dependent on the size and growth of the globe, anophthalmic orbits are small, with hypoplastic eyelids and orbital adnexal structures.

Microphthalmia

Microphthalmia is much more common than anophthalmia and is defined as the presence of a small eye. Eyes vary in size depending on the severity of the defect. Most infants with a unilateral small orbit and no visible eye actually have a microphthalmic globe.

All children with microphthalmia have hypoplastic orbits. Most microphthalmic eyes have no potential for vision, and treatment focuses on achieving a cosmetically acceptable appearance that is reasonably symmetrical. Treatment begins shortly after birth and consists of socket expansion with progressively larger conformers, which are used until the patient can be fitted with a prosthesis at around age 3–4 months. In cases of severe bony asymmetry, intraorbital tissue expanders may be progressively inflated to enlarge the hypoplastic orbit.

Enucleation is usually not necessary for the fitting of a conformer or an ocular prosthesis and is ordinarily avoided because it may worsen the bony hypoplasia. However, in some cases of early enucleation, dermis-fat grafts have been used successfully as orbital implants. These grafts appear to grow along with the patient, resulting in progressive socket expansion. For older microphthalmic children, craniofacial techniques have been used to reposition and resize the orbit. Such repairs are complex, as noted in the following discussion of craniofacial clefting.

Microphthalmia with orbital cyst results from the failure of the choroidal fissure to close in the embryo. This condition is usually unilateral but may be bilateral. The presence of an orbital cyst may be beneficial for stimulating normal growth of the involved orbital bone and eyelids. In some cases, the orbital cyst may have to be removed to allow for fitting of an ocular prosthesis.

Craniofacial Clefting

Craniofacial clefts occur as a result of a developmental arrest. Etiologic theories include a failure of neural crest cell migration and a failure of fusion of facial processes. Facial clefts in the skeletal structures are distributed around the orbit and maxilla; clefts in the soft tissues are most apparent around the eyelids and lips. Examples of clefting syndromes affecting the orbit and eyelids are mandibulofacial dysostosis (Treacher Collins–Franceschetti syndrome; Fig 3-1), oculoauricular dysplasia (Goldenhar syndrome), and some forms of midline clefts with hypertelorism.

The bones of the skull or orbit may also have congenital clefts through which the intracranial contents can herniate. These protruding contents can be the meninges

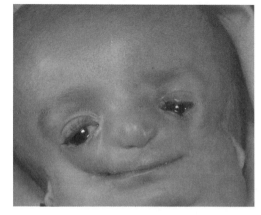

Figure 3-1 Treacher Collins–Franceschetti syndrome (mandibulofacial dysostosis). *(Courtesy of James Garrity, MD.)*

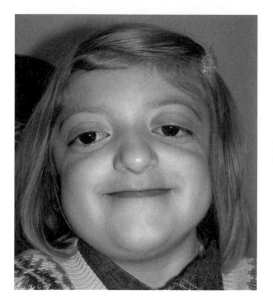

Figure 3-2 Crouzon syndrome (craniofacial dysostosis). *(Courtesy of Jill Foster, MD.)*

(meningocele), brain tissue *(encephalocele)*, or both meninges and brain tissue *(meningo-encephalocele)*. When these herniations involve the orbit, they most commonly present anteriorly with a protrusion subcutaneously near the medial canthus or over the bridge of the nose. Straining or crying may increase the size of the mass, and the globe may be displaced temporally and downward (inferolaterally). Such herniations less commonly move into the posterior orbit; these lesions may cause anterior displacement and pulsation of the globe. Treatment is surgical and should be carried out in collaboration with a neurosurgeon. Meningoceles and encephaloceles adjacent to the orbit are frequently associated with anomalies of the optic disc, such as morning glory disc.

Craniosynostosis, the premature closure of 1 or more sutures in the bones of the skull, results in various skeletal deformities. Secondary intracranial hypertension can be a complication. Hypertelorism and proptosis are frequently observed in craniosynostosis syndromes such as Crouzon syndrome (craniofacial dysostosis; Fig 3-2) and Apert syndrome (acrocephalosyndactyly).

The severe orbital and facial defects associated with craniofacial deformities can sometimes be corrected with surgery. Bony and soft-tissue reconstruction is generally needed. Such operations are often staged and usually require a team approach with multiple subspecialists.

Congenital Orbital Tumors

Hamartomas and Choristomas

Hamartomas are anomalous growths of tissue consisting only of mature cells normally found at the involved site. Classic examples are capillary hemangiomas and the characteristic lesions of neurofibromatosis. *Choristomas* are tissue anomalies characterized by types of cells not normally found at the involved site. Classic examples are dermoid cysts, epidermoid cysts, dermolipomas, and teratomas. These congenital and juvenile tumors are discussed further in BCSC Section 6, *Pediatric Ophthalmology and Strabismus.*

Dermoid cyst

Dermoid and epidermoid cysts are among the most common orbital tumors of childhood. These cysts are present congenitally and enlarge progressively. The more superficial cysts usually become symptomatic in childhood, but deeper orbital dermoids may not become clinically evident until adulthood. *Dermoid cysts* are lined by keratinizing epidermis with dermal appendages, such as hair follicles and sebaceous glands. They contain an admixture of oil and keratin. In contrast, *epidermoid cysts* are lined by epidermis only and are usually filled with keratin; they do not contain dermal appendages.

Preseptal orbital dermoid cysts occur most commonly in the area of the lateral brow adjacent to the frontozygomatic suture (Fig 3-3); less often they may be found in the medial upper eyelid adjacent to the frontoethmoidal suture. Dermoid cysts commonly present as palpable smooth, painless, oval masses that enlarge slowly. They may be freely mobile or they may be fixed to periosteum at the underlying suture. If the dermoid occurs more posteriorly, in the temporal fossa, computed tomography (CT) is often indicated to rule out dumbbell expansion through the suture into the underlying orbit. Medial lesions in the infant should be distinguished from congenital encephaloceles and dacryoceles.

Dermoid cysts that do not present until adulthood often are not palpable because they are situated posteriorly in the orbit, usually in the superior and temporal portions adjacent to the bony sutures. The globe and adnexa may be displaced, causing progressive proptosis, and erosion or remodeling of bone can occur. Long-standing dermoids in the superior orbit may completely erode the orbital roof and become adherent to the dura mater. An uncommon variant is the *intradiploic epidermoid cyst,* which tends to present late, after it has broken through and expanded the bony perimeter. Less commonly, the clinical presentation may be orbital inflammation, which is incited by leakage of oil and keratin from the cyst. Expansion of the dermoid cyst and inflammatory response to leakage may result in an orbitocutaneous fistula, which may also occur following incomplete surgical removal.

Management Dermoid cysts are usually removed surgically. Because dermoids that present in childhood are often superficial, they can be excised through an incision placed in the upper eyelid crease or directly over the lesion. If possible, the cyst wall should be

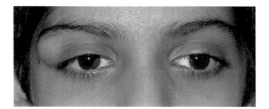

Figure 3-3 Child with a typical laterally located dermoid tumor (epithelial choristoma). *(Courtesy of Roberta Gausas, MD.)*

maintained during surgery. Rupture of the cyst can lead to an acute inflammatory process if part of the cyst wall or any of the contents remain within the eyelid or orbit. If the cyst wall is ruptured, the surgeon should remove the entire wall and then thoroughly irrigate the wound to remove all cyst contents. Surgical removal may be difficult if the cyst has leaked preoperatively and adhesions have developed.

Kersten RC. The eyelid crease approach to superficial lateral dermoid cysts. *J Pediatr Ophthalmol Strabismus.* 1988;25(1):48–51.

Shields JA, Kaden IH, Eagle RC Jr, Shields CL. Orbital dermoid cysts: clinicopathologic correlations, classification, and management. *Ophthal Plast Reconstr Surg.* 1997;13(4):265–276.

Dermolipomas

Dermolipomas are solid tumors usually located beneath the conjunctiva over the globe's lateral surface (Fig 3-4). These benign lesions may have deep extensions that can extend to the levator and extraocular muscles. Superficially, dermolipomas may have fine hairs that can be irritating to patients. These tumors typically require no treatment. If the lesion is large and cosmetically objectionable, only the anterior, visible portion should be excised; if possible, the overlying conjunctiva should be preserved. Care must be taken to avoid damage to the lacrimal gland ducts, extraocular muscles, and the levator aponeurosis. Lesions that may simulate dermolipomas include prolapsed orbital fat, prolapsed palpebral lobe of the lacrimal gland, and lymphomas (such processes are generally found only in adults).

Fry CL, Leone CR Jr. Safe management of dermolipomas. *Arch Ophthalmol.* 1994;112(8):1114–1116.

Teratoma

Teratomas are rare tumors that arise from all 3 germinal layers (ectoderm, mesoderm, and endoderm). These tumors are usually cystic and can cause dramatic proptosis at birth. As a consequence, the globe and optic nerve may be maldeveloped. If malignant, exenteration may be necessary. However, some cystic teratomas can be removed and ocular function preserved.

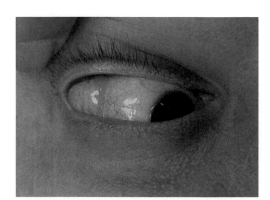

Figure 3-4 Dermolipoma of right lateral orbit. *(Courtesy of Vikram Durairaj, MD.)*

CHAPTER 4

Orbital Inflammatory and Infectious Disorders

Orbital inflammatory disease comprises a broad range of disorders that can be divided conceptually into specific and nonspecific inflammations; in other words, those that have an identifiable cause and those that do not. For example, an infection or autoimmune disease can be considered a specific cause of orbital inflammation. In contrast, *nonspecific orbital inflammation (NSOI)* is defined as a benign inflammatory process of the orbit without a known local or systemic cause. It is therefore a diagnosis of exclusion arrived at after all specific causes of inflammation have been eliminated. Table 4-1 shows a limited differential diagnosis of orbital inflammatory disease. This chapter presents an overview of the major causes of specific and nonspecific orbital inflammation, with the goal of providing a working knowledge of the most common of these disorders.

Gordon LK. Orbital inflammatory disease: a diagnostic and therapeutic challenge. *Eye (Lond).* 2006;20(10):1196–1206.

Table 4-1 Differential Diagnosis of Major Orbital Inflammations

---

Infectious (identify the anatomic location as preseptal or orbital cellulitis)
  Bacterial (identify the source)
    Direct inoculation (trauma, surgery)
    Spread from adjacent tissue (sinusitis, dacryocystitis)
    Spread from distant focus (bacteremia, pneumonia)
    Opportunistic (necrotizing fasciitis, tuberculosis)
  Fungal
    Zygomycosis
    Aspergillosis
  Parasitic
    Echinococcosis
    Cysticercosis
Autoimmune
  Thyroid eye disease (TED)
Vasculitic
  Giant cell arteritis
  Wegener granulomatosis
  Polyarteritis nodosa
  Vasculitis associated with connective tissue disorders
Granulomatous
  Sarcoidosis
Nonspecific orbital inflammation (NSOI) (diagnosis of exclusion)

Infectious Inflammation

Cellulitis

The most common cause of cellulitis is bacterial infection. However, in each clinical setting, the physician must first define the etiology of the cellulitis; failure to do so may result in delays both in the identification of noninfectious (ie, autoimmune, malignant, foreign body) etiologies and in their effective treatment.

Bacterial infections of the orbit or periorbital soft tissues originate from 3 primary sources:

- direct spread from adjacent sinusitis or dacryocystitis
- direct inoculation following trauma or skin infection
- bacteremic spread from a distant focus (otitis media, pneumonia)

Although periorbital infections are typically classified as being either preseptal (all findings anterior to the orbital septum) or orbital cellulitis (involvement posterior to the septum), they often represent a continuum, with common underlying causes requiring similar treatment regimens. It must be emphasized that infectious cellulitis—whether preseptal or orbital—is most commonly caused by underlying sinusitis if no obvious source of inoculation is noted.

Preseptal cellulitis

Preseptal cellulitis occurs anterior to the septum. Eyelid edema, erythema, and inflammation may be severe, but the globe is uninvolved. Therefore, pupillary reaction, visual acuity, and ocular motility are not disturbed; and pain on eye movement and chemosis are absent.

Although preseptal cellulitis in adults is usually due to penetrating cutaneous trauma or dacryocystitis, in children the most common cause is underlying sinusitis. Historically, preseptal cellulitis in infants and children younger than 5 years was often associated with bacteremia, septicemia, and meningitis caused by *Haemophilus influenzae.* However, the introduction of the *H influenzae* B (Hib) vaccine has virtually eliminated this etiology. Now, most pediatric cases are the result of gram-positive cocci infection. Because some children have not received appropriate immunization, the clinician should discuss the child's vaccination history with the parents to determine whether all vaccinations are current.

Treatment Workup should proceed quickly, particularly in children, and include computed tomography (CT) of the orbit and sinuses if the eyelid swelling is profound enough to preclude examination of the globe and thereby exclude orbital cellulitis.

The patient should be treated in consultation with a primary care physician. In children, oral antibiotics (such as cephalexin or ampicillin) and nasal decongestants (such as oxymetazoline nasal spray), in cases of associated sinusitis, are typically effective therapy; this approach is chosen if the examination of the child is reliable and follow-up examinations can be ensured. Hospitalization and intravenous (IV) antibiotics (such as ceftriaxone and vancomycin) are indicated if the cellulitis progresses despite outpatient therapy, as cases of preseptal infection can progress to orbital cellulitis.

In teenagers and adults, preseptal cellulitis usually arises from a superficial source and responds quickly to appropriate oral antibiotics (such as ampicillin-sulbactam, trimethoprim-sulfamethoxazole, or clindamycin) and warm compresses. Initial antibiotic selection is based on the history, clinical findings, and initial laboratory studies. Prompt sensitivity studies are indicated so that the antibiotic selection can be revised, if necessary. *Staphylococcus aureus* is the most common pathogen in patients with preseptal cellulitis resulting from trauma. The infection usually responds rapidly to a penicillinase-resistant penicillin, such as methicillin or ampicillin-sulbactam. However, methicillin-resistant *S aureus (MRSA)*, previously recognized as a cause of severe nosocomial infections, is now increasingly encountered in the community setting as well. Community-associated MRSA (CA-MRSA) infections tend to present as a fluctuant abscess with surrounding cellulitis. The pain associated with the lesion is often out of proportion to its appearance. CA-MRSA is often susceptible to a range of antibiotics (including trimethoprim-sulfamethoxazole, rifampin, or clindamycin), whereas hospital-associated MRSA is sensitive only to vancomycin and linezolid. However, both types of MRSA may result in acute morbidity and long-term disability. MRSA has also been associated with necrotizing fasciitis, orbital cellulitis, endogenous endophthalmitis, panophthalmitis, and cavernous sinus thrombosis. Because of the potentially aggressive nature of this pathogen, successful management demands a high degree of clinical suspicion and prompt medical and surgical intervention. In addition, consultation with infectious disease specialists may be warranted.

In elderly patients, infections behave differently. These patients may not manifest the typical signs of inflammation, increased erythema and calor, as seen in younger patients. Furthermore, more severe infections may not be associated with febrile reactions. Response to antibiotics may also be delayed, and surgical intervention to excise devitalized tissue may be necessary to clear an infection.

Imaging studies should be performed to rule out underlying sinusitis if no direct inoculation site is identified. If the patient does not respond within a day to oral antibiotics or if orbital involvement becomes evident, prompt hospital admission, CT, and IV antibiotics are usually indicated.

Surgical drainage may be necessary if preseptal cellulitis progresses to a localized abscess. Incision and drainage can usually be performed directly over the abscess, but care should be taken to avoid damaging the levator aponeurosis in the upper eyelid. To avoid contaminating the orbital soft tissues, the surgeon should not open the orbital septum.

Pelton RW, Klapper SR. Preseptal and orbital cellulitis. *Focal Points: Clinical Modules for Ophthalmologists.* San Francisco: American Academy of Ophthalmology; 2009, module 11.

Rutar T, Chambers HF, Crawford JB, et al. Ophthalmic manifestations of infections caused by the USA300 clone of community-associated methicillin-resistant *Staphylococcus aureus*. *Ophthalmology.* 2006;113(8):1455–1462.

Orbital cellulitis

Orbital cellulitis involves structures posterior to the orbital septum; and in more than 90% of cases, it occurs as a secondary extension of acute or chronic bacterial sinusitis (Table 4-2). Clinical findings include fever, leukocytosis (75% of cases), proptosis, chemosis, ptosis, and restriction of and pain with ocular movement (Fig 4-1). Decreased visual acuity, impaired color vision, restricted visual fields, and pupillary abnormalities suggest

Rarely, contralateral ophthalmoplegia has been reported as well. Meningitis and frank brain abscess may develop. A lumbar puncture may reveal acute inflammatory cells and the causative organism on stain and culture.

Garcia GH, Harris GJ. Criteria for nonsurgical management of subperiosteal abscess of the orbit: analyses of outcomes 1988–1998. *Ophthalmology.* 2000;107(8):1454–1458.

Harris GJ. Subperiosteal abscess of the orbit: age as a factor in the bacteriology and response to treatment. *Ophthalmology.* 1994;101(3):585–595.

Necrotizing Fasciitis

Necrotizing fasciitis is a severe, potentially vision- or life-threatening bacterial infection involving the subcutaneous soft tissues, particularly the superficial and deep fasciae. Group A β-hemolytic *Streptococcus* is the organism most commonly responsible, although a variety of organisms, including aerobic and anaerobic, gram-positive and gram-negative bacteria, may cause this disorder.

This infection develops rapidly and requires immediate attention because it is potentially fatal. Although most patients are immunocompromised by conditions such as diabetes mellitus or alcoholism, it may also occur in immunocompetent patients. The initial clinical presentation is similar to that of orbital or preseptal cellulitis, with swelling, erythema, and pain; but it may be accompanied by a shocklike syndrome. Because necrotizing fasciitis tends to track along avascular tissue planes, an early sign may be anesthesia over the affected area caused by involvement of deep cutaneous nerves. In addition, disproportionate complaints of pain may suggest the possibility of necrotizing fasciitis, as do typical changes in skin color progressing from rose to blue-gray with bullae formation and frank cutaneous necrosis. Usually, the course is rapid and the patient requires treatment in an intensive care unit.

Treatment includes early surgical debridement along with IV antibiotics. If the involved pathogen is unknown, broad-spectrum coverage for gram-positive and gram-negative as well as anaerobic organisms is indicated. Clindamycin is of particular value, as it is uniquely effective against the toxins produced by group A *Streptococcus*. To limit the inflammatory damage associated with the toxins, adjunctive corticosteroid therapy after the start of antibiotic therapy has been advocated. Some cases of necrotizing fasciitis limited to the eyelids can be cautiously followed with systemic antibiotic therapy and little or no debridement; this approach should be considered only in cases that rapidly demarcate and show no signs of toxic shock.

Patients may experience rapid deterioration, culminating in hypotension, renal failure, and adult respiratory distress syndrome. Clinical series from all body sites report up to a 30% mortality rate, usually due to toxic shock syndrome, but this occurs less commonly in the periocular region.

Lazzeri D, Lazzeri S, Figus M, et al. Periorbital necrotizing fasciitis. *Br J Ophthalmol.* 2009 Nov 5 [Epub ahead of print].

Luksich JA, Holds JB, Hartstein ME. Conservative management of necrotizing fasciitis of the eyelids. *Ophthalmology.* 2002;109(11):2118–2122.

Orbital Tuberculosis

Although previously recognized mostly in endemic areas of the developing world, tuberculosis has recently reemerged as a public health threat in developed countries as well. Orbital tuberculosis occurs most commonly as a result of hematogenous spread from a pulmonary focus, which is often subclinical. Less often, spread occurs from an adjacent tuberculous sinusitis. Proptosis, motility dysfunction, bone destruction, and chronic draining fistulas may be the presenting findings. In the developed world, this disease is most often associated with human immunodeficiency virus and inner-city poverty. The majority of recent orbital cases have been reported in children, and the infection is often mistaken for an orbital malignancy. The disease is usually unilateral. Acid-fast bacilli may be difficult to detect in pathologic specimens, which usually show caseating necrosis, epithelioid cells, and Langhans giant cells. Skin testing and fine-needle aspiration biopsy with culture early in the course of the disease may help establish the diagnosis. Antituberculous therapy is usually curative.

Khalil M, Lindley S, Matouk E. Tuberculosis of the orbit. *Ophthalmology*. 1985;92(11): 1624–1627.

Zygomycosis

Zygomycosis (also known as *phycomycosis* or *mucormycosis*) is the most common and the most virulent fungal disease involving the orbit. The specific fungal genus involved is usually *Mucor* or *Rhizopus*. These fungi, belonging to the class Zygomycetes, almost always extend into the orbit from an adjacent sinus or the nasal cavity. The fungi invade blood vessel walls, producing thrombosing vasculitis. The resultant tissue necrosis promotes further fungal invasion.

Patients commonly present with proptosis and an orbital apex syndrome (internal and external ophthalmoplegia, ptosis, decreased corneal sensation, and decreased vision). Elderly patients may be relatively immunosuppressed compared to younger patients and therefore are at risk for these virulent infections.

Predisposing factors include systemic disease with associated metabolic acidosis, diabetes mellitus, malignancies, and treatment with antimetabolites or steroids. Diagnosis is confirmed by a biopsy of the necrotic-appearing tissues in the nasopharynx or the involved sinus or orbit. The histology of zygomycosis shows nonseptate large branching hyphae that stain with hematoxylin-eosin, unlike most fungi (see the discussion of fungal infections in BCSC Section 5, *Neuro-Ophthalmology*).

Therapeutic measures should be aimed at both systemic control of the underlying metabolic or immunologic abnormality and local surgical debridement. Antifungal therapy should be given via IV administration of amphotericin B or liposomal amphotericin B. Alternatively, other lipid-encapsulated antifungal agents, which permit a higher cumulative dose with a reduced level of toxicity, may be considered. Some authors have proposed adjunctive hyperbaric oxygen therapy. The role of primary exenteration has decreased, but it is unclear whether patient survival (typically poor) has been adversely affected by less-aggressive surgical excision.

Ferry AP, Abedi S. Diagnosis and management of rhino-orbitocerebral mucormycosis (phyco-mycosis). A report of 16 personally observed cases. *Ophthalmology.* 1983;90(9):1096–1104.

Kronish JW, Johnson TE, Gilberg SM, Corrent GF, McLeish WM, Scott KR. Orbital infections in patients with human immunodeficiency virus infection. *Ophthalmology.* 1996;103(9): 1483–1492.

Aspergillosis

The fungus *Aspergillus* can affect the orbit in several distinct clinical entities. *Acute as-pergillosis* is a fungal disease characterized by fulminant sinus infection with secondary orbital invasion. Patients present with severe periorbital pain, decreased vision, and prop-tosis. Diagnosis is confirmed by 1 or more biopsies. Grocott-Gomori methenamine–silver nitrate stain shows septate branching hyphae of uniform width (see the discussion of fun-gal infections in BCSC Section 5, *Neuro-Ophthalmology*). Therapy consists of aggressive surgical excision of all infected tissues and administration of amphotericin B, flucytosine, rifampin, or a combination thereof.

Chronic aspergillosis is an indolent infection resulting in slow destruction of the si-nuses and adjacent structures. Although the prognosis is much better than for acute ful-minant disease, intraorbital and intracranial extension can occur in the chronic invasive form of fungal sinusitis as well and result in significant morbidity.

Chronic localized noninvasive aspergillosis also involves the sinuses and occurs in immunocompetent patients who may not have a history of atopic disease. Often, there is a history of chronic sinusitis, and proliferation of saprophytic organisms results in a tightly packed fungus ball. This type of aspergillosis is characterized by a lack of either inflam-mation or bone erosion.

Allergic aspergillosis sinusitis occurs in immunocompetent patients with nasal pol-yposis and chronic sinusitis. Patients may have peripheral eosinophilia; elevated total im-munoglobulin E level, fungus-specific immunoglobulin E, and immunoglobulin G levels; or positive skin test results for fungal antigens. CT scanning reveals thick allergic mucin within the sinus as mottled areas of increased attenuation on nonenhanced images. Bone erosion and remodeling are frequently present but do not signify actual tissue invasion. Magnetic resonance imaging (MRI) may be more specific, showing signal void areas on T2-weighted scans. Sinus biopsy results reveal thick, peanut butter–like or green mucus, pathologic study of which reveals numerous eosinophils and eosinophil degradation products, as well as extramucosal fungal hyphae. Endoscopic debridement of the involved sinuses is indicated. Treatment with systemic and topical corticosteroids is also recom-mended. Up to 17% of patients with allergic fungal sinusitis present first with orbital signs.

Como JA, Dismukes WE. Oral azole drugs as systemic antifungal therapy. *N Engl J Med.* 1994;330(4):263–272.

Klapper SR, Lee AG, Patrinely JR, Stewart M, Alford EL. Orbital involvement in allergic fungal sinusitis. *Ophthalmology.* 1997;104(12):2094–2100.

Levin LA, Avery R, Shore JW, Woog JJ, Baker AS. The spectrum of orbital aspergillosis: a clini-copathological review. *Surv Ophthalmol.* 1996;41(2):142–154.

Parasitic Diseases

Parasitic diseases of the orbit are generally limited to developing countries and include trichinosis and echinococcosis. *Trichinosis* is caused by ingestion of the nematode *Trichinella spiralis*. The eyelids and extraocular muscles may be inflamed by migration of the larvae. *Echinococcosis* is caused by the dog tapeworm *Echinococcus granulosus*. A hydatid cyst containing tapeworm larvae may form in the orbit. Rupture of such a cyst may cause progressive inflammation and a severe immune response. *Taenia solium,* the pork tapeworm, may also encyst and progressively enlarge in the orbital tissues, causing a condition known as *cysticercosis.*

Noninfectious Inflammation

Thyroid Eye Disease

Thyroid eye disease (TED; also known as *Graves ophthalmopathy, dysthyroid ophthalmopathy, thyroid-associated orbitopathy, thyroid orbitopathy, thyrotoxic exophthalmos,* and other terms) is an autoimmune inflammatory disorder whose underlying cause continues to be elucidated. The clinical signs, however, are characteristic and include 1 or more of the following: eyelid retraction, lid lag, proptosis, restrictive extraocular myopathy, and compressive optic neuropathy (Figs 4-3 through 4-5). TED was originally described as part of the triad comprising Graves disease, which includes the aforementioned orbital signs, hyperthyroidism, and pretibial myxedema. Though typically associated with Graves hyperthyroidism, TED may also occur with Hashimoto thyroiditis (immune-induced hypothyroidism) or in the absence of thyroid dysfunction. The course of the eye disease does not necessarily parallel the activity of the thyroid gland or the treatment of thyroid abnormalities.

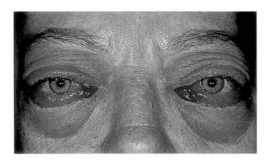

Figure 4-3 Signs of active inflammation in a patient with TED include bilateral proptosis, chemosis, and eyelid swelling. *(Courtesy of Jeffrey A. Nerad, MD.)*

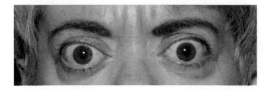

Figure 4-4 TED, showing bilateral proptosis and eyelid retraction. *(Courtesy of Roberta E. Gausas, MD.)*

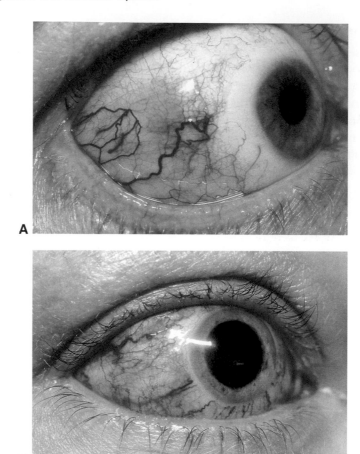

Figure 4-5 **A,** Conjunctival erythema over the insertions of the rectus muscles is a frequent sign of TED. Typically, there is a clear zone between the anterior extent of the abnormally dilated blood vessels and the corneoscleral limbus. **B,** In contrast, the arterialization of blood vessels that occurs with a dural shunt is usually more diffuse and extends to the limbus. *(Courtesy of George B. Bartley, MD.)*

Diagnosis

The diagnosis of TED is made when 2 of the following 3 signs of the disease are present:

1. Concurrent or recently treated immune-related thyroid dysfunction (1 or more of the following):

   a. Graves hyperthyroidism
   b. Hashimoto thyroiditis
   c. Presence of circulating thyroid antibodies without a coexisting dysthyroid state (partial consideration given): TSH-receptor (TSH-R) antibodies, thyroid-binding inhibitory immunoglobulins (TBII), thyroid-stimulating immunoglobulins (TSI), antimicrosomal antibody

2. Typical orbital signs (1 or more of the following):

   a. Unilateral or bilateral eyelid retraction with typical temporal flare (with or without lagophthalmos)
   b. Unilateral or bilateral proptosis (as evidenced by comparison with patient's old photos)
   c. Restrictive strabismus in a typical pattern
   d. Compressive optic neuropathy
   e. Fluctuating eyelid edema/erythema
   f. Chemosis/caruncular edema

3. Radiographic evidence of TED—unilateral/bilateral fusiform enlargement of 1 or more of the following (Figs 4-6, 4-7):

   a. Inferior rectus muscle
   b. Medial rectus muscle
   c. Superior rectus/levator complex
   d. Lateral rectus muscle

If only orbital signs are present, the patient should continue to be observed for other orbital diseases and for the future development of a dysthyroid state.

Gerding MN, van der Meer JW, Broenink M, Bakker O, Wiersinga WM, Prummel MF. Association of thyrotrophin receptor antibodies with the clinical features of Graves' ophthalmopathy. *Clin Endocrinol.* 2000;52(3):267–271.

Mourits MP, Prummel MF, Wiersinga WM, Koornneef L. Clinical activity score as a guide in the management of patients with Graves' ophthalmopathy. *Clin Endocrinol.* 1997;47(1):9–14.

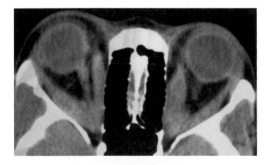

Figure 4-6 Axial orbital CT scan of TED shows characteristic fusiform extraocular muscle enlargement that spares the tendons. Marked enlargement of the extraocular muscles with effacement of the perioptic fat is consistent with compressive optic neuropathy. *(Courtesy of Roberta E. Gausas, MD.)*

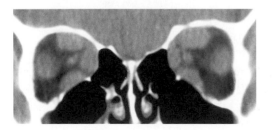

Figure 4-7 Coronal orbital CT scan shows bilateral enlargement of extraocular muscles in TED. *(Courtesy of Roberta E. Gausas, MD.)*

Pathogenesis

Over the last decade, the focus of in vitro research has shifted away from the extraocular muscles/myocytes to the orbital fibroblasts as the primary target of the inflammatory process associated with TED. Of particular importance is the recognition that orbital fibroblasts are phenotypically different from fibroblasts derived from other sites in the body. Orbital fibroblasts—through the expression of characteristic surface receptors, gangliosides, and proinflammatory genes—play an active role in modulating the inflammatory process. Unlike fibroblasts from other parts of the body, orbital fibroblasts express CD40 receptors, generally found on B cells. When engaged by T-cell–bound CD154, several fibroblast proinflammatory genes are up-regulated, including interleukin-6 (IL-6), IL-8, and prostaglandin E_2 (PGE$_2$). In turn, synthesis of hyaluronan and glycosaminoglycan (GAG) is increased. The up-regulation of GAG synthesis is known to be essential in the pathology of TED, and it occurs at a rate that is 100-fold greater in orbital fibroblasts derived from patients with TED than in abdominal fibroblasts in the same patients. This cascade of up-regulation is dampened by the addition of therapeutic levels of corticosteroids.

Orbital fibroblasts are embryologically derived from the neural crest and, as such, possess developmental plasticity. A subpopulation of orbital fibroblasts appears capable of undergoing adipocyte differentiation. It is believed that this response to the inflammatory matrix is responsible for the fatty hypertrophy that predominates in some patients, particularly those younger than 40 years.

The role of TSH-R in this process has been investigated extensively. Though studies demonstrate the expression of TSH-R on nearly all cells in the body, the unique response of orbital fibroblasts to TSH-R–mediated signaling may be due to up-regulation of TSH-R–mRNA synthesis in this cell population. It is thought that enhanced signaling through this receptor on orbital fibroblasts may promote adipogenesis, thereby stimulating the expansion of the orbital fat compartments seen in patients with TED.

Recent studies have also identified a circulating immunoglobulin (IgG) that recognizes and activates the insulin-like growth factor I receptor expressed on the surface of numerous cell types, including fibroblasts. These autoantibodies have been found in a majority of patients with Graves disease and may contribute to orbital pathogenesis by stimulating orbital fibroblasts to secrete glycosaminoglycans, cytokines, and chemoattractants. These latter signaling families may contribute to orbital inflammation and congestion. Manipulation of this pathway by available biologic agents (eg, rituximab) has recently emerged as a promising therapeutic strategy for treating patients with severe or refractory TED.

Kazim M, Goldberg RA, Smith TJ. Insights into the pathogenesis of thyroid-associated orbitopathy: evolving rationale for therapy. *Arch Ophthalmol.* 2002;120(3):380–386.

Naik V, Khadavi N, Naik MN, et al. Biologic therapeutics in thyroid-associated ophthalmopathy: translating disease mechanism into therapy. *Thyroid.* 2008;18(9):967–971.

Tsui S, Naik V, Hoa N, et al. Evidence for an association between thyroid-stimulating hormone and insulin-like growth factor 1 receptors: a tale of two antigens implicated in Graves' disease. *J Immunol.* 2008;181(6):4397–4405.

Epidemiology

A 1996 epidemiologic study of white American patients with TED determined that the overall age-adjusted incidence rate for women was 16 cases per 100,000 population per year, whereas the rate for men was 3 cases per 100,000 population per year. TED affects women approximately 6 times more frequently than men (86% versus 14% of cases, respectively). The peak incidence rates occurred in the age groups 40–44 years and 60–64 years in women and 45–49 years and 65–69 years in men. The median age at the time of diagnosis of TED was 43 years (range, 8–88 years). Smokers are up to 7 times more likely than nonsmokers to develop TED.

Clinical features

Among patients with TED, approximately 90% have Graves hyperthyroidism, 1% have primary hypothyroidism, 3% have Hashimoto thyroiditis, and 6% are euthyroid. There is a close temporal relationship between the development of hyperthyroidism and TED: in about 20% of patients, the diagnoses are made at the same time; in approximately 60% of patients, the eye disease occurs within 1 year of onset of the thyroid disease. Of those patients who have no history of abnormal thyroid function or regulation at the time of diagnosis of TED, the risk of developing thyroid disease is approximately 25% within 1 year and 50% within 5 years. Although most patients with TED have or will develop hyperthyroidism, only about 30% of patients with autoimmune hyperthyroidism have or will develop TED.

Eyelid retraction is the most common ophthalmic feature of TED, being present either unilaterally or bilaterally in more than 90% of patients at some point in their clinical course (see Chapter 11, Fig 11-17). Exophthalmos of 1 or both eyes affects approximately 60% of patients, restrictive extraocular myopathy is apparent in about 40% of patients, and optic nerve dysfunction occurs in 1 or both eyes in approximately 5% of patients with TED. Only 5% of patients have the complete constellation of classic findings: eyelid retraction, exophthalmos, optic nerve dysfunction, extraocular muscle involvement, and hyperthyroidism.

Upper eyelid retraction, either unilateral or bilateral, is documented in approximately 75% of patients at the time of diagnosis of TED. Lid lag in downgaze also is a frequent early sign, being present either unilaterally or bilaterally in 50% of patients at the initial examination. The most frequent ocular symptom when TED is first confirmed is dull, deep orbital pain or discomfort, which affects 30% of patients. Some degree of diplopia is noted by approximately 17% of patients, lacrimation or photophobia by 15%–20% of patients, and blurred vision by 7.5% of patients. Decreased vision attributable to optic neuropathy is present in less than 2% of eyes at the time of diagnosis of TED.

Pretibial myxedema and acropachy (soft-tissue swelling and periosteal changes affecting the distal extremities, principally fingers and toes) accompany TED in approximately 4% and 1% of patients, respectively, and are associated with a poor prognosis for the orbitopathy. Myasthenia gravis occurs in less than 1% of patients.

Bartley GB, Fatourechi V, Kadrmas EF, et al. Clinical features of Graves' ophthalmopathy in an incidence cohort. *Am J Ophthalmol.* 1996;121(3):284–290.

Holds JB, Buchanan AG. Graves orbitopathy. *Focal Points: Clinical Modules for Ophthalmologists.* San Francisco: American Academy of Ophthalmology; 2010, module 11.

Treatment and prognosis

TED is a self-limiting disease that on average lasts 1 year in nonsmokers and between 2 and 3 years in smokers. After the active disease plateaus, a quiescent burnt-out phase ensues. Reactivation of inflammation occurs in approximately 5%–10% of patients over their lifetime.

Treatment of patients with TED follows a stepwise, graded approach based on patient-reported symptoms, clinical examination, and ancillary testing (Tables 4-3, 4-4). Most patients with TED require only supportive care, including use of topical ocular lubricants; in some cases, topical cyclosporine has helped to reduce ocular surface irritation. Patients may also find certain lifestyle changes helpful. For example, eating a reduced-salt diet limits water retention and orbital edema, and sleeping with the head of the bed elevated specifically reduces fluid retention within the orbit. Wearing wraparound sunglasses relieves symptoms of dry eye and photophobia. If diplopia is present, use of temporary prism lenses helps maintain binocular fusion during the active phase of the disease.

Poor prognostic features include smoking, rapidly progressive (typically congestive) TED, and the presence of myxedema.

If orbital inflammation is severe, intervention may be necessary to prevent or ameliorate corneal exposure, globe subluxation, or optic neuropathy. Therapy usually is directed toward either decreasing orbital congestion and inflammation (through use of periocular corticosteroids or, if response is inadequate, by administration of systemic corticosteroids or periocular radiotherapy) or expanding the orbital bony volume (by surgical orbital decompression).

Establishing a euthyroid state is an important part of the care of patients with TED. Hyperthyroidism is most commonly treated with antithyroid drugs. If the patient does not tolerate the medications or if the medications fail to restore a persistent euthyroid state, the clinician usually tries radioactive iodine (RAI) as the next treatment modality. In some studies, TED has been demonstrated to worsen after RAI treatment, presumably because

---

Table 4-3 Evaluation of Thyroid Eye Disease

Clinical examination
Best-corrected visual acuity
Color vision
Pupillary examination
Ocular motility
Hertel exophthalmometry
Intraocular pressure (in primary gaze and upgaze)
Adnexal examination
Slit-lamp examination
Dilated fundus examination
Laboratory studies
T_3, free T_4, TSH, TSI
Imaging studies
Orbital ultrasound (assessment of extraocular muscle size and reflectivity)
Orbital CT scan or MRI (including coronal imaging)

Table 4-4 Management of Thyroid Eye Disease

Mild disease
  Observation
  Patient education/lifestyle changes
    Smoking cessation
    Salt restriction
    Elevation of head of bed
    Wearing sunglasses
  Ocular surface lubrication
Moderate disease
  Topical cyclosporine
  Eyelid taping at night
  Moisture goggles/chambers
  Prism glasses or selective ocular patching
  Moderate-dose oral steroid therapy
Severe disease
  High-dose oral steroid therapy or intravenous steroid therapy
  Surgical orbital decompression (followed by strabismus surgery and/or eyelid surgery)
  Periocular radiotherapy
Refractory disease
  Steroid-sparing immunomodulators (rituximab, others)

---

of the release of TSH-R antigens, which incite an enhanced immune response. In addition, hypothyroidism occurring after RAI treatment may exacerbate TED via stimulation of TSH-R. Hyperthyroid patients with severe, active TED; those with elevated T_3 levels; and smokers appear to be at greatest risk for exacerbation of eye disease after RAI treatment. Consequently, some patients are treated concurrently with oral corticosteroids. Although this may be a reasonable strategy for high-risk patients, the regular use of moderate-dose prednisone for 3 months, during which time the thyroid gland involutes, is not indicated for the average patient. Block-and-replace therapy with iodine 131, methimazole, and thyroxine may prevent exacerbation of eye findings by limiting posttreatment TSH spikes. Patients with severe TED (rapidly progressive and congestive, with compressive optic neuropathy) may, as an alternative to RAI, benefit from thyroidectomy, which renders them hypothyroid without extended antigen release.

Approximately 20% of patients with TED undergo surgical treatment. In 1 review, 7% of patients underwent orbital decompression; 9%, strabismus surgery; and 13%, eyelid surgery. Only 2.5% required all 3 types of surgery. Men and older patients are more likely to have more severe TED requiring surgical intervention. Surgery should be delayed until the disease has stabilized, unless urgent intervention is required to reverse visual loss due to compressive optic neuropathy or corneal exposure unresponsive to maximal medical measures. Elective orbital decompression, strabismus surgery, and eyelid retraction repair are usually not considered until a euthyroid state has been maintained and the ophthalmic signs have been confirmed to be stable for 6–9 months.

Acute-phase TED featuring compressive optic neuropathy is typically treated with oral corticosteroids. The usual starting dose is 1 mg/kg of prednisone. This dose is maintained for 2–4 weeks until a clinical response is apparent. The dose is then reduced as rapidly as can be tolerated by the patient, based on the clinical response of optic nerve function. In the setting of more severe inflammation or rapid disease progression, treatment with intravenous methylprednisolone may be considered. Liver function tests should be checked prior to initial administration and monitored frequently throughout treatment because of the reported association of fatal hepatotoxicity with this agent. Though effective at reversing optic nerve compression, high-dose corticosteroids are poorly tolerated and are associated with an extensive list of potential systemic adverse effects, which limit their long-term use. Thus, some authors have advocated the adjunctive use of orbital radiotherapy (2000 cGy). The mechanism for radiotherapy's effect on the orbit is not well understood, but beyond temporary lymphocyte sterilization, there is evidence that this dose induces terminal differentiation of fibroblasts and kills tissue-bound monocytes, which play an important role in antigen presentation. It is important to note, however, that radiation therapy should be avoided in patients with diabetes or vasculitic disease, as the radiation may exacerbate retinopathy.

A number of studies have demonstrated the effectiveness of orbital radiotherapy in the treatment of compressive optic neuropathy in reducing the need for acute-phase surgical decompression. However, a large, prospective clinical trial designed to assess the efficacy of periocular radiotherapy versus sham treatment demonstrated no statistically significant effect of treatment as compared with the natural history of TED. However, an important limitation of this trial is that it excluded patients with optic neuropathy. Critics of the study have also suggested that, because the median time from onset of TED to radiation therapy was 1.3 years, the lack of apparent benefit could be ascribed to the inclusion of patients with inactive disease. Furthermore, the sham-treated orbits also failed to show any change in clinically measured parameters for the duration of the study, which, critics suggest, indicates a stable phase of disease.

Orbital decompression, though historically used to treat optic neuropathy, severe orbital congestion, and advanced proptosis, has been used increasingly in recent years as an elective procedure to restore normal globe position in patients without sight-threatening ophthalmopathy. In the stable phase of disease, the surgical plan for decompression should be graded to achieve the greatest return to the premorbid state at the least possible risk. Preoperative review of the patient's old photos allows the surgeon to determine the amount of decompressive effect desired. The preoperative CT scan details the relative contributions of extraocular muscle enlargement and fat expansion to the proptosis (see Figs 4-6, 4-7). Typically, there is a difference in the phenotype of the orbital involvement based on the patient's age. Patients younger than 40 years demonstrate enlargement of the orbital fat compartment, whereas those older than 40 typically show more significant extraocular muscle enlargement. This difference determines the effectiveness of bone versus fat decompression surgery. Orbital decompression may alter extraocular motility and, if indicated, should precede strabismus surgery.

If intractable diplopia persists in primary gaze or in the reading position, strabismus surgery may be helpful in restoring single vision. In addition, procedures to correct eyelid retraction may decrease corneal exposure and help improve appearance. Because extraocular muscle surgery may affect eyelid retraction, eyelid surgery should be undertaken last.

Alternatively, botulinum toxin may rarely be employed to temporarily paralyze a tight extraocular muscle in restrictive strabismus or to weaken the levator palpebrae superioris muscle to treat eyelid retraction. Due to technical and practical limitations (the difficulty of titrating the effect and precisely delivering the agent within the orbit, the unpredictability and frequent ineffectiveness of botulinum toxin on fibrotic muscles, and the need for indefinite readministration), this therapeutic approach is infrequently employed. However, it may be of benefit in patients who are poor surgical candidates.

A long-term follow-up study of patients in an incidence cohort demonstrated that visual loss from optic neuropathy was uncommon and that persistent diplopia usually could be treated with prism spectacles. Subjectively, however, more than 50% of patients thought that their eyes looked abnormal, and 38% of patients were dissatisfied with the appearance of their eyes. Thus, although few patients experience long-term functional impairment from TED, the psychological and aesthetic sequelae of the disease are considerable. Orbital decompression surgery is discussed in Chapter 7.

See Key Points 4-1.

Bartalena L, Marcocci C, Bogazzi F, et al. Relation between therapy for hyperthyroidism and the course of Graves' ophthalmopathy. *N Engl J Med.* 1998;338(2):73–78.

Bartley GB, Fatourechi V, Kadrmas EF, et al. Long-term follow-up of Graves ophthalmopathy in an incidence cohort. *Ophthalmology.* 1996;103(6):958–962.

Gorman CA, Garrity JA, Fatourechi V, et al. A prospective, randomized, double-blind, placebo-controlled study of orbital radiotherapy for Graves' ophthalmopathy. *Ophthalmology.* 2001;108(9):1523–1534 [erratum in *Ophthalmology.* 2004;111(7):1306].

Kazim M. Perspective—Part II: radiotherapy for Graves orbitopathy: the Columbia University experience. *Ophthal Plast Reconstr Surg.* 2002;18(3):173–174.

Morgenstern KE, Evanchan J, Foster JA, et al. Botulinum toxin type A for dysthyroid upper eyelid retraction. *Ophthal Plast Reconstr Surg.* 2004;20(3):181–185.

Mourits MP, van Kempen-Harteveld ML, Garcia MB, Koppeschaar HP, Tick L, Terwee CB. Radiotherapy for Graves' orbitopathy: randomized placebo-controlled study. *Lancet.* 2000;355(9412):1505–1509.

Trokel S, Kazim M, Moore S. Orbital fat removal. Decompression for Graves orbitopathy. *Ophthalmology.* 1993;100(5):674–682.

Vasculitis

The vasculitides are inflammatory conditions in which the vessel walls are infiltrated by inflammatory cells. These lesions represent a type III hypersensitivity reaction to circulating immune complexes and usually lead to significant ocular or orbital morbidity. They are often associated with systemic vasculitis. The following discussion focuses mainly on the orbital manifestations of the vasculitides. See also BCSC Section 1, *Update on General Medicine,* and Section 5, *Neuro-Ophthalmology.*

Giant cell arteritis

Although the orbital vessels are inflamed in giant cell arteritis (GCA; also known as *temporal arteritis*), it is not typically thought of as an orbital disorder. The vasculitis affects the aorta and branches of the external and internal carotid arteries and vertebral arteries but

KEY POINTS 4-1

Thyroid eye disease (TED) The following list highlights the essential points for the ophthalmologist to remember about TED.

- Eyelid retraction is the most common clinical feature of TED (and TED is the most common cause of eyelid retraction).
- TED is the most common cause of unilateral or bilateral proptosis.
- TED may be markedly asymmetric.
- TED is associated with hyperthyroidism in 90% of patients, but 6% of patients may be euthyroid.
- Severity of TED usually does not parallel serum levels of T_4 or T_3.
- TED is 6 times more common in women than in men.
- Smoking is associated with increased risk and severity of TED.
- Urgent care may be required for optic neuropathy or severe proptosis with corneal decompensation.
- If surgery is needed, the usual order is orbital decompression, followed by strabismus surgery, followed by eyelid retraction repair (see Chapter 7).

usually spares the intracranial carotid branches, which lack an elastic lamina. Symptoms of visual loss are caused by central retinal artery occlusion or ischemic optic neuropathy, and diplopia may result from ischemic dysfunction of other cranial nerves. Symptoms of headache, scalp tenderness, jaw claudication, or malaise are often present. The erythrocyte sedimentation rate (ESR) is markedly elevated in 90% of patients, and diagnostic confidence is increased if the C-reactive protein level and the platelet count are elevated. Temporal artery biopsy usually provides a definitive diagnosis, although bilateral biopsies are sometimes necessary due to intervals of normal tissue between affected segments. GCA should be managed as an ophthalmic emergency. Failure to diagnose and treat GCA immediately after loss of vision in 1 eye is particularly tragic because timely treatment with corticosteroids usually prevents an attack in the second eye. Generalized orbital ischemia resulting from temporal arteritis is a rare manifestation of the disease.

Goodwin JA. Temporal arteritis: diagnosis and management. *Focal Points: Clinical Modules for Ophthalmologists.* San Francisco: American Academy of Ophthalmology; 1992, module 2.

Wegener granulomatosis

Wegener granulomatosis is characterized by necrotizing granulomatous vasculitis, lesions of the upper and lower respiratory tract, necrotizing glomerulonephritis, and a small-vessel vasculitis that can affect any organ system, including the orbit. Clinically, the full-blown syndrome includes sinus mucosal involvement with bone erosion, tracheobronchial necrotic lesions, cavitary lung lesions, and glomerulonephritis (Fig 4-8). The orbit and nasolacrimal drainage system may be involved by extension from the surrounding sinuses. Up to 25% of patients with Wegener granulomatosis have associated scleritis.

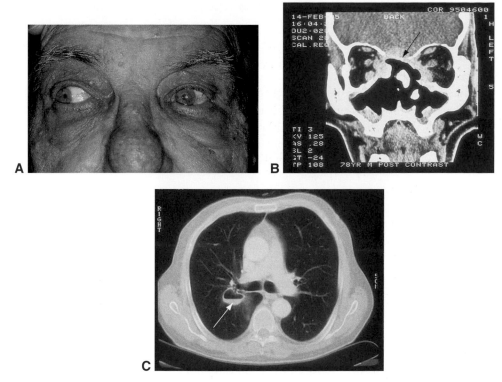

Figure 4-8 Wegener granulomatosis. **A,** Restrictive strabismus OS due to inflammatory tissue extending into medial aspects of orbit. **B,** Coronal CT scan showing extensive destruction of the nasal and sinus cavities with inflammatory tissue extending into orbits and brain *(arrow).* **C,** CT of chest showing cavitary lung lesions *(arrow). (Courtesy of Jeffrey Nerad, MD.)*

Limited forms of the disease have been described in which the renal component is absent or in which there is solitary orbital involvement by a granulomatous and lymphocytic vasculitis. Such isolated orbital involvement may be unilateral or bilateral; may lack frank necrotizing vasculitis on histologic examination; and, in the absence of respiratory tract and renal findings, may be difficult to diagnose.

Characteristic pathologic findings consist of the triad of vasculitis, granulomatous inflammation (with or without giant cells), and tissue necrosis. Often, only 1 or 2 of these 3 are present on extrapulmonary biopsies. Antineutrophil cytoplasmic antibody (ANCA) titers measured by serum immunofluorescence have been shown to be associated with certain systemic vasculitides. The ANCA test distinguishes 2 types of immunofluorescence patterns. Diffuse granular fluorescence within the cytoplasm (c-ANCA) is highly specific for Wegener granulomatosis. This pattern is caused by autoantibodies directed against proteinase 3, which can also be detected by enzyme-linked immunosorbent assay (ELISA). Fluorescence surrounding the nucleus (p-ANCA) is an artifact of ethanol fixation and can be caused by autoantibodies against many different target antigens. This finding is therefore nonspecific and needs to be confirmed by ELISA for ANCA reacting with myeloperoxidase (MPO-ANCA). MPO-ANCA testing has a high specificity for small-vessel vasculitis. Absolute levels of ANCA do not define disease severity or activity, but changing titers can give a general idea of disease activity or response to therapy. The c-ANCA findings may be negative early in the course of the disease, especially in the absence of multisystem involvement.

Wegener granulomatosis may proceed to a fulminant, life-threatening course. Treatment relies on immunosuppression, usually with cyclophosphamide, and should be coordinated with a rheumatologist. Treatment with corticosteroids alone is associated with a significantly higher rate of mortality. Long-term treatment with trimethoprim-sulfamethoxazole appears to suppress disease activity in some patients.

Polyarteritis nodosa

Like giant cell arteritis, polyarteritis nodosa is a vasculitis that may affect orbital vessels but does not usually cause orbital disease. Instead, the ophthalmic manifestations are the result of retinal and choroidal infarction. In this multisystem disease, small- and medium-sized arteries are affected by inflammation characterized by the presence of neutrophils and eosinophils, with necrosis of the muscularis layer.

Vasculitis associated with connective tissue disorders

A number of connective tissue disorders may be associated with systemic vasculitis, most commonly systemic lupus erythematosus, dermatomyositis, and rheumatoid arthritis. In these entities, vasculitis primarily affects retinal vessels and, less often, involves conjunctival vessels. Symptomatic orbital vasculitis is rare.

Sarcoidosis

Sarcoidosis is a multisystem disease of unknown origin. It occurs most commonly in persons of African or Scandinavian descent. The lungs are most commonly involved, but the orbit may be affected. Histologically, the lesions are composed of noncaseating collections of epithelioid histiocytes in a granulomatous pattern. A mononuclear inflammation often appears at the periphery of the granuloma. The lacrimal gland is the site most frequently affected within the orbit, and the inflammation is typically bilateral. Gallium scanning of the lacrimal glands is nonspecific but has been reported to demonstrate lacrimal gland involvement in 80% of patients with systemic sarcoidosis, although only 7% of patients have clinically detectable enlargement of the lacrimal glands. Other orbital soft tissues, including the extraocular muscles and optic nerve, may very rarely be involved. Infrequently, sinus involvement with associated lytic bone lesions invades into the adjacent orbit.

A biopsy specimen of the affected lacrimal gland or of a suspicious conjunctival lesion may establish the diagnosis. Random conjunctival biopsies have a low yield. Chest radiography or CT to detect hilar adenopathy or pulmonary infiltrates, blood tests for angiotensin-converting enzyme, and measurement of serum lysozyme and serum calcium levels may be used to establish the diagnosis of sarcoidosis. Because gallium scanning is nonspecific, bronchoscopy with washings and biopsy may be needed to confirm the diagnosis.

Isolated orbital lesions demonstrating noncaseating granulomas can occur without associated systemic disease. This condition is called orbital sarcoid.

See BCSC Section 5, *Neuro-Ophthalmology,* and Section 9, *Intraocular Inflammation and Uveitis,* for more extensive discussion and clinical photographs of sarcoidosis.

Nonspecific Orbital Inflammation

Nonspecific orbital inflammation (NSOI) is defined as a benign inflammatory process of the orbit characterized by a polymorphous lymphoid infiltrate with varying degrees of fibrosis, without a known local or systemic cause. It is a diagnosis of exclusion that should be used only after all specific causes of inflammation have been eliminated. It has previously been called *orbital pseudotumor* or *idiopathic orbital inflammatory syndrome.*

The pathogenesis of NSOI remains controversial, although it is generally believed to be an immune-mediated process because it is often associated with systemic immunologic disorders including Crohn disease, systemic lupus erythematosus, rheumatoid arthritis, diabetes mellitus, myasthenia gravis, and ankylosing spondylitis. Additionally, NSOI typically has a rapid and favorable response to systemic corticosteroid treatment, as well as to other immunosuppressive agents, indicating a cell-mediated component.

The symptoms and clinical findings in NSOI may vary widely but are dictated by the degree and anatomical location of the inflammation. NSOI tends to occur in 5 orbital locations or patterns. In order of frequency, the most common are the extraocular muscles *(myositis),* the lacrimal gland *(dacryoadenitis),* the anterior orbit (eg, *scleritis*), the orbital apex, or diffuse inflammation throughout the orbit. Although NSOI is usually limited to the orbit, it may also extend into the adjacent sinuses or intracranial space.

Symptoms depend on the location of the involved tissue; however, deep-rooted, boring pain is a typical feature. Extraocular muscle restriction, proptosis, conjunctival inflammation, and chemosis are common, as are eyelid erythema and soft-tissue swelling. Pain associated with ocular movement suggests myositis. Visual acuity may be impaired if the optic nerve or posterior sclera is involved. In dacryoadenitis, CT reveals diffuse enlargement of the lacrimal gland (the most common target area in this type). CT, MRI, and ultrasonography reveal thickening of the extraocular muscles if the inflammatory response has a myositic component. The extraocular muscle tendons of insertion may be thickened in up to 50% of patients with NSOI; in contrast, TED typically spares the muscle insertions. An inflammatory infiltrate of the retrobulbar fat pad is commonly seen, and contrast enhancement of the sclera may be caused by tenonitis (producing the *ring sign*). B-scan ultrasonography often shows an acoustically hollow area corresponding to an edematous Tenon capsule.

Peripheral blood eosinophilia, elevated erythrocyte sedimentation rate and antinuclear antibody levels, and mild cerebrospinal fluid pleocytosis can be found.

These typical clinical presentations, combined with orbital imaging, strongly suggest the diagnosis of NSOI (Fig 4-9). Prompt response to systemic steroids supports the diagnosis, although the physician must be aware that the inflammation associated with other orbital processes (eg, metastases, ruptured dermoid cysts, infections) may also improve with systemic steroid administration. A thorough systemic evaluation should be undertaken if there is any uncertainty regarding the diagnosis.

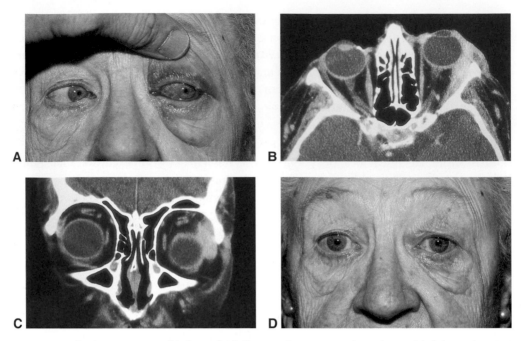

Figure 4-9 **A,** Acute onset of left eyelid inflammation, proptosis, pain, and left lateral rectus paresis. **B,** Axial CT scan demonstrating left eye proptosis and hazy inflammatory swelling of lateral rectus and lacrimal gland suggestive of the diagnosis of nonspecific orbital inflammation. **C,** Coronal CT scan demonstrating inflammatory process adjacent to the lateral rectus. **D,** Marked improvement of inflammatory changes following a 48-hour course of oral prednisone. *(Courtesy of Robert C. Kersten, MD.)*

Not all patients with NSOI present with the classic signs and symptoms. There may be atypical pain, limited inflammatory signs, or presence of a fibrotic variant called *sclerosing NSOI*. Such lesions more commonly require biopsy for diagnosis. Simultaneous bilateral orbital inflammation in adults suggests the possibility of systemic vasculitis. In children, however, approximately one-third of cases of NSOI are bilateral and are rarely associated with systemic disorders, although half of the children have headache, fever, vomiting, abdominal pain, and lethargy. Uveitis, elevated ESR, and eosinophilia may also be more common in children.

Histologically, NSOI is characterized by a pleomorphic cellular infiltrate consisting of lymphocytes, plasma cells, and eosinophils with variable degrees of reactive fibrosis. The fibrosis becomes more marked as the process becomes more chronic, and early or acute cases are usually more responsive to steroids than are the advanced stages associated with fibrosis. The sclerosing subtype demonstrates a predominance of fibrosis with sparse inflammation. Although, historically, hypercellular lymphoid proliferations were often grouped with the pseudotumors, it is now recognized that such proliferations are different clinical and histologic entities from NSOI.

Mottow-Lippa L, Jakobiec FA, Smith M. Idiopathic inflammatory orbital pseudotumor in childhood. II. Results of diagnostic tests and biopsies. *Ophthalmology.* 1981;88(6):565–574.

Treatment

Once other diagnoses have been excluded, initial therapy for NSOI consists of systemic corticosteroids. Initial daily adult dosage is typically 1 mg/kg of prednisone. Acute cases generally respond rapidly, with an abrupt resolution of the associated pain. Steroids can be tapered as soon as the clinical response is complete, but this tapering should proceed more slowly below about 40 mg/day and very slowly below 20 mg/day, based on the clinical response. Rapid reduction of systemic steroids may cause a recurrence of inflammatory symptoms and signs. Some investigators believe that the use of pulse-dosed IV dexamethasone followed by oral prednisone may produce clinical improvement when oral prednisone alone fails to control the inflammation.

Because other pathologic orbital processes may be masked by steroids, an incomplete therapeutic response or recurrent disease suggests the need for orbital biopsy, which can provide histologic confirmation and exclude specific inflammatory diseases. Thus, other investigators advise biopsy before initiating empiric steroids to avoid delayed or missed diagnoses. Biopsy allows identification of specific disease and possible systemic implications and thereby enables the clinician to develop a better-targeted treatment plan. In 1 study, 50% of biopsied inflammatory lacrimal gland lesions were associated with systemic disease, including Wegener granulomatosis, sclerosing inflammation, Sjögren syndrome, sarcoidal reactions, and autoimmune disease.

Given the low morbidity of the procedure and the high incidence of systemic disease involving the lacrimal gland, biopsy is recommended for isolated inflammation of the lacrimal gland. Many advocate biopsy of almost all infiltrative lesions, except for 2 clinical scenarios: orbital myositis and orbital apex syndrome. In these situations, characteristic clinical and radiographic findings may strongly support the presumed diagnosis, and the risk of biopsy may outweigh the risk of a missed diagnosis. However, cases of recurrent or nonresponsive orbital myositis or orbital apex syndrome warrant a biopsy.

Sclerosing NSOI is a distinct subtype of the disease, with predominant fibrosis and minimal cellular inflammation. It responds poorly to steroids and to low-dose (2000 cGy) radiotherapy and typically requires more aggressive immunosuppression with cyclosporine, methotrexate, or cyclophosphamide.

Mombaerts I, Goldschmeding R, Schlingemann RO, Koornneef L. What is orbital pseudotumor? *Surv Ophthalmol.* 1996;41(1):66–78.

Rootman J. *Orbital Disease—Present Status and Future Challenges.* Boca Raton, FL: Taylor & Francis; 2005:1–13.

Rootman J, McCarthy M, White V, Harris G, Kennerdell J. Idiopathic sclerosing inflammation of the orbit: a distinct clinicopathologic entity. *Ophthalmology.* 1994;101(3):570–584.

Rootman J, Nugent R. The classification and management of acute orbital pseudotumors. *Ophthalmology.* 1982;89(9):1040–1048.

CHAPTER 5

Orbital Neoplasms and Malformations

Vascular Tumors, Malformations, and Fistulas

Capillary Hemangiomas

Capillary hemangiomas are common primary benign tumors of the orbit in children (Fig 5-1). These lesions may be present at birth or appear in the first few weeks after birth, enlarging dramatically over the first 6–12 months of life, and involuting after the first year; 75% of lesions resolve during the first 4–5 years of life. Premature infants and newborns whose mothers had chorionic villus sampling are at risk of developing capillary hemangiomas.

Congenital capillary hemangiomas may be superficial, in which case they involve the skin and appear as a bright red, soft mass with a dimpled texture; or they may be subcutaneous and bluish in color. Hemangiomas located deeper within the orbit may present merely as a progressively enlarging mass without any overlying skin change. The ophthalmologist should always be aware, however, that a rapidly growing mass may suggest a malignant tumor, rhabdomyosarcoma in particular. Magnetic resonance imaging (MRI) may be used to help distinguish capillary hemangiomas from other vascular malformations by demonstrating characteristic fine intralesional vascular channels and high blood flow.

In the periocular area, capillary hemangiomas have a propensity for the superonasal quadrant of the orbit and the medial upper eyelid. They are commonly associated with hemangiomas on other parts of the body; lesions that involve the neck can compromise the airway and lead to respiratory obstruction, and multiple large visceral lesions can produce thrombocytopenia *(Kasabach-Merritt syndrome)*.

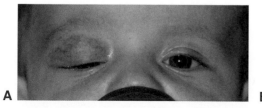 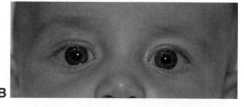

Figure 5-1 **A,** Capillary hemangioma of right upper eyelid. **B,** Marked regression of capillary hemangioma 6 weeks after propranolol therapy. *(Courtesy of William R. Katowitz, MD.)*

Management

The main ocular complications of capillary hemangiomas are amblyopia, strabismus, and anisometropia. Severe disfigurement may necessitate therapy, but treatment should be deferred until it is clear that the natural course of the lesion will not lead to the desired result.

Most lesions will regress spontaneously; therefore, observation, refractive correction, and amblyopia therapy are the first line of management. When therapy is indicated, treatment consists of steroids, administered either topically, by local injection, or orally (see the section Capillary hemangioma in Chapter 10). Adverse effects of steroid injection include necrosis of the skin, subcutaneous fat atrophy, systemic growth retardation, and risk of orbital hemorrhage and retinal embolic visual loss with injection into the orbit.

Recently, successful management of these lesions with systemic beta-blockers has been described. Because of the risk of side effects accompanying systemic treatment with either steroids or beta-blockers, such treatment in children must proceed in close collaboration with the pediatrician. Surgical excision may be considered for lesions that are smaller, subcutaneous, or refractory to steroids. Meticulous hemostasis must be maintained during such surgery. The use of systemic interferon-α has been reported; however, the systemic side effects have been significant and poorly tolerated in most cases. Radiation therapy has also been used, but it has the potential to cause cataract formation, bony hypoplasia, and future malignancy. Pulsed-dye laser therapy has not been shown to have any efficacy. High-potency topical corticosteroid (clobetasol) has shown efficacy in the treatment of superficial lesions. Sclerosing solutions are not recommended because of the severe scarring that results.

Cruz OA, Zarnegar SR, Myers SE. Treatment of periocular capillary hemangioma with topical clobetasol propionate. *Ophthalmology.* 1995;102(12):2012–2015.

Haik BG, Karcioglu ZA, Gordon RA, Pechous BP. Capillary hemangioma (infantile periocular hemangioma). *Surv Ophthalmol.* 1994(5);38:399–426.

Walker RS, Custer PL, Nerad JA. Surgical excision of periorbital capillary hemangiomas. *Ophthalmology.* 1994(8);101:1333–1340.

Cavernous Hemangioma

Cavernous hemangiomas are the most common benign neoplasm of the orbit in adults (Fig 5-2). Women are affected more often than men. The principal finding is slowly progressive proptosis, although growth may accelerate during pregnancy. Other findings may include retinal striae, hyperopia, optic nerve compression, increased intraocular pressure, and strabismus. Orbital imaging shows a homogeneously enhancing, well-encapsulated mass that, on MRI, demonstrates small intralesional vascular channels containing slowly flowing blood. Chronic lesions may contain radiodense phleboliths. Arteriography and venography usually are not useful in diagnosis because the lesion has a very limited communication with the systemic circulation.

Histologically, the lesions are encapsulated and are composed of large cavernous spaces containing red blood cells. The walls of the spaces contain smooth muscle.

Management

Treatment consists of surgical excision if the lesion compromises ocular function. The surgical approach is dictated by the location of the lesion. Coronal imaging is important in

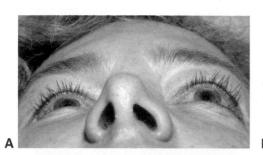

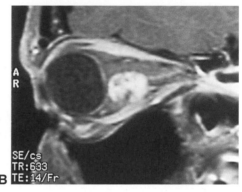

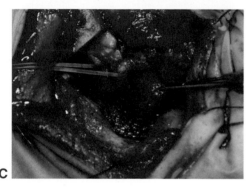

Figure 5-2 **A,** Left axial proptosis. **B,** Sagittal CT scan showing large, well-circumscribed cavernous hemangioma within the muscle cone. **C,** Lateral orbitotomy through an upper eyelid crease incision allows complete removal of the cavernous hemangioma. *(Courtesy of Roberta E. Gausas, MD.)*

determining the position of the cavernous hemangioma relative to the optic nerve. These tumors rarely undergo spontaneous involution.

Hemangiopericytoma

Hemangiopericytomas are uncommon encapsulated, hypervascular, hypercellular lesions that appear in midlife. These lesions resemble cavernous hemangiomas on both CT and MRI, but they appear bluish intraoperatively. Hemangiopericytomas are composed of plump pericytes that surround a rich capillary network. Histologically, these lesions are unique in that microscopically "benign" lesions may recur and metastasize, whereas microscopically "malignant" lesions may remain localized. There is no correlation between the mitotic rate and the clinical behavior. Treatment consists of complete excision because they may recur, undergo malignant degeneration, or metastasize.

Lymphatic Malformation

Lymphatic malformations (LMs; previously called *lymphangiomas*) are believed to represent vascular dysgenesis. They result from a disruption of the initially pluripotent vascular anlage, which leads to aberrant development and congenital malformation. In the orbit, they usually become apparent in the first decade of life; they may also occur in the conjunctiva, eyelids, oropharynx, or sinuses. LMs often contain both venous and lymphatic components. They may enlarge during upper respiratory tract infections, probably because of the response of the lymphoid tissues within the lesion. In such cases, they may present with sudden proptosis caused by spontaneous intralesional hemorrhage.

Histologically, LMs are characterized by large, serum-filled channels that are lined by flat endothelial cells that have immunostaining patterns consistent with lymphatic capillaries. Because their endothelial cells do not proliferate, they are not neoplasms. Scattered follicles of lymphoid tissues are found in the interstitium. These lesions have an infiltrative pattern and are not encapsulated.

The natural history of LMs varies and is unpredictable. Some are localized and slowly progressive, whereas others may diffusely infiltrate orbital structures and inexorably enlarge. Sudden hemorrhage from interstitial capillaries may present as abrupt proptosis or as a mass lesion. MRI may demonstrate pathognomonic features (multiple grapelike cystic lesions with fluid–fluid layering of the serum and red blood cells), confirming the diagnosis (Fig 5-3).

Management

Surgical intervention should be deferred unless vision is affected, due to the risk of hemorrhage. Because of the infiltrating nature of LMs, a subtotal resection is generally needed to avoid sacrificing important structures.

Orbital hemorrhage occurring in an LM should first be allowed to resorb spontaneously; but if optic neuropathy or corneal ulceration threatens vision, aspiration of blood through a hollow-bore needle or by open surgical exploration can be attempted.

Noncontiguous intracranial vascular malformations have been reported to occur in up to 25% of patients with orbital LMs. These lesions have a low rate of spontaneous hemorrhage and are not treated prophylactically.

Harris GJ. Orbital vascular malformations: a consensus statement on terminology and its clinical implications. Orbital Society. *Am J Ophthalmol.* 1999(4);127:453–455.

Harris GJ, Sakol PJ, Bonavolonta G, De Conciliis C. An analysis of thirty cases of orbital lymphangioma: pathophysiologic considerations and management recommendations. *Ophthalmology.* 1990;97(12):1583–1592.

Kazim M, Kennerdell JS, Rothfus W, Marquardt M. Orbital lymphangioma: correlation of magnetic resonance images and intraoperative findings. *Ophthalmology.* 1992;99(10):1588–1594.

Rootman J, Hay E, Graeb D, Miller R. Orbital-adnexal lymphangiomas. A spectrum of hemodynamically isolated vascular hamartomas. *Ophthalmology.* 1986;93(12):1558–1570.

Venous Malformation

Venous malformations of the orbit (also known as *orbital varices*) are low-flow vascular lesions resulting from vascular dysgenesis. Patients may exhibit enophthalmos at rest, when

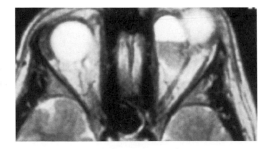

Figure 5-3 T2-weighted axial MRI of a large lymphatic malformation of the left orbit demonstrating fluid–fluid layering. *(Courtesy of Roberta E. Gausas, MD.)*

the lesion is not engorged. Proptosis that increases when the patient's head is dependent or after a Valsalva maneuver suggests the presence of a venous malformation. The diagnosis can be confirmed via contrast-enhanced rapid spiral CT during a Valsalva maneuver (or other means of decreasing venous return) showing characteristic enlargement of the engorged veins. Phleboliths may be present on imaging.

Treatment is usually conservative. Biopsy should be avoided because of the risk of hemorrhage. Surgery is reserved for relief of significant pain or for cases in which the venous malformation causes vision-threatening compressive optic neuropathy. Complete surgical excision is difficult, as these lesions often intertwine with normal orbital structures and directly communicate with the abundant venous reservoir in the cavernous sinus. Intraoperative embolization of the lesion may aid surgical removal. Embolization with coils inserted through a distal venous cutdown has also been reported to diminish symptoms.

Arteriovenous Malformations

Arteriovenous malformations (AVMs) are high-flow developmental anomalies also resulting from vascular dysgenesis. They are composed of abnormally formed anastomosing arteries and veins without an intervening capillary bed. Dilated corkscrew episcleral vessels may be prominent. After these lesions are studied by arteriography, they may be treated by selective occlusion of the feeding vessels, followed by surgical excision of the malformations. However, exsanguinating arterial hemorrhage may occur with surgical intervention.

Arteriovenous Fistula

Arteriovenous fistulas are acquired lesions caused by abnormal direct communication between an artery and a vein. Blood flows directly from artery to vein without passing through an intervening capillary bed. An arteriovenous fistula may be caused by trauma or degeneration (Figs 5-4, 5-5). There are 2 forms: the *carotid cavernous fistula,* which typically occurs after a basal skull fracture; and the spontaneous *dural cavernous fistula,* which forms most often as a degenerative process in older patients with systemic hypertension and atherosclerosis.

Carotid cavernous fistulas, which have a high blood-flow rate, produce characteristic tortuous epibulbar vessels and a bruit that may be audible to the examiner and the patient. Pulsatile proptosis may also be present. Ischemic ocular damage results from diversion of arterialized blood into the venous system, which causes venous outflow obstruction. This in turn results in elevated intraocular pressure (IOP), choroidal effusions, blood in the Schlemm canal, and nongranulomatous iritis. Increased pressure in the cavernous sinus can cause compression of cranial nerves III, IV, or, most commonly, VI, with associated extraocular muscle palsies.

A *dural cavernous fistula* occurs when small meningeal arterial branches communicate with venous drainage. Because dural fistulas generally produce less blood flow than carotid cavernous fistulas, their onset can be insidious with only mild orbital congestion, proptosis, and pain. Arterialization of the conjunctival veins causes chronic red eye. Increased episcleral venous pressure results in asymmetric elevation of IOP on the ipsilateral

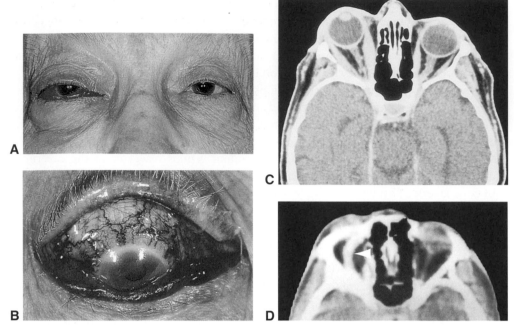

Figure 5-4 **A,** Carotid cavernous fistula, right eye, in elderly woman. **B,** Arterialization of epi-scleral and conjunctival vessels and chemosis of conjunctiva. **C,** CT scan demonstrating prop-tosis of right eye secondary to congested orbital tissues. Note enlarged medial rectus and lateral rectus muscles. **D,** Axial CT scan showing dilated superior ophthalmic vein *(arrowhead)*, typical of carotid cavernous fistula. *(Parts A–C courtesy of Jeffrey A. Nerad, MD.)*

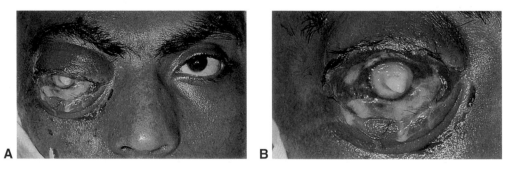

Figure 5-5 High-flow carotid cavernous fistula in a young man following head trauma. Note marked proptosis and exposure of eye **(A)** with resulting corneal perforation **(B)**. *(Courtesy of Robert C. Kersten, MD.)*

side, and patients with chronic fistulas are at risk for glaucomatous optic disc damage. CT scans show diffuse enlargement of all the extraocular muscles resulting from venous engorgement and a characteristically enlarged superior ophthalmic vein.

Small dural cavernous fistulas often close spontaneously. Recent data suggest that pa-tients with dural cavernous fistulas are at higher risk for intracranial hemorrhage because of the arterialization of the venous system; therefore, some investigators have recom-mended more aggressive management of these lesions.

Selective arteriography is used to evaluate arteriovenous fistulas of the orbit and cavernous sinus. Embolization using coils to obstruct the fistula is generally accomplished through an endovascular transarterial route. Occasionally, a transvenous approach is utilized to access the cavernous sinus, but it is more typically reached by transcutaneous canalization of the superior ophthalmic vein.

Meyers PM, Halbach VV, Dowd CF, et al. Dural carotid cavernous fistula: definitive endovascular management and long-term follow-up. *Am J Ophthalmol.* 2002;134(1):85–92.

Spinelli HM, Falcone S, Lee G. Orbital venous approach to the cavernous sinus: an analysis of the facial and orbital venous system. *Ann Plast Surg.* 1994;33(4):377–383.

Orbital Hemorrhage

An orbital hemorrhage may result from trauma or spontaneous bleeding from vascular malformations. Rarely, a spontaneous hemorrhage may be caused by a sudden increase in venous pressure (eg, a Valsalva maneuver). An orbital hemorrhage almost always occurs in the superior subperiosteal space. It should be allowed to spontaneously resorb unless there is associated visual compromise, in which case urgent drainage is indicated. See also Chapter 6, in the section Orbital Hemorrhage.

Atalla ML, McNab AA, Sullivan TJ, Sloan B. Nontraumatic subperiosteal orbital hemorrhage. *Ophthalmology.* 2001;108(1):183–189.

Neural Tumors

The neural tumors include optic nerve gliomas, neurofibromas, meningiomas, and schwannomas.

Optic Nerve Glioma

Optic nerve gliomas are uncommon, usually benign, tumors that occur predominantly in children in the first decade of life (Fig 5-6). *Malignant optic nerve gliomas (glioblastomas)* are very rare and tend to affect adult males. Initial signs and symptoms of malignant gliomas include severe retro-orbital pain, unilateral or bilateral vision loss, and, typically, massive swelling and hemorrhage of the optic nerve head (although disc pallor may also be observed with posterior lesions). Despite treatment, including high-dose radiotherapy and chemotherapy, these tumors usually result in death within 6–12 months.

Up to half of optic nerve gliomas are associated with neurofibromatosis. The chief clinical feature is gradual, painless, unilateral axial proptosis associated with loss of vision and an afferent pupillary defect. Other ocular findings may include optic atrophy, optic disc swelling, nystagmus, and strabismus. The chiasm is involved in roughly half of cases of optic nerve glioma. Intracranial involvement may be associated with intracranial hypertension as well as decreased function of the hypothalamus and pituitary gland.

Gross pathology of resected tumors reveals a smooth, fusiform intradural lesion. Microscopically, the benign tumors in children are considered to be juvenile pilocytic (hairlike) astrocytomas. Other histologic findings include arachnoid hyperplasia, mucosubstance, and Rosenthal fibers (see the discussion of the pathologic features of glioma in BCSC Section 4, *Ophthalmic Pathology and Intraocular Tumors*). Optic gliomas arising

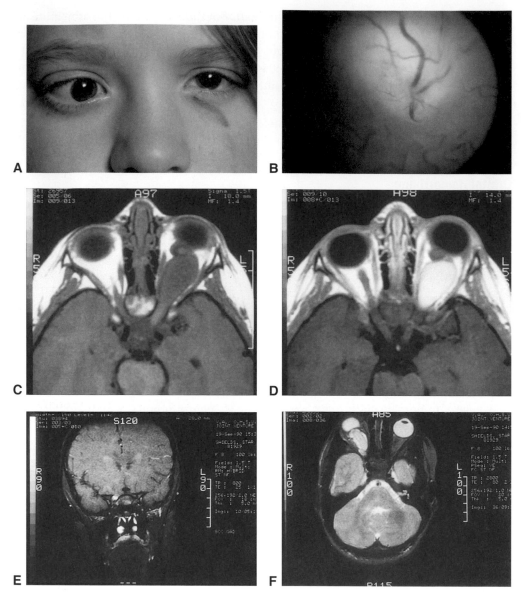

Figure 5-6   A, Clinical photograph of a child with right optic nerve glioma displaying proptosis with esotropia. **B,** Funduscopic view of same patient. Note swollen disc with obscured disc margins. **C,** T1-weighted axial MRI of optic nerve glioma demonstrating kinking of the optic nerve. **D,** T1-weighted image with contrast of the same patient. **E,** Coronal MRI demonstrating involvement of the optic nerve near the chiasm. **F,** T2-weighted axial MRI demonstrating enlargement of the right optic nerve with apparent kink. Note that the central enlarged optic nerve is surrounded by tumor in the perineural space. *(Courtesy of Roger A. Dailey, MD.)*

in patients with neurofibromatosis often proliferate in the subarachnoid space. Those occurring in patients without neurofibromatosis usually expand within the optic nerve substance without invasion of the dura mater.

Optic nerve gliomas can usually be diagnosed by means of orbital imaging. CT and MRI usually show fusiform enlargement of the optic nerve, often with stereotypical kinking of the nerve. MRI may also show cystic degeneration, if present, and may be more accurate in defining the extent of an optic canal lesion and intracranial disease.

It is usually unnecessary to perform a biopsy of a suspected lesion, as neuroimaging is frequently diagnostic. Moreover, biopsy tissue obtained from too peripheral a portion of the optic nerve may capture reactive meningeal hyperplasia adjacent to the optic nerve glioma and lead to the misdiagnosis of fibrous meningioma, and biopsy of the optic nerve itself may produce additional loss of visual field or acuity.

Management

The treatment of optic nerve gliomas is controversial. Although most cases remain stable or progress very slowly, leading some authors to consider them benign hamartomas, the occasional case behaves aggressively. There are rare reports of spontaneous regression of optic nerve and visual pathway gliomas. Cystic enlargement of the lesions associated with sudden visual loss can occur even without true cellular growth. A treatment plan must be carefully individualized for each patient. The following options may be considered.

Observation only Presumed optic nerve glioma, particularly with good vision on the involved side, may be carefully followed if the radiographic evidence is characteristic of this type of tumor and if the glioma is confined to the orbit. Follow-up examinations and appropriate radiographic studies, preferably MRI, must be performed at regular intervals. Many patients maintain good vision and never require surgery.

Surgical excision Rapid intraorbital tumor growth may prompt surgical resection in an effort to isolate the tumor from the optic chiasm and thus prevent chiasmal invasion. The surgeon should use an intracranial approach to obtain tumor-free surgical margins. Additional surgical indications for excision of tumors confined to the orbit include corneal exposure and compromised cosmesis unacceptable to the patient. Removal through an intracranial approach may also be indicated at the time of initial diagnosis or after a short period of observation if the tumor involves the prechiasmal intracranial portion of the optic nerve. Complete excision is possible if the tumor ends 2–3 mm anterior to the chiasm. Excision may also be required if the glioma causes an increase in intracranial pressure.

Radiation therapy Radiation therapy as the sole treatment is considered if the tumor cannot be resected (usually chiasmal or optic tract lesions) and if symptoms (particularly neurological) progress. Postoperative radiation of the chiasm and optic tract may also be considered if good radiographic studies document subsequent growth of the tumor within the chiasm or if chiasmal and optic tract involvement is extensive. Because of debilitating side effects (including mental retardation, growth retardation, and secondary tumors within the radiation field), radiation is generally held as a last resort for children who have not completed growth and development.

Chemotherapy Combination chemotherapy using actinomycin D, vincristine, etoposide, and other agents has also been reported to be effective in patients with progressive chiasmal/hypothalamic gliomas. Chemotherapy may delay the need for radiation therapy and thus enhance long-term intellectual development and preservation of endocrine function in children. However, chemotherapy may also carry long-term risks of blood-borne cancers.

In summary, any treatment plan must be carefully individualized. Therapeutic decisions must be based on the tumor growth characteristics, the extent of optic nerve and chiasmal involvement as determined by clinical and radiographic evaluation, the visual acuity of the involved and uninvolved eye, the presence or absence of concomitant neurological or systemic disease, and the history of previous treatment. (See additional discussion of optic nerve glioma in BCSC Section 5, *Neuro-Ophthalmology*.)

Dutton JJ. Gliomas of the anterior visual pathway. *Surv Ophthalmol.* 1994;38(5):427–452.

Jenkin D, Angyalfi S, Becker L, et al. Optic glioma in children: surveillance, resection, or irradiation? *Int J Radiat Oncol Biol Phys.* 1993;25(2):215–225.

Massry GG, Morgan CF, Chung SM. Evidence of optic pathway gliomas after previously negative neuroimaging. *Ophthalmology.* 1997;104(6):930–935.

Pepin SM, Lessell S. Anterior visual pathway gliomas: the last 30 years. *Semin Ophthalmol.* 2006;21(3):117–124.

Neurofibroma

Neurofibromas are tumors composed chiefly of proliferating Schwann cells within the nerve sheaths (Figs 5-7, 5-8). Axons, endoneural fibroblasts, and mucin are also noted histologically. *Plexiform neurofibromas* consist of diffuse proliferations of Schwann cells within nerve sheaths, and they usually occur in neurofibromatosis 1 (NF1). They are well vascularized and infiltrative lesions, making complete surgical excision difficult. *Discrete neurofibromas* are less common than the plexiform type, and they can usually be excised surgically without recurrence. In either instance, surgery is limited to tumors that compromise vision or produce disfigurement.

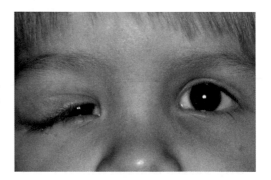

Figure 5-7 Ptosis of right upper eyelid, with S-shaped deformity characteristic of plexiform neurofibroma infiltration. *(Courtesy of Roberta E. Gausas, MD.)*

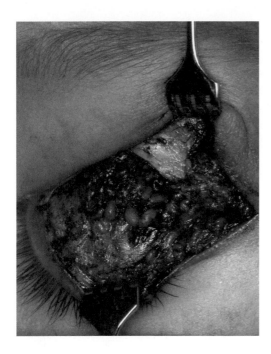

Figure 5-8 Plexiform neurofibroma excision during ptosis surgery. Percutaneous palpation of the subcutaneous fibrous neoplastic cords visible here produces a "bag-of-worms" consistency. *(Courtesy of Roberta E. Gausas, MD.)*

Neurofibromatosis 1

Also known as *von Recklinghausen disease,* NF1 is inherited through an autosomal dominant gene with incomplete penetrance. Because NF1 is characterized by the presence of hamartomas involving the skin, eye, central nervous system, and viscera, it is classified as a phakomatosis. Neurofibromatosis 1 is the most common phakomatous disorder. Significant orbital features that can be seen in NF1 include plexiform neurofibromas involving the lateral aspect of the upper eyelid and causing an S-shaped contour of the eyelid margin (see Fig 5-7), pulsating proptosis secondary to sphenoid bone dysplasia, and optic nerve glioma. (See BCSC Section 6, *Pediatric Ophthalmology and Strabismus,* for further discussion of neurofibromatosis and other phakomatoses.)

Farris SR, Grove AS Jr. Orbital and eyelid manifestations of neurofibromatosis: a clinical study and literature review. *Ophthal Plast Reconstr Surg.* 1996;12(4):245–259.

Meningioma

Meningiomas are invasive tumors that arise from the arachnoid villi. They usually originate intracranially along the sphenoid wing with secondary extension into the orbit through the bone, the superior orbital fissure, or the optic canal (Fig 5-9), or they may arise primarily in the optic nerve (Fig 5-10). Ophthalmic manifestations are related to the location of the primary tumor. Meningiomas arising near the sella and optic nerve cause early visual field defects and papilledema or optic atrophy. Tumors arising near the pterion (posterior end of the parietosphenoid fissure, at the lateral portion of the sphenoid bone) often produce a temporal fossa mass and may be associated with proptosis or nonaxial

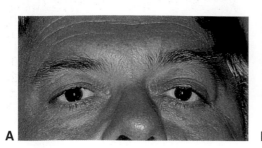

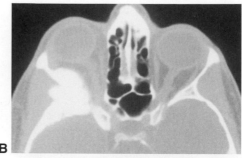

Figure 5-9 **A,** Left proptosis and fullness of left temple secondary to sphenoid wing meningioma. CT scan **(B)** and T1-weighted MRI **(C)** of another orbital menigioma arising from the sphenoid wing. Note hyperostosis of the sphenoid bone. *(Part A courtesy of Jeffrey A. Nerad, MD. Parts B and C courtesy of Roberta E. Gausas, MD.)*

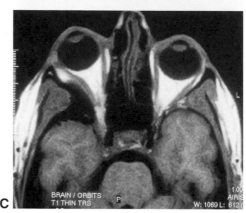

displacement of the globe. Eyelid edema (especially of the lower eyelid) and chemosis are common. Interestingly, while primary optic nerve meningiomas can rarely produce axial proptosis with preserved vision, depending on their anatomic location, small *en plaque* meningiomas can produce early profound visual loss without any proptosis.

Sphenoid wing meningiomas produce hyperostosis of the involved bone and hyperplasia of associated soft tissues. When contrast enhancement is used, MRI helps define the extent of meningiomas along the dura. The presence of a dural tail helps distinguish a meningioma from fibrous dysplasia.

Primary orbital meningiomas usually originate in the arachnoid of the optic nerve sheath. They occur most commonly in women in their third and fourth decades of life. Symptoms usually include a gradual, painless, unilateral loss of vision. Examination typically shows decreased visual acuity and a relative afferent pupillary defect. Proptosis and ophthalmoplegia may also be present. The optic nerve head may appear normal, atrophic, or swollen; and optociliary shunt vessels may be visible. Occasionally, optic nerve sheath meningiomas occur bilaterally and are associated with neurofibromatosis.

Imaging characteristics are usually sufficient to allow diagnosis of optic nerve sheath meningiomas. Both CT and MRI show diffuse tubular enlargement of the optic nerve with contrast enhancement. In some cases, CT can show calcification within the meningioma, referred to as *tram-tracking*. MRI reveals a fine pattern of enhancing striations emanating from the lesion in a longitudinal fashion. These striations represent the infiltrative nature of what otherwise appears to be an encapsulated lesion. As with the sphenoid wing meningiomas, MRI can show dural extension into the chiasm and the intracranial space. The

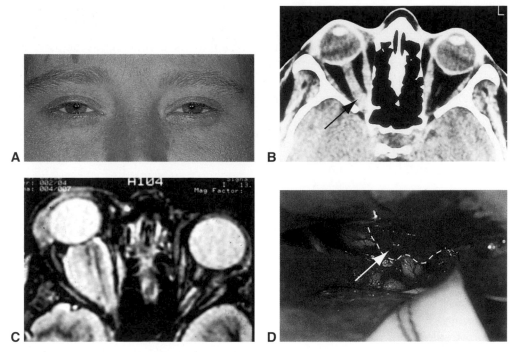

Figure 5-10   A, Primary optic nerve meningioma of right optic nerve, with minimal proptosis.
B, CT scan showing thickened right optic nerve with calcification *(arrow)*. **C,** MRI showing a
fusiform enlargement of the right optic nerve sheath with preservation of the centrally located
optic nerve in a different patient. **D,** The meningioma is exposed through a craniotomy and
superior orbitotomy. Intraoperative view shows intracranial prechiasmal optic nerve. Note cuff
(arrow, dashes) of meningioma wrapping around optic nerve extending out from optic canal.
(Parts A, B, and D courtesy of Jeffrey A. Nerad, MD. Part C courtesy of Michael Kazim, MD.)

en plaque variant appears as a focal knobby excrescence of the optic nerve that enhances
with both CT and MRI.

Malignant meningioma is rare and results in rapid tumor growth that is not responsive to surgical resection, radiotherapy, or chemotherapy. Histologically, malignant meningiomas are indistinguishable from the more common benign group.

Management

Sphenoid wing meningiomas are typically observed until they cause functional deficits,
such as profound proptosis, compressive optic neuropathy, motility impairment, or cerebral edema. Treatment includes subtotal resection of the tumor through a combined
approach to the intracranial and orbital component. Complete surgical resection is not
a practical goal because the dural tail of the tumor extends far beyond the surgical field.
Rather, the goal of surgery is to reverse the volume-induced compressive effects of the lesion. Postoperative radiotherapy is advocated to reduce the risk of recurrence and spread
of the residual tumor.

Treatment of optic nerve sheath meningiomas must be individualized. Both the extent of visual loss and the presence of intracranial extension are important factors in treatment planning. Observation is indicated if vision is minimally affected and no intracranial

extension is present. If the tumor is confined to the orbit and visual loss is significant or progressive, radiation therapy should be considered. Fractionated stereotactic radiotherapy often results in stabilization or improvement of visual function. If the patient is observed or treated with radiation, periodic MRI examination is necessary to carefully monitor for possible posterior or intracranial extension. With rare exceptions, attempts to surgically excise optic nerve sheath meningiomas result in irreversible visual loss due to compromise of the optic nerve blood supply. Thus, surgery is reserved for patients with severe visual loss and profound proptosis. In such cases, the optic nerve is excised with the tumor, from the back of the globe to the chiasm, if preoperative MRI suggests the opportunity for complete resection.

Andrews DW, Faroozan R, Yang BP, et al. Fractionated stereotactic radiotherapy for the treatment of optic nerve sheath meningiomas: preliminary observations of 33 optic nerves in 30 patients with historical comparison to observation with or without prior surgery. *Neurosurgery*. 2002;51(4):890–904.

Dutton JJ. Optic nerve sheath meningiomas. *Surv Ophthalmol*. 1992;37(3):167–183.

Lesser RL, Knisely JP, Wang SL, Yu JB, Kupersmith MJ. Long-term response to fractionated radiotherapy of presumed optic nerve sheath meningioma. *Br J Ophthalmol*. 2010;94(5): 559–563.

Turbin RE, Thompson CR, Kennerdell JS, Cockerham KP, Kupersmith MJ. A long-term visual outcome comparison in patients with optic nerve sheath meningioma managed with observation, surgery, radiotherapy, or surgery and radiotherapy. *Ophthalmology*. 2002;109(5): 890–899.

Schwannoma

Schwannomas, sometimes known as *neurilemomas,* are proliferations of Schwann cells that are encapsulated by perineurium. These tumors have a characteristic biphasic pattern of solid areas with nuclear palisading *(Antoni A pattern)* and myxoid areas *(Antoni B pattern).* Hypercellular schwannomas sometimes recur even after what is thought to be complete removal, but they seldom undergo malignant transformation. These tumors are usually well encapsulated and can be excised with relative ease.

Mesenchymal Tumors

Rhabdomyosarcoma

Rhabdomyosarcoma is the most common primary orbital malignancy of childhood (Fig 5-11). The average age of onset is 8–10 years. The classic clinical picture is that of a child with sudden onset and rapid progression of unilateral proptosis. However, patients in their early teens may experience a less dramatic course, with gradually progressive proptosis lasting from weeks to more than a month. There is often a marked adnexal response with edema and discoloration of the eyelids. Ptosis and strabismus may also be present. A mass may be palpable, particularly in the superonasal quadrant of the eyelid. However, the tumor may be retrobulbar, involve any quadrant of the orbit, and may rarely arise from the conjunctiva. The patient sometimes has an unrelated history of trauma to the orbital area that can lead to a delay in diagnosis and treatment.

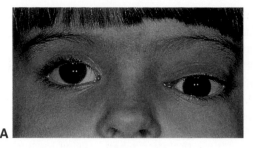 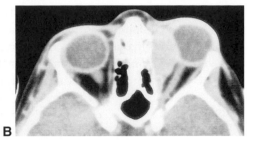

Figure 5-11 **A,** Six-year-old girl with rapid onset of axial proptosis, lateral and downward displacement of left eye. **B,** CT scan demonstrating a medial orbital mass proven by biopsy to be rhabdomyosarcoma. *(Courtesy of Jeffrey A. Nerad, MD.)*

If a rhabdomyosarcoma is suspected, the workup should proceed on an urgent basis. CT and MRI can be used to define the location and extent of the tumor. A biopsy should be undertaken, usually through an anterior orbitotomy. It is often possible to completely remove a rhabdomyosarcoma if it has a pseudocapsule. If this is not practical, there is some indication that the smaller the volume of residual tumor, the more effective is the combination of adjuvant radiation and chemotherapy in achieving a cure. In diffusely infiltrating tumors, a large biopsy specimen should be obtained so that adequate material is available for frozen sections, permanent light-microscopy sections, electron microscopy, and immunohistochemistry. Cross-striations are often not visible on light microscopy and may be more readily apparent on electron microscopy.

The physician should palpate the cervical and preauricular lymph nodes of the patient with orbital rhabdomyosarcoma to rule out regional metastases. A chest radiograph, bone marrow aspirate and biopsy, and lumbar puncture should be obtained to search for more distant metastases. Sampling of the bone marrow and the cerebrospinal fluid is best performed, if possible, with the patient under anesthesia at the time of the initial orbital biopsy.

Rhabdomyosarcomas arise from undifferentiated pluripotential mesenchymal elements in the orbital soft tissues and not from the extraocular muscles. They may be grouped into the following 4 categories:

- *Embryonal.* This is by far the most common type, accounting for more than 80% of cases. The embryonal form has a predilection for the superonasal quadrant of the orbit. The tumor is composed of loose fascicles of undifferentiated spindle cells, only a minority of which show cross-striations in immature rhabdomyosarcomas on trichrome staining. Embryonal rhabdomyosarcomas are associated with a good (94%) survival rate.
- *Alveolar.* This form has a predilection for the inferior orbit and accounts for 9% of orbital rhabdomyosarcomas. The tumor displays regular compartments composed of fibrovascular strands in which rounded rhabdomyoblasts either line up along the connective tissue strands or float freely in the alveolar spaces. This is the most malignant form of rhabdomyosarcoma, with a 10-year survival rate of 10%.
- *Pleomorphic.* Pleomorphic rhabdomyosarcoma is the least common and most differentiated form. In this type, many of the cells are straplike or rounded, and

cross-striations are easily visualized with trichrome stain. The pleomorphic variety has the best prognosis (97% survival rate).

- *Botryoid.* This rare variant of embryonal rhabdomyosarcoma appears grapelike. It is not found in the orbit as a primary tumor; rather, the botryoid variant occurs as a secondary invader from the paranasal sinuses or from the conjunctiva.

Management

Before 1965, the standard treatment of orbital rhabdomyosarcoma was orbital exenteration, and the survival rate was poor. Since 1965, radiation therapy and systemic chemotherapy have become the mainstays of primary treatment, based on the guidelines set forth by the Intergroup Rhabdomyosarcoma Studies I–IV. Exenteration is reserved for recurrent cases. The total dose of local radiation varies from 4500 to 6000 cGy, given over a period of 6 weeks. The goal of systemic chemotherapy is to eliminate microscopic cellular metastases. Survival rates with radiation and chemotherapy are better than 90% if the orbital tumor has not invaded or extended beyond the bony orbital walls. Adverse effects of radiation are common in children and include cataract, radiation dermatitis, and bony hypoplasia if orbital development has not been completed.

Kodet R, Newton WA Jr, Hamoudi AB, Asmar L, Wharam MD, Maurer HM. Orbital rhabdomyosarcomas and related tumors in childhood: relationship of morphology to prognosis—an Intergroup Rhabdomyosarcoma Study. *Med Pediatr Oncol.* 1997;29(1):51–60.

Mannor GE, Rose GE, Plowman PN, Kingston J, Wright JE, Vardy SJ. Multidisciplinary management of refractory orbital rhabdomyosarcoma. *Ophthalmology.* 1997;104(7):1198–1201.

Shields CL, Shields JA, Honavar SG, Demirci H. Clinical spectrum of primary ophthalmic rhabdomyosarcoma. *Ophthalmology.* 2001;108(12):2284–2292.

Miscellaneous Mesenchymal Tumors

Tumors of fibrous connective tissue, cartilage, and bone are uncommon lesions that may involve the orbit. A number of these mesenchymal tumors were likely incorrectly classified before the availability of immunohistochemical staining, which has allowed them to be differentiated and classified accurately.

Fibrous histiocytoma is the most common of these tumors. It is characteristically very firm and displaces normal structures. Both fibroblastic and histiocytic cells in a storiform (matlike) pattern are found in these locally aggressive tumors. Fewer than 10% have metastatic potential. This tumor is sometimes difficult to distinguish clinically and histologically from hemangiopericytoma.

A more recently described entity, *solitary fibrous tumor,* is composed of spindle-shaped cells that are strongly CD34-positive on immunohistochemical studies. It can occur anywhere in the orbit. It may recur, undergo malignant degeneration, and metastasize if incompletely excised.

Fibrous dysplasia (Fig 5-12) is a benign developmental disorder of bone that may involve a single region or be polyostotic. CT shows hyperostotic bone, and MRI shows the lack of dural enhancement that distinguishes this condition from meningioma. When associated with cutaneous pigmentation and endocrine disorders, the condition is known as *Albright syndrome.* Resection or debulking is performed when the lesion results in disfigurement or visual loss due to stricture of the optic canal.

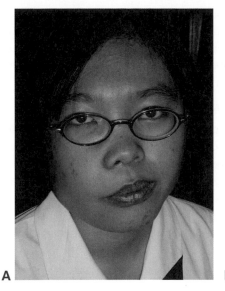
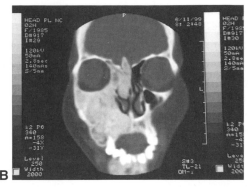

Figure 5-12 Fibrous dysplasia. **A,** This young woman manifests facial asymmetry due to fibrous dysplasia. **B,** CT scan shows characteristic hyperostosis of involved facial bones. *(Courtesy of Jerry Popham, MD.)*

Osteomas are benign tumors that can involve any of the periorbital sinuses. CT scans show dense hyperostosis with well-defined margins. The lesions can produce proptosis, compressive optic neuropathy, and orbital cellulitis secondary to obstructive sinusitis. Most are incidental, slow-growing lesions that require no treatment. Complete excision is advised when the tumor is symptomatic.

Malignant mesenchymal tumors such as *liposarcoma, fibrosarcoma, chondrosarcoma,* and *osteosarcoma* rarely appear in the orbit. When chondrosarcomas and osteosarcomas are present, they usually destroy normal bone and have characteristic calcifications visible in radiographs and CT scans. Children with a history of bilateral retinoblastoma are at higher risk for osteosarcoma, chondrosarcoma, or fibrosarcoma, even if they have not been treated with therapeutic radiation.

Katz BJ, Nerad JA. Ophthalmic manifestations of fibrous dysplasia: a disease of children and adults. *Ophthalmology.* 1998;105(12):2207–2215.

Lymphoproliferative Disorders

Lymphoid Hyperplasia and Lymphoma

Lymphoproliferative lesions of the ocular adnexa constitute a heterogeneous group of neoplasms that are defined by clinical, histologic, immunologic, molecular, and genetic characteristics. Lymphoproliferative neoplasms account for more than 20% of all orbital tumors.

Most orbital lymphoproliferative lesions are non-Hodgkin lymphomas. The incidence of non-Hodgkin lymphoma of all anatomical sites has been increasing at a rate of 3%–4%

per year (representing a 50% increase over the last 15 years), and non-Hodgkin lymphoma is now the fourth most common malignancy among men and women. The incidence of orbital lymphomas has been increasing at an even greater rate. Workers with long-term exposure to bioactive solvents and reagents are at increased risk for non-Hodgkin lymphoma, as are older persons and patients with chronic autoimmune diseases.

Identification and classification of lymphoproliferative disorders

Classification of non-Hodgkin lymphomas is evolving and largely based on nodal architecture. Extranodal sites, including the orbit, have been included in the Revised European American Lymphoma (REAL) classification. However, orbital extranodal disease appears to represent a biological continuum and to behave unpredictably. Often, patients with orbital lymphoid infiltrates that appear benign histologically eventually develop extraorbital lymphoma, whereas others with malignant lymphoma of the ocular adnexa may respond satisfactorily to local therapy without subsequent systemic involvement. Currently, 70%–80% of orbital lymphoproliferative lesions are designated as malignant lymphomas on the basis of monoclonal cell-surface markers, whereas 90% are found to be malignant on the basis of molecular genetic studies. The significance of this discrepancy is not yet clear, as polymerase chain reaction studies have shown that, over time, some conjunctival lymphoid lesions fluctuate between being monoclonal and polyclonal.

The vast majority of orbital lymphomas are derived from B cells. T-cell lymphoma is rare and more lethal. B-cell lymphoma is divided into Hodgkin and non-Hodgkin tumors, with the former rarely metastasizing to the orbit. Malignant non-Hodgkin B-cell lymphoma accounts for more than 90% of orbital lymphoproliferative disease. The 4 most common types of orbital lymphomas, based on the REAL classification, are discussed in the following paragraphs.

1. *Mucosa-associated lymphoid tissue (MALT) lymphomas* account for 40%–60% of orbital lymphomas. MALT lesions were originally described as occurring in the gastrointestinal tract, where approximately 50% of MALT lymphomas arise. Studies have suggested that proliferation of early MALT tumors may be antigen driven. Therapy directed at the antigen (eg, against *Helicobacter pylori* in gastric lymphomas) may result in regression of early lesions. There is evidence to suggest that some conjunctival MALT lymphomas are associated with chronic chlamydial infection. In contrast to MALT lymphomas occurring in other areas of the body, those in the ocular adnexa do not appear to be preferentially associated with mucosal tissue (ie, conjunctiva or lacrimal gland).

   Although MALT lymphomas have a low grade of malignancy, long-term follow-up has demonstrated that at least 50% of patients will develop systemic disease at 10 years. MALT lymphomas may undergo spontaneous remission in 5%–15% of cases. They may undergo histologic transformation to a higher-grade lesion, usually of a large cell type, in 15%–20% of cases. Such transformation usually occurs after several years and is not related to therapy.

2. *Chronic lymphocytic lymphoma (CLL)* also represents a low-grade lesion of small, mature-appearing lymphocytes.

3. *Follicular center lymphoma* represents a low-grade lesion with follicular centers.
4. *High-grade lymphomas* include large cell lymphoma, lymphoblastic lymphoma, and Burkitt lymphoma.

See also BCSC Section 4, *Ophthalmic Pathology and Intraocular Tumors.*

Clinical presentation

The typical lymphoproliferative lesion presents as a gradually progressive, painless mass. These tumors are often located anteriorly in the orbit (Fig 5-13) or beneath the conjunctiva, where they may show the typical salmon-patch appearance (Fig 5-14). Lymphoproliferative lesions, whether benign or malignant, usually mold to surrounding orbital structures rather than invade them; consequently, disturbances of extraocular motility or visual function are unusual. Reactive lymphoid hyperplasias and low-grade lymphomas often have a history of slow expansion over a period of months to years. Orbital imaging reveals a characteristic puttylike molding of the tumor to normal structures. Bone erosion

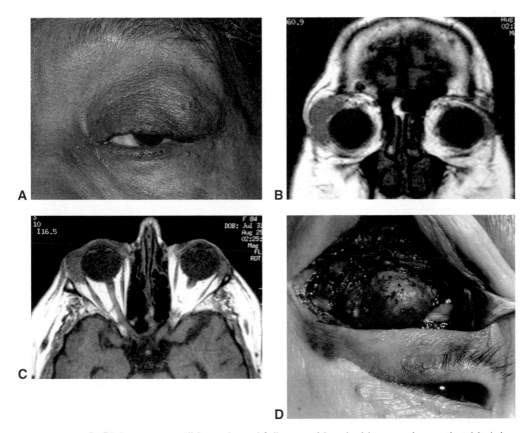

Figure 5-13   A, Right upper eyelid ptosis and fullness with palpable mass beneath orbital rim. **B,** Coronal MRI demonstrating right lacrimal gland enlargement with infiltration of anterior orbital tissues. **C,** Axial MRI showing characteristic molding of lesion to adjacent structures. **D,** Incisional biopsy of the abnormal infiltration of lacrimal gland reveals orbital lymphoma. *(Courtesy of Roberta E. Gausas, MD.)*

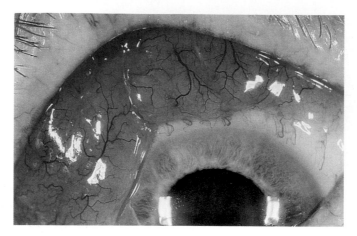

Figure 5-14 Subconjunctival lymphoma. Note classic salmon-patch appearance of lesion. *(Courtesy of Jeffrey A. Nerad, MD.)*

or infiltration is usually not seen except with high-grade malignant lymphomas. Up to 50% of orbital lymphoproliferative lesions arise in the lacrimal fossa. Lymphomas in the retrobulbar fat may appear more infiltrative. Approximately 17% of orbital lymphoid lesions occur bilaterally, but this does not necessarily indicate the presence of extraorbital disease.

Diagnosis

For all lymphoproliferative lesions, an open biopsy is preferred to obtain an adequate tissue specimen, which is used to establish a diagnosis and to characterize the lesion's morphologic, immunologic, cytogenetic, and molecular properties under the REAL classification. A portion of the tissue should be placed in a suitable fixative for light microscopy. The majority of the specimen should be sent fresh to a molecular diagnostics laboratory for possible flow cytometry and polymerase chain reaction analysis. Alternatively, fine-needle aspiration biopsy can provide adequate sample volume to establish all but the morphologic characteristics of the lesion.

Both reactive hyperplasia and malignant lymphoma are hypercellular proliferations with sparse or absent stromal components. Histologically, light microscopy may reveal a continuum from reactive hyperplasia to low-grade lymphoma to higher-grade malignancy. Within this spectrum, it may be difficult to characterize a given lesion by light microscopy alone. In such cases, immunopathology and molecular diagnostic studies have been proposed to aid further categorization.

Malignant lymphomas are thought to represent clonal expansions of abnormal precursor cells. Immunologic identification of cell-surface markers on lymphocytes can be used to classify tumors as containing B cells or T cells and as being either monoclonal or polyclonal in origin. Specific monoclonal antibodies directed against surface light-chain (κ or λ) immunoglobulins are used to study cells in smears, histologic sections, or cell suspensions to determine whether the cells represent monoclonal (ie, malignant) proliferations.

Newer techniques of molecular analysis allow more precise identification of tumor clonality by extracting, amplifying, and hybridizing tumor DNA with radioactively labeled nucleotide probes. DNA hybridization is more sensitive than cell-surface marker typing in detecting clonality, but this technique is also more time-consuming and expensive. DNA genetic studies have demonstrated that most lymphoproliferative lesions that appear to be immunologically polyclonal actually harbor small monoclonal proliferations of B lymphocytes. The finding of monoclonality, established by either immunophenotype or molecular genetics, does not predict which tumors will ultimately result in systemic disease.

Approximately 90% of orbital lymphoproliferations prove monoclonal and 10% polyclonal by molecular genetic studies; but both types of lesions may have prior, concurrent, or future systemic spread. This occurs in greater than half of periocular lymphomas, with 20%–30% of periocular lymphoproliferative lesions having a history of previous or concomitant systemic disease and an additional 30% developing it over 5 years. The anatomical site of origin offers some prediction of the risk of having or developing systemic non-Hodgkin lymphoma. The risk is lowest for conjunctival lesions, greater for orbital lesions, and highest for lesions arising in the eyelid. Lymphoid lesions developing in the lacrimal fossa may carry a greater risk of systemic disease than those occurring elsewhere in the orbit. Bilateral periocular involvement markedly increases the risk of systemic disease, but such involvement is not definitive evidence of systemic disease. It is also clear that the risk of systemic disease increases for decades after the original lesion is diagnosed, regardless of the initial lesion's location in the orbit or its clonality.

Management

Because the various lymphoproliferative lesions show great overlap in terms of clinical behavior, all patients with hypercellular lymphoid lesions (whether monoclonal or polyclonal) should be examined by an oncologist. Depending on the histologic type of the lesion, the examination may include a general physical examination, a complete blood count, a bone marrow biopsy, a liver and spleen scan, a chest radiograph, and serum immunoprotein electrophoresis. The oncologist may also recommend CT of the thorax and abdomen to check for mediastinal and retroperitoneal lymph node involvement. The patient should be reexamined periodically because systemic lymphoma may occur many years after the presentation of an isolated orbital lymphoid neoplasm.

Although systemic corticosteroids are useful in nonspecific orbital inflammation, they are not recommended in the treatment of lymphoproliferative lesions. Radiotherapy is the treatment of choice for patients with localized ocular adnexal lymphoproliferative disease. A dose of 2000–3000 cGy is typically administered. This regimen achieves local control in virtually all cases and, if the lesion is isolated, may prevent systemic spread. A surgical cure usually cannot be achieved because of the infiltrative nature of lymphoid tumors.

The treatment of low-grade lymphoid lesions that have already undergone systemic dissemination is somewhat controversial because indolent lymphomas are generally refractory to chemotherapy and are associated with long-term survival, even if untreated. Many oncologists take a watchful waiting approach and treat only symptomatic disease. Lymphomas that are more aggressive require radiation, aggressive chemotherapy, or both; up to one-third of these lesions can be cured.

Sullivan TJ, Whitehead K, Williamson R, et al. Lymphoproliferative disease of the ocular adnexa: a clinical and pathologic study with statistical analysis of 69 patients. *Ophthal Plast Reconstr Surg.* 2005;21(3):177–188.

White WL, Ferry JA, Harris NL, Grove AS Jr. Ocular adnexal lymphoma: a clinicopathologic study with identification of lymphomas of mucosa-associated lymphoid tissue type. *Ophthalmology.* 1995;102(12):1994–2006.

Plasma Cell Tumors

Lesions composed predominantly of mature plasma cells may be plasmacytomas or localized plasma cell–rich pseudotumors. Multiple myeloma should be ruled out, particularly if there is bone destruction or any immaturity or mitotic activity among the plasmacytic elements. Some lesions are composed of lymphocytes and lymphoplasmacytoid cells that combine properties of both lymphocytes and plasma cells. Plasma cell tumors display the same spectrum of clinical involvement as do lymphoproliferative lesions but are much less common.

Histiocytic Disorders

Langerhans cell histiocytosis, formerly known as *histiocytosis X,* is a collection of rare disorders of the mononuclear phagocytic system. These disorders are now thought to result from abnormal immune regulation. All subtypes are characterized by an accumulation of proliferating dendritic histiocytes. The disease occurs most commonly in children, with a peak incidence between 5 and 10 years of age, and varies in severity from benign lesions with spontaneous resolution to chronic dissemination resulting in death. Older names representing the various manifestations of histiocytic disorders (*eosinophilic granuloma of bone, Hand-Schüller-Christian syndrome,* and *Letterer-Siwe disease*) are being displaced by the terms *unifocal* and *multifocal eosinophilic granuloma of bone* and *diffuse soft tissue histiocytosis.*

The most frequent presentation in the orbit is a lytic defect, usually affecting the superotemporal orbit or sphenoid wing and causing relapsing episodes of orbital inflammation often misinterpreted initially as infectious orbital cellulitis. Ultimately, the mass may cause proptosis. Younger children more often present with significant overlying soft-tissue inflammation; they are also more likely to have evidence of multifocal or systemic involvement. Even if the initial workup shows no evidence of systemic dissemination, younger patients require regular observation for detection of subsequent multiorgan involvement.

Histiocytic disorders have a reported survival rate of only 50% in patients presenting under 2 years of age; if the disease develops after age 2, the survival rate rises to 87%. Treatment of localized orbital disease consists of confirmatory biopsy with debulking, which may be followed by intralesional steroid injection or low-dose radiation therapy. Spontaneous remission has also been reported. Although destruction of the orbital bone may be extensive at the time of presentation, the bone usually reossifies completely. Children with systemic disease are treated aggressively with chemotherapy.

Woo KI, Harris GJ. Eosinophilic granuloma of the orbit: understanding the paradox of aggressive destruction responsive to minimal intervention. *Ophthal Plast Reconstr Surg.* 2003;19(6):429–439.

Xanthogranuloma

Adult xanthogranuloma of the adnexa and orbit is often associated with systemic manifestations. These manifestations are the basis for classification into the following 4 syndromes, presented in their order of frequency:

1. necrobiotic xanthogranuloma (NBX)
2. adult-onset asthma with periocular xanthogranuloma (AAPOX)
3. Erdheim-Chester disease (ECD)
4. adult-onset xanthogranuloma (AOX)

NBX is characterized by the presence of subcutaneous lesions in the eyelids and anterior orbit; the lesions may also occur throughout the body. Although skin lesions are seen in all of these syndromes, the lesions in NBX have a propensity to ulcerate and fibrose. Frequent systemic findings include paraproteinemia and multiple myeloma.

AAPOX is a syndrome that includes periocular xanthogranuloma, asthma, lymphadenopathy, and, often, increased IgG levels.

ECD, the most devastating of the adult xanthogranulomas, is characterized by dense, progressive, recalcitrant fibrosclerosis of the orbit and internal organs, including the mediastinum; pericardium; and the pleural, perinephric, and retroperitoneal spaces. Whereas xanthogranuloma of the orbit and adnexa tends to be anterior in NBX, AAPOX, and AOX, it is often diffuse in ECD and leads to visual loss. Bone involvement is common and death frequent, despite aggressive therapies.

AOX is an isolated xanthogranulomatous lesion without systemic involvement. *Juvenile xanthogranuloma* is a separate non-Langerhans histiocytic disorder that occurs as a self-limited, corticosteroid-sensitive, and usually focal subcutaneous disease of childhood. See BCSC Section 6, *Pediatric Ophthalmology and Strabismus,* for additional discussion of juvenile xanthogranuloma.

Sivak-Callcott JA, Rootman J, Rasmussen SL, et al. Adult xanthogranulomatous disease of the orbit and ocular adnexa: new immunohistochemical findings and clinical review. *Br J Ophthalmol.* 2006;90(5):602–608.

Lacrimal Gland Tumors

Most lacrimal gland masses represent nonspecific inflammation (dacryoadenitis). They present with acute inflammatory signs and usually respond to anti-inflammatory medication (see the section Nonspecific Orbital Inflammation in Chapter 4). Of those lacrimal gland tumefactions not presenting with inflammatory signs and symptoms, the majority represent lymphoproliferative disorders (discussed previously): up to 50% of orbital lymphomas develop in the lacrimal fossa. Only a minority of lacrimal fossa lesions are epithelial neoplasms of the lacrimal gland.

Imaging is helpful in evaluating lesions in the lacrimal gland region. Inflammatory and lymphoid proliferations within the lacrimal gland tend to cause it to expand diffusely and appear elongated, whereas epithelial neoplasms tend to appear as isolated globular masses. Inflammatory and lymphoproliferative lesions usually mold around the globe, whereas epithelial neoplasms tend to displace and indent it. The bone of the lacrimal fossa is remodeled in response to a slowly growing benign epithelial lesion of the lacrimal gland, whereas there is typically no bony change due to a lymphoproliferative lesion.

Epithelial Tumors of the Lacrimal Gland

Approximately 50% of epithelial tumors are benign mixed tumors (pleomorphic adenomas) and about 50% are carcinomas. Approximately half of the carcinomas are adenoid cystic, and the remainder are malignant mixed-tumor primary adenocarcinoma, mucoepidermoid carcinoma, or squamous carcinoma.

Pleomorphic adenoma

Shown in Figure 5-15, *pleomorphic adenoma (benign mixed tumor)* is the most common epithelial tumor of the lacrimal gland. This tumor usually occurs in adults during the fourth and fifth decades of life and affects slightly more men than women. Patients present with a progressive, painless downward and inward displacement of the globe with axial proptosis. Symptoms are usually present for more than 12 months.

A firm, lobular mass may be palpated near the superolateral orbital rim, and orbital imaging often reveals enlargement or expansion of the lacrimal fossa. On imaging, the lesion appears well circumscribed but may have a slightly nodular configuration.

Microscopically, benign mixed tumors have a varied cellular structure consisting primarily of a proliferation of benign epithelial cells and a stroma composed of spindle-shaped cells with occasional cartilaginous, mucinous, or even osteoid degeneration or

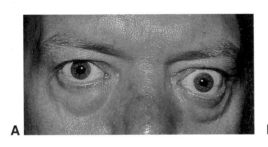

A

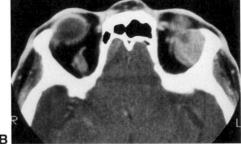

B

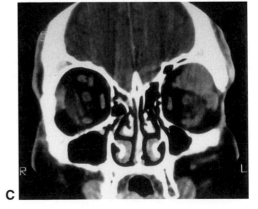

C

Figure 5-15 A, Proptosis and downward displacement of left eye in a man with benign mixed tumor of lacrimal gland. **B,** Axial CT scan showing tumor in lacrimal fossa. No bony remodeling is present in this case. **C,** Coronal CT scan showing rounded mass in lacrimal gland consistent with benign mixed tumor. *(Courtesy of Robert C. Kersten, MD.)*

metaplasia. This variability accounts for the designation *mixed tumor*. The lesion is circumscribed by a pseudocapsule.

Management Treatment is complete removal of the tumor with its pseudocapsule and a surrounding margin of orbital tissue. Surgery should be performed without a preliminary biopsy: in an early study, the recurrence rate was 32% when the capsule of the pleomorphic adenoma was incised for direct biopsy. In recurrences, the risk of malignant degeneration is 10% per decade.

Rose GE, Wright JE. Pleomorphic adenoma of the lacrimal gland. *Br J Ophthalmol.* 1992;76(7): 395–400.

Adenoid cystic carcinoma

Also known as *cylindroma,* adenoid cystic carcinoma is the most common malignant tumor of the lacrimal gland. This highly malignant tumor may cause pain because of perineural invasion and bone destruction. The relatively rapid course, with a history of generally less than 1 year, and early onset of pain help differentiate this malignant tumor from benign mixed tumor, which tends to show progressive proptosis for more than a year and is painless. The tumor usually extends into the posterior orbit because of its capacity to infiltrate and its lack of true encapsulation.

Microscopically, this tumor is made of disarmingly benign-appearing cells that grow in tubules, solid nests, or a cribriform Swiss-cheese pattern. The basaloid morphology is associated with worse survival than the cribriform variant. Infiltration of the orbital tissues, including perineural invasion, is often seen in microscopic sections.

Malignant mixed tumor

These lesions are histologically similar to benign mixed tumors, but they have areas of malignant change, usually poorly differentiated adenocarcinomas. They typically arise from long-standing primary benign mixed tumors or from a benign mixed tumor that has recurred following initial incomplete excision or violation of the pseudocapsule (see the section Pleomorphic adenoma).

Management of malignant lacrimal gland tumors

Suspicion of a malignant lacrimal gland tumor warrants biopsy with permanent histologic confirmation. Exenteration and radical orbitectomy with removal of the roof, lateral wall, and floor along with the overlying soft tissues and anterior portion of the temporalis muscle have failed to produce improvement in long-term survival rates. High-dose radiation therapy (conventional electrons, photons, and neutrons have all been used), in conjunction with surgical debulking, may be offered as an alternative. Intracarotid chemotherapy followed by exenteration has also been advocated; however, the duration of follow-up is not yet adequate to prove the efficacy of this treatment. Despite these measures, perineural extension into the cavernous sinus often occurs, and the typical clinical course is that of multiple painful recurrences with ultimate mortality from intracranial extension or, less commonly, from systemic metastases (which are managed by local resection), usually occurring a decade or more after the initial presentation.

Bartley GB, Harris GJ. Adenoid cystic carcinoma of the lacrimal gland: is there a cure . . . yet? *Ophthal Plast Reconstr Surg.* 2002;18(5):315–318.

Bernardini FP, Devoto MH, Croxatto JO. Epithelial tumors of the lacrimal gland: an update. *Curr Opin Ophthalmol.* 2008;19(5):409–413.

Font RL, Smith SL, Bryan RG. Malignant epithelial tumors of the lacrimal gland. A clinico-pathologic study of 21 cases. *Arch Ophthalmol.* 1998;116(5):613–616.

Nonepithelial Tumors of the Lacrimal Gland

Most of the nonepithelial lesions of the lacrimal gland represent lymphoid proliferation or inflammations. Up to 50% of orbital lymphoproliferative lesions occur in the lacrimal gland. Inflammatory conditions such as nonspecific orbital inflammation and sarcoidosis are covered in Chapter 4. Lymphoepithelial lesions may also occur either in Sjögren syndrome or as a localized lacrimal gland and salivary gland lesion (the so-called *Mikulicz syndrome*).

Benign lymphocytic infiltrates may be seen in patients, particularly women, who develop bilateral swellings of the lacrimal gland, producing a dry-eye syndrome. This condition can occur insidiously or following a symptomatic episode of lacrimal gland inflammation. The enlargement of the lacrimal glands may not be clinically apparent. Biopsy specimens of the affected glands show a spectrum of lymphocytic infiltration, from scattered patches of lymphocytes to lymphocytic replacement of the lacrimal gland parenchyma, with preservation of the inner duct cells, which are surrounded by proliferating myoepithelial cells *(epimyoepithelial islands)*. This combination of lymphocytes and epimyoepithelial islands has led some authors to designate this manifestation as a lymphoepithelial lesion. Some patients with lymphocytic infiltrates may also have systemic rheumatoid arthritis and, therefore, have classic Sjögren syndrome. These lesions may develop into low-grade B-cell lymphoma (see earlier discussion in the section Lymphoproliferative Disorders). Associated dry-eye symptoms may improve with the use of topical cyclosporine.

Secondary Orbital Tumors

Secondary orbital tumors are those that extend into the orbit from contiguous structures, such as the globe, the eyelids, the sinuses, or the brain.

Globe and Eyelid Origin

Tumors and inflammations from within the eye (especially from choroidal melanomas and retinoblastomas) or from the eyelid (eg, sebaceous gland carcinoma, squamous cell carcinoma, and basal cell carcinoma) can invade the orbit. Primary eyelid tumors are discussed in Chapter 10. Retinoblastoma, choroidal melanoma, and other ocular neoplasms are covered in BCSC Section 4, *Ophthalmic Pathology and Intraocular Tumors;* and Section 6, *Pediatric Ophthalmology and Strabismus.*

Sinus Origin

Tumors from the nose or the paranasal sinuses may secondarily invade the orbit. Proptosis and globe displacement are common. The diagnosis is made by imaging, which must be carried to the base of the sinuses for the proper evaluation.

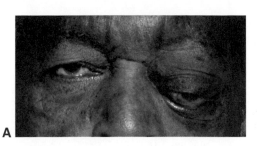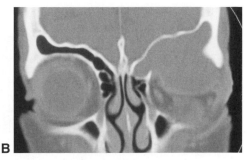

Figure 5-16 **A,** Marked proptosis and inferior displacement of the globe in a man with a large frontal mucocele. **B,** CT scan demonstrating frontal sinus mucocele expansion into superior orbit. *(Courtesy of Roberta E. Gausas, MD.)*

Mucoceles and *mucopyoceles* of the sinuses (Fig 5-16) are cystic structures with pseudostratified ciliated columnar (respiratory) epithelium resulting from obstruction of the sinus excretory ducts. These lesions may invade the orbit by expansion and erosion of the bones of the orbital walls. In the case of mucoceles, the cysts are usually filled with thick mucoid secretions; and in the case of pyoceles, they are filled with pus. Most mucoceles arise from the frontal or ethmoidal sinuses. Surgical treatment includes evacuation of the mucocele and reestablishment of drainage of the affected sinus or obliteration of the sinus by mucosal stripping and packing with bone or fat.

Another result of sinus outflow pathology is the *silent sinus syndrome.* Chronic subclinical sinusitis presumably causes thinning of the bone of the involved sinus, leading to enophthalmos due to collapse of the orbital floor. This collapse may occur in association with a recent significant change in atmospheric pressure as occurs, for example, during airplane travel or scuba diving. The upper eyelid may appear relatively retracted and there may be transient diplopia. Treatment includes restoration of normal sinus drainage and reconstruction of the orbital floor.

Squamous cell carcinoma is the most common epithelial tumor secondarily invading the orbit (Fig 5-17). These malignancies usually arise within the maxillary sinuses, followed by the nasopharynx or the oropharynx. Nasal obstruction, epistaxis, or epiphora may be associated with the growth of such tumors. Treatment is usually a combination of surgical excision and radiation therapy and often includes exenteration if the periorbita is traversed by tumor.

Nonepithelial tumors that can invade the orbit from the sinuses, nose, and facial bones include a wide variety of benign and malignant lesions. Among the most common of these are *osteomas, fibrous dysplasia,* and miscellaneous *sarcomas.*

Johnson LN, Krohel GB, Yeon EB, Parnes SM. Sinus tumors invading the orbit. *Ophthalmology.* 1984;91(3):209–217.

Soparkar CN, Patrinely JR, Cuaycong MJ, et al. The silent sinus syndrome. A cause of spontaneous enophthalmos. *Ophthalmology.* 1994;101(4):772–778.

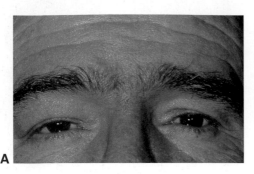
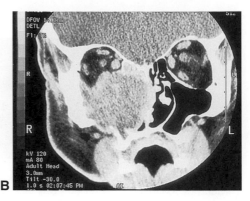

Figure 5-17 Squamous cell carcinoma of the sinus extending into the orbit. **A,** Clinical photo; note minimal proptosis despite large tumor of the sinus extending into the orbit. **B,** CT scan; sinus cancers typically do not show early clinical signs, usually presenting after the tumor has grown to a large size. *(Courtesy of Jeffrey Nerad, MD.)*

Metastatic Tumors

Metastatic Tumors in Children

In children, distant tumors metastasize to the orbit more frequently than to the globe (in contrast to adults, who more frequently have metastases to the choroid).

Neuroblastoma

Metastatic orbital neuroblastoma typically produces an abrupt ecchymotic proptosis that may be bilateral. A deposition of blood in the eyelids may lead to the mistaken impression of injury. Horner syndrome may also be apparent in some cases. Commonly, bone destruction is apparent, particularly in the lateral orbital wall or sphenoid marrow (Fig 5-18). Metastases typically occur late in the course of the disease, when the primary tumor can be detected readily in the abdomen, mediastinum, or neck. Treatment is primarily chemotherapy; radiotherapy is reserved for cases of impending visual loss due to compressive optic neuropathy. The survival rate is related to the patient's age at diagnosis. Patients diagnosed before 1 year of age have a 90% survival rate. Only 10% of those diagnosed at an older age survive. Congenital neuroblastoma of the cervical ganglia may produce an ipsilateral Horner syndrome with heterochromia.

   Miller NR, ed. *Walsh and Hoyt's Neuro-Ophthalmology.* 4th ed. Baltimore: Williams & Wilkins; 1988;3:1296–1300.

Leukemia

In advanced stages, leukemia may produce unilateral or bilateral proptosis. *Acute lymphoblastic leukemia* is the type of leukemia most likely to metastasize to the orbit. A primary leukemic orbital mass, called *granulocytic sarcoma,* or *chloroma,* is a rare variant of myelogenous leukemia. Least common are metastases to the subarachnoid space of the optic nerve. These cases present with sudden visual loss and swelling of the optic nerve.

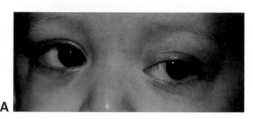
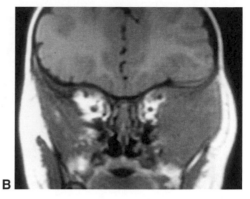

A   B

Figure 5-18   **A,** Child with a metastatic left orbital neuroblastoma. **B,** MRI demonstrates a large infiltrating lesion of the left sphenoid wing extending into the orbital soft tissues and the temporalis fossa. *(Courtesy of Michael Kazim, MD.)*

They constitute an emergency and are treated with orbital radiotherapy. Typically, orbital lesions present in advance of blood or bone marrow signs of leukemia, which almost invariably follow within several months. Special stains for cytoplasmic esterase in the cells (Leder stain) indicate that these are granulocytic precursor cells. Chances for survival are improved if chemotherapy is instituted before the discovery of leukemic involvement in bone marrow or peripheral blood.

Stockl FA, Dolmetsch AM, Saornil MA, Font RL, Burnier MN Jr. Orbital granulocytic sarcoma. *Br J Ophthalmol.* 1997;81(12):1084–1088.

Metastatic Tumors in Adults

Although virtually any carcinoma of the internal organs and cutaneous melanoma can metastasize to the orbit, breast and lung tumors account for the majority of orbital metastases. The presence of pain, proptosis, inflammation, bone destruction, and early ophthalmoplegia suggests the possibility of metastatic carcinoma.

Some 75% of patients have a history of a known primary tumor, but in 25% the orbital metastasis may be the presenting sign. The extraocular muscles are frequently involved because of their abundant blood supply. The second most common site is the bone marrow space of the sphenoid bone because of the relatively high volume of low-flow blood in this site (Fig 5-19). Lytic destruction of this part of the lateral orbital wall is highly suggestive of metastatic disease. Elevation of serum carcinoembryonic antigen levels also may suggest a metastatic process. Fine-needle aspiration biopsy can be performed in the office and may obviate the need for orbitotomy and open biopsy.

Breast carcinoma

The most common primary source of orbital metastases in women is breast cancer. Metastases may occur many years after the breast has been removed; thus, a history should always include inquiries about previous cancer surgery. Breast metastasis to the orbit may elicit a fibrous response that causes enophthalmos and possibly restriction of ocular motility (Fig 5-20).

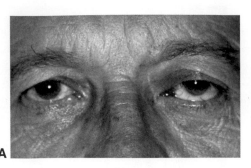
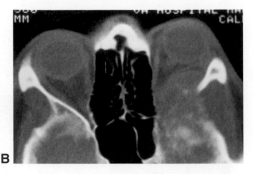

A

B

Figure 5-19 **A,** Left proptosis and orbital congestion in an elderly man with prostate carcinoma. **B,** CT scan showing left posterior orbital mass with adjacent bony destruction proven by biopsy to be metastatic prostate cancer. *(Courtesy of Roberta E. Gausas, MD.)*

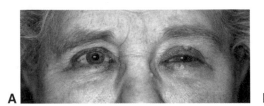
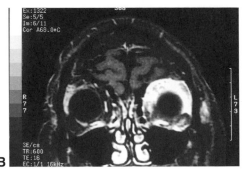

A

B

Figure 5-20 **A,** Woman with enophthalmos and motility restriction secondary to metastatic breast carcinoma to the orbit. **B,** T1-weighted MRI showing diffuse inferior infiltration of orbit. *(Courtesy of John B. Holds, MD.)*

Some patients with breast cancer respond favorably to hormonal therapy. This response usually correlates with the presence of estrogen and other hormone receptors found in the tumor tissue. If metastatic breast cancer is found at the time of orbital exploration, fresh tissue should be submitted for estrogen-receptor assay even if this test was previously performed because estrogen-receptor content may differ between the primary and the metastatic lesion. Hormone therapy is most likely to help patients whose tumors are receptor-positive.

Bronchogenic carcinoma

The most frequent origin of orbital metastasis in men is bronchogenic carcinoma. The primary lesion may be quite small, and CT of suspicious lung lesions may be performed in patients suspected of having orbital metastases.

Prostate carcinoma

Metastatic prostate carcinoma can produce a clinical picture resembling that of acute nonspecific orbital inflammation. Typically, a lytic bone lesion is identified on imaging.

Management of Orbital Metastases

The treatment of metastatic tumors of the orbit is usually palliative, consisting of local radiation therapy. Some metastatic tumors, such as carcinoids and renal cell carcinomas, may be candidates for wide excision of the orbital lesion because some patients may survive for many years following resection of isolated metastases from these primary tumors. Consultation with the patient's oncologist should identify candidates who might benefit from wide excision.

Char DH, Miller T, Kroll S. Orbital metastases: diagnosis and course. *Br J Ophthalmol.* 1997; 81(5):386–390.

Henderson JW, Campbell RJ, Farrow GM, et al. *Orbital Tumors.* 3rd ed. New York: Raven; 1994.

Rootman J, ed. *Diseases of the Orbit: A Multidisciplinary Approach.* Philadelphia: Lippincott; 1988.

CHAPTER 6

Orbital Trauma

Orbital trauma can damage the facial bones and adjacent soft tissues. Fractures may be associated with injuries to orbital contents, intracranial structures, and paranasal sinuses. Orbital hemorrhage and embedded foreign bodies may also be present and have secondary effects on the orbit. Decreased visual acuity, intraocular injuries, strabismus, eyelid malpositions, and ptosis may occur.

Because of the high incidence of concomitant intraocular injury, an ocular examination must always be performed on patients who have sustained orbital trauma. Ocular damage accompanying orbital trauma may include hyphema, angle recession, corneoscleral laceration, retinal tear, retinal dialysis, and vitreous hemorrhage.

Midfacial (Le Fort) Fractures

Le Fort fractures involve the maxilla and are often complex and asymmetric (Figs 6-1, 6-2). By definition, Le Fort fractures must extend posteriorly through the pterygoid plates. Treatment may include dental stabilization with arch bars and open reduction of the fracture with rigid fixation using miniplating and microplating systems. These fractures may be divided into 3 categories, *although clinically they often do not conform precisely to these groupings.*

- *Le Fort I* is a low transverse maxillary fracture above the teeth with no orbital involvement.
- *Le Fort II* fractures generally have a pyramidal configuration and involve the nasal, lacrimal, and maxillary bones as well as the medial orbital floor.
- *Le Fort III* fractures cause craniofacial disjunction in which the entire facial skeleton is completely detached from the base of the skull and suspended only by soft tissues. The orbital floor and medial and lateral orbital walls are involved.

Orbital Fractures

Zygomatic Fractures

Zygomaticomaxillary complex (ZMC) fractures are called *tripod fractures* (Fig 6-3), which is a misnomer because the zygoma is usually fractured at 4 of its articulations with the adjacent bones (lateral orbital rim, inferior orbital rim, zygomatic arch, and lateral wall

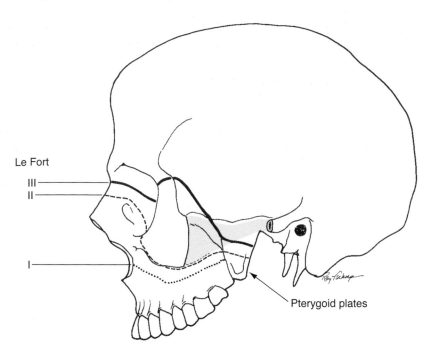

Le Fort

III
II

I

Pterygoid plates

Figure 6-1 Le Fort fractures (lateral view). Note that all the fractures extend posteriorly through the pterygoid plates *(arrow). (Modified from Converse JM, ed.* Reconstructive Plastic Surgery: Principles and Procedures in Correction, Reconstruction, and Transplantation. *2nd ed. Philadelphia: Saunders; 1977:2. Used with permission.)*

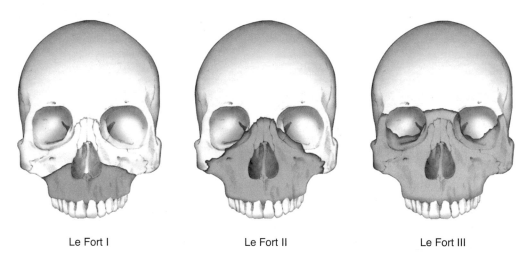

Le Fort I   Le Fort II   Le Fort III

Figure 6-2 Le Fort's classification of midfacial fractures. Le Fort I, horizontal fracture of the maxilla, also known as Guérin fracture. Le Fort II, pyramidal fracture of the maxilla. Le Fort III, craniofacial dysjunction. *(Modified from Converse JM, ed.* Reconstructive Plastic Surgery: Principles and Procedures in Correction, Reconstruction, and Transplantation. *2nd ed. Philadelphia: Saunders; 1977:2. Used with permission. Illustration by Cyndie C. H. Wooley.)*

of the maxillary sinus). ZMC fractures involve the orbital floor to varying degrees. If the zygoma is not significantly displaced, treatment may not be necessary. ZMC fractures can cause globe displacement, cosmetic deformity, diplopia, and trismus (limitation of mandibular opening) due to fracture impingement on the coronoid process of the mandible.

When treatment is indicated, the best results are obtained with open reduction of the fracture and fixation with miniature metal plates that are attached with bone screws (see Fig 6-3). Exact realignment and stabilization of the maxillary buttress and the lateral orbital wall are essential for accurate fracture reduction and can be achieved through a sublabial or buccal sulcus incision. It is not always necessary to explore the orbital floor unless there is concern that orbital contents might have been entrapped in fracture reduction.

Shumrick KA, Kersten RC, Kulwin DR, Smith CP. Criteria for selective management of the orbital rim and floor in zygomatic complex and midface fractures. *Arch Otolaryngol Head Neck Surg.* 1997;123(4):378–384.

Orbital Apex Fractures

Orbital apex fractures usually occur in association with other fractures of the face, orbit, or skull and may involve the optic canal, superior orbital fissure, and structures that pass through them. Possible associated complications include damage to the optic nerves, with

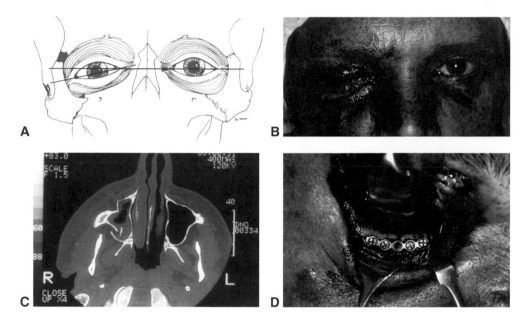

Figure 6-3 **A,** Zygomatic fracture (anterior view). Downward displacement of the globe and lateral canthus as a result of frontozygomatic separation and downward displacement of the zygoma and the floor of the orbit. **B,** Globe ptosis and lateral canthal dystopia due to depressed zygomaticomaxillary complex (ZMC) fracture. **C,** Axial CT scan showing depression of malar prominence and telescoping of bone fragment into the maxillary sinus. **D,** Intraoperative view showing rigid plate fixation of orbital rim fracture in prior patient. *(Part A modified from Converse JM, ed.* Reconstructive Plastic Surgery: Principles and Procedures in Correction, Reconstruction, and Transplantation. *2nd ed. Philadelphia: Saunders; 1977:2. Used with permission. Parts B, C, and D courtesy of John B. Holds, MD.)*

decreased visual acuity; cerebrospinal fluid leaks; and carotid cavernous sinus fistulas. Indirect traumatic optic neuropathy usually results from stretching, tearing, twisting, or bruising of the fixed canalicular portion of the nerve as the cranial skeleton suffers sudden deceleration. In most patients, thin-section computed tomography (CT) through the orbital apex and anterior clinoid processes demonstrates fractures at or adjacent to the optic canal. The management of neurogenic visual loss after blunt head trauma is discussed later in this chapter in the section Traumatic Visual Loss With Clear Media.

Orbital Roof Fractures

Orbital roof fractures are usually caused by blunt trauma or missile injuries and are more common in young children, in whom the frontal sinus has not yet pneumatized. The brain and cribriform plate may be involved. In older patients, frontal trauma tends to be absorbed by the frontal sinus, which acts as a crumple zone, preventing extension along the orbital roof. Complications include intracranial injuries, cerebrospinal fluid rhinorrhea, pneumocephalus, subperiosteal hematoma, ptosis, and extraocular muscle imbalance. The entrapment of extraocular muscles is rare, with most early diplopia resulting from hematoma, edema, or contusion of the orbital structures. In severely comminuted fractures, pulsating exophthalmos may occur as a delayed complication. Young children may develop nondisplaced linear roof fractures after fairly minor trauma, which may present with delayed ecchymosis of the upper eyelid. Most roof fractures do not require repair. Indications for surgery are generally neurosurgical, and treatment often involves a team approach with a neurosurgeon and an orbital surgeon.

Medial Orbital Fractures

Direct (naso-orbital-ethmoidal) fractures (Fig 6-4) usually result from the face striking solid surfaces. These fractures commonly involve the frontal process of the maxilla, the lacrimal bone, and the ethmoid bones along the medial wall of the orbit. Patients characteristically have a depressed bridge of the nose and traumatic telecanthus. These fractures are categorized as types I–III, with type I being a central fragment of bone attached to canthal tendon, type II having comminuted fracture of the central fragment, and type III having a comminuted tendon attachment or avulsed tendon.

Complications include cerebral and ocular damage, severe epistaxis due to avulsion of the anterior ethmoidal artery, orbital hematoma, cerebrospinal fluid rhinorrhea, damage to the lacrimal drainage system, lateral displacement of the medial canthus, and associated fractures of the medial orbital wall and floor. Treatment includes repair of the nasal fracture and miniplate stabilization. Transnasal wiring of the medial canthus is used less frequently, as miniplate fixation often allows precise bony reduction.

Indirect (blowout) fractures are frequently extensions of blowout fractures of the orbital floor. Isolated blowout fractures of the medial orbital wall may also occur. Surgical intervention is unnecessary unless the medial rectus muscle or its associated tissues are entrapped. Significant enophthalmos is uncommon after isolated medial wall blowout fractures.

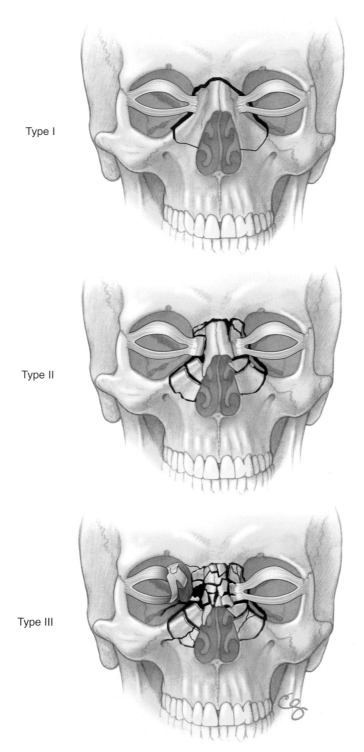

Type I

Type II

Type III

Figure 6-4   Naso-orbital-ethmoidal fractures result in traumatic telecanthus with rounding of the medial canthus. Types I–III are described depending on the severity of the injury. *(Illustration by Christine Gralapp.)*

Large, isolated medial wall fractures may result in cosmetically noticeable enophthalmos; however, the risk of enophthalmos is greatest when both the floor and the medial wall are fractured. If surgery is required, the medial orbital wall may be approached by continuing the exploration of the floor up along the medial wall via the eyelid or transconjunctival approach. An alternative approach is a medial orbitotomy through the skin or a transcaruncular approach.

Markowitz BL, Manson PN, Yaremchuk M, Glassman D, Kawamoto H. High-energy orbital dislocations: the possibility of traumatic hypertelorbitism. *Plast Reconstr Surg.* 1991;88(1): 20–28.

Nolasco FP, Mathog RH. Medial orbital wall fractures: classification and clinical profile. *Otolaryngol Head Neck Surg.* 1995;112(4):549–556.

Shorr N, Baylis HI, Goldberg RA, Perry JD. Transcaruncular approach to the medial orbit and orbital apex. *Ophthalmology.* 2000;107(8):1459–1463.

Orbital Floor Fractures

Direct fractures of the orbital floor can extend from fractures of the inferior orbital rim. Indications for repair of the orbital floor in these cases are the same as those for indirect (blowout) fractures. Indirect fractures of the orbital floor are not associated with fracture of the inferior orbital rim.

Past theory held that blowout fractures were caused by increased intraorbital pressure when the impact of a blunt object rapidly occluded the orbital aperture. According to this theory, the contents of the orbit are compressed posteriorly toward the apex of the orbit, and the orbital bones break at their weakest point, usually the posterior medial part of the floor in the maxillary bone. The orbital contents prolapse through the fracture into the maxillary sinus and may be entrapped. More recently, however, it has been suggested that an impacting object may compress the inferior rim, directly buckling the orbital floor. In this case, the degree of increased orbital pressure determines whether orbital tissues are pushed down through the fracture into the maxillary antrum.

The diagnosis of a blowout fracture of the orbital floor is suggested by the patient's history, physical examination, and radiographs. There is a history of the orbital entrance being struck by an object, usually one larger than the diameter of the orbital opening (eg, a ball, an automobile dashboard, or a fist). An orbital blowout fracture should be suspected in any patient who has received a periorbital blow forceful enough to cause ecchymosis. Physical examination typically reveals the following:

- *Eyelid signs.* Ecchymosis and edema of the eyelids may be present, but other external signs of injury can be absent *(white-eyed blowout).*
- *Diplopia with limitation of upgaze, downgaze, or both.* Limited vertical movement of the globe, vertical diplopia, and pain in the inferior orbit on attempted vertical movement of the globe are consistent with entrapment of the inferior rectus muscle or its adjacent septa in the fracture. Orbital edema and hemorrhage or damage to the extraocular muscles or their innervation can also limit movement of the globe. A significant limitation of both horizontal and vertical eye movements may indicate nerve damage or generalized soft-tissue injury. Limitations of globe movements

caused by hemorrhage or edema generally improve during the first 1–2 weeks after injury. If entrapment is present, a *forced duction test (traction test)* shows restriction of passive movement of the eye; however, restriction can also result from edema and hemorrhage. This test is performed most easily with the instillation of anesthetic eyedrops followed by a cotton pledget of topical anesthetic in the inferior cul-de-sac for several minutes. Using a toothed forceps, the examiner grasps the insertion of the inferior rectus muscle through the conjunctiva and attempts to rotate the globe gently up and down. Comparing the intraocular pressure (IOP) as measured in primary position and in upgaze usually shows a significant increase in upgaze if the inferior rectus is entrapped.

- *Enophthalmos and ptosis of the globe.* These findings occur with large fractures in which the orbital soft tissues prolapse into the maxillary sinus. A medial wall fracture, if associated with the orbital floor fracture, may significantly contribute to enophthalmos because of prolapse of the orbital tissues into both the ethmoidal and the maxillary sinuses. Enophthalmos may be masked by orbital edema immediately following the injury, but it becomes more apparent as the orbital edema subsides. Globe ptosis is often a sign of a sizable fracture.
- *Hypoesthesia in the distribution of the infraorbital nerve.*
- *Emphysema of the orbit and eyelids.* Any fracture that extends into a sinus may allow air to escape into the subcutaneous tissues. This occurs most commonly with medial wall fractures.

In patients with orbital floor fractures, visual loss can result from globe trauma, injury to the optic nerve, or increased orbital pressure causing a *compartment syndrome* (discussed in the section Traumatic Visual Loss With Clear Media). An orbital hemorrhage should be suspected if loss of vision is associated with proptosis and increased IOP. Injuries to the globe and ocular adnexa may also be present.

CT scans with coronal or sagittal views help guide treatment. They allow evaluation of fracture size and extraocular muscle relationships, providing information that can be used to help predict enophthalmos and muscle entrapment. Despite the publication of multiple studies suggesting neuroimaging criteria for associated extraocular muscle entrapment, restrictive strabismus related to blowout fracture remains a clinical diagnosis.

The majority of blowout or other orbital floor fractures do not require surgical intervention. Orbital blowout fractures are usually observed for 5–10 days to allow swelling and orbital hemorrhage to subside. Oral steroids (1 mg/kg per day for the first 7 days) decrease edema and may limit the risk of diplopia from inferior rectus contracture and fibrosis.

An exception to initial observation occurs in pediatric patients, in whom the inferior rectus muscle may become tightly trapped beneath a trapdoor fracture (Fig 6-5). In these patients, vertical globe excursion is significantly limited, and CT reveals the inferior rectus muscle within the maxillary sinus. Eye movement may stimulate the oculocardiac reflex, causing pain, nausea, and bradycardia. Urgent repair should be undertaken in these cases. Release of the entrapped muscle without delay may improve the final ocular motility result by limiting fibrosis.

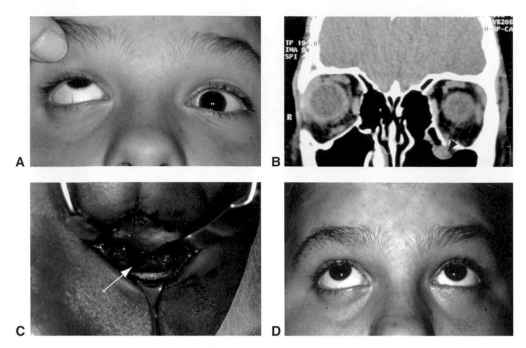

Figure 6-5 A, 13-year-old patient following blunt trauma to eye and orbit. Attempted gaze up and left. Left eye unable to elevate to midline. (Note: The pupillary dilation is pharmacologic). **B,** Coronal CT of orbit showing small orbital floor fracture and inferior rectus muscle prolapsing into maxillary sinus *(arrow)*. **C,** Intraoperative view of similar case showing orbital floor defect *(arrow)* enlarged surgically to release and extract inferior rectus muscle. **D,** 2 months postoperatively, the patient demonstrates resolution of upgaze limitation. *(Courtesy of John B. Holds, MD.)*

Although the indications for surgery are controversial, certain guidelines are helpful in determining when surgery is advisable:

- *Diplopia with limitation of upgaze and/or downgaze within 30° of the primary position with a positive forced duction test result 7–10 days after injury and with radiologic confirmation of a fracture of the orbital floor.* These findings indicate functional entrapment of tissues affecting the inferior rectus muscle. Diplopia may improve significantly over the course of the first 2 weeks as orbital edema, hemorrhage, or both resolve and as some of the entrapped tissues stretch. However, if the findings are still present after 2 weeks and if the entrapped tissues are not freed, vertical diplopia is likely to persist. As mentioned previously, tight entrapment of the inferior rectus muscle with a frozen globe is an indication for immediate repair.

- *Enophthalmos that exceeds 2 mm and is cosmetically unacceptable to the patient.* Enophthalmos is usually masked by orbital edema immediately after the trauma, and several weeks may pass before the extent of this problem is fully appreciated. Appropriate measurements must be taken at the initial evaluation and at subsequent visits. If significant enophthalmos is present within the first 2 weeks in association with a large orbital floor fracture, even greater enophthalmos can be anticipated in the future.

- *Large fractures involving at least half of the orbital floor, particularly when associated with large medial wall fractures (determined by CT).* Orbital fractures of this size have a high incidence of subsequent significant enophthalmos.

Burnstine MA. Clinical recommendations for repair of isolated orbital floor fractures: an evidence-based analysis. *Ophthalmology.* 2002;109(7):1207–1210.

Egbert JE, May K, Kersten RC, Kulwin DR. Pediatric orbital floor fracture: direct extraocular muscle involvement. *Ophthalmology.* 2000;107(10):1875–1879.

Harris GJ, Garcia GH, Logani SC, Murphy ML. Correlation of preoperative computed tomography and postoperative ocular motility in orbital blowout fractures. *Ophthal Plast Reconstr Surg.* 2000;16(3):179–187.

Hawes MJ, Dortzbach RK. Surgery on orbital floor fractures: influence of time of repair and fracture size. *Ophthalmology.* 1983;90(9):1066–1070.

Jordan DR, Allen LH, White J, Harvey J, Pashby R, Esmaile B. Intervention within days for some orbital floor fractures: the white-eyed blowout. *Ophthal Plast Reconstr Surg.* 1998;14(6):379–390.

Kersten RC. Blowout fracture of the orbital floor with entrapment caused by isolated trauma to the orbital rim. *Am J Ophthalmol.* 1987;103(2):215–220.

Rhee JS, Kilde J, Yoganadan N, Pintar F. Orbital blowout fractures: experimental evidence for the pure hydraulic theory. *Arch Facial Plast Surg.* 2002;4(2):98–101.

Rubin PAD, Bilyk JR, Shore JW. Management of orbital trauma: fractures, hemorrhage, and traumatic optic neuropathy. *Focal Points: Clinical Modules for Ophthalmologists.* San Francisco: American Academy of Ophthalmology; 1994, module 7.

Management

When surgery is indicated for blowout fractures of the orbital floor, it generally is preferable to proceed with the repair within 2 weeks of the initial trauma. Formation of scar tissue and contracture of the prolapsed tissue make later correction of entrapment and diplopia difficult. Larger fractures in which eventual enophthalmos is anticipated are also more easily repaired within the first 2 weeks of the trauma; however, satisfactory correction of enophthalmos is often obtainable even if surgery is delayed.

The surgical approach to blowout fractures of the orbital floor can be made through an infraciliary incision or a conjunctival (inferior fornix) incision combined with or without a lateral cantholysis. The approaches through the lower eyelid have the following steps in common: elevation of the periorbita from the orbital floor, release of the prolapsed tissues from the fracture, and, usually, placement of an implant over the fracture to prevent recurrent adhesions and prolapse of the orbital tissues.

The development of miniplating and microplating systems and their various metallic orbital implants has significantly improved the management of large, unstable orbital floor fractures. Orbital implants can be alloplastic (porous polyethylene, Supramid, Gore-Tex, Teflon, silicone sheet, or titanium mesh) or autogenous (split cranial bone, iliac crest bone, or fascia). The harvesting of autogenous grafts requires an additional operative site, and bone grafts are rarely indicated.

Delayed treatment of blowout fractures to correct debilitating strabismus and diplopia or cosmetically unacceptable enophthalmos may include exploration of the orbital floor in an attempt to free the scarred tissues entrapped or prolapsed through the fracture and to replace them in the orbit. Other treatment options include strabismus surgery and procedures to camouflage the narrowed palpebral fissure and deep superior sulcus associated with enophthalmos.

Complications of blowout fracture surgery include decreased visual acuity or blindness, diplopia, undercorrection or overcorrection of enophthalmos, lower eyelid retraction, infraorbital nerve hypoesthesia, infection, extrusion of the implant, lymphedema, and damage to the lacrimal drainage system.

Intraorbital Foreign Bodies

If foreign bodies within the orbit are radiopaque, they can be localized by plain-film radiographs or by CT or magnetic resonance imaging (MRI). Some wooden foreign bodies may be missed on CT and are seen better on MRI. However, MRI should be avoided if there is a possibility that the foreign object is ferromagnetic. If an embedded foreign body causes an orbital infection that drains to the skin surface, it is sometimes possible to locate the object by surgically following the fistulous tract posteriorly. Treatment of orbital foreign bodies initially involves culturing the wound (or the foreign body if it is removed) and administering antibiotics. Foreign bodies should be removed if they are composed of vegetable matter or if they are easily accessible in the anterior orbit. In many cases, objects can be safely observed without surgery if they are inert and have smooth edges or are located in the posterior orbit. BBs are common intraorbital foreign bodies and are usually best left in place. MRI can be safely performed with a BB in the orbit.

Finkelstein M, Legmann A, Rubin PA. Projectile metallic foreign bodies in the orbit: a retrospective study of epidemiologic factors, management, and outcomes. *Ophthalmology.* 1997;104(1):96–103.

McGuckin JF Jr, Akhtar N, Ho VT, Smergel EM, Kubacki EJ, Villafana T. CT and MR evaluation of a wooden foreign body in an in vitro model of the orbit. *Am J Neuroradiol.* 1996;17(1):129–133.

Orbital Hemorrhage

Hemorrhage into the orbit can arise after trauma or surgery or occur spontaneously in association with an underlying orbital lymphangioma or varix. Lateral canthotomy and cantholysis, orbital decompression, or surgical drainage is seldom necessary unless visual function is compromised by compression of the optic nerve or by increased orbital pressure that impedes arterial perfusion. Occasionally, a hematic cyst may form following accidental trauma, usually beneath the periosteum.

Traumatic Visual Loss With Clear Media

Many patients complain of decreased vision following periocular trauma. The decrease may be due to associated injuries of the cornea, lens, vitreous, or retina. Patients without globe damage may also complain of decreased vision because of serosanguinous drainage obscuring incident light. In addition, swelling of the eyelids may cause difficulty in opening the eyes sufficiently to clear the visual axis. However, a small percentage of patients have true visual loss without any evidence of globe injury. Visual loss in this setting suggests traumatic dysfunction of the optic nerve *(traumatic optic neuropathy)*. Such visual loss usually results from 1 of 3 mechanisms:

- direct injury to the optic nerve from a penetrating wound
- disruption of the blood supply to the optic nerve due to a compartment syndrome, in which posttraumatic orbital edema or hemorrhage causes orbital pressure to increase above arterial perfusion pressure
- indirect injury caused by force from a frontal blow transmitted to the optic nerve in the orbital apex and optic canal

All patients with decreased visual acuity following periorbital trauma should be immediately examined for evidence of direct globe injury. Two key diagnostic questions should be answered when the patient has reduced vision with an apparently normal globe:

- Is an afferent pupillary defect present?
- Is there a "tight" orbit?

Detection of an afferent pupillary defect in the presence of an intact globe strongly suggests traumatic optic neuropathy. However, the examiner must remember that detection of an afferent defect may be difficult if the patient has received narcotics that cause pupillary constriction. The second key diagnostic indicator is intraorbital pressure. Periorbital trauma may cause significant retrobulbar hemorrhage or edema, which can lead to proptosis, ptosis, and limitation of extraocular motility. A Schiøtz tonometer or Tono-Pen may be used in the emergency room to measure IOP, which is increased in the tight orbit in response to the underlying increased orbital pressure. Although fundus examination may reveal a central retinal artery occlusion, visual loss is more often caused by occlusion of the posterior ciliary arteries, which have a lower perfusion pressure than the central retinal artery.

Patients with a tight orbit, increased IOP, and decreased visual acuity with afferent pupillary defect should undergo emergent decompression of the orbit. This is most easily achieved by disinsertion of the lids from the lateral canthus (lateral canthotomy and cantholysis), allowing the orbital volume to expand anteriorly. Lateral canthotomy alone does not sufficiently increase the orbital volume; inferior cantholysis and sometimes superior cantholysis are also required. Surgical relief of the increased orbital pressure is a priority. Although IOP is elevated in the setting of traumatic orbital hemorrhage, the elevation reflects the increased orbital pressure and is not indicative of glaucoma (although angle-closure glaucoma occurs rarely following retrobulbar hemorrhages).

If a tight orbit has been ruled out, then a mechanism other than an ischemic compartment syndrome should be sought to explain the visual loss. The circumstances suggest indirect trauma to the optic nerve. The shock wave from trauma is transmitted through the orbital contents and can result in significant injury. Patients with this disorder usually have a history of blunt trauma to the frontal region or rapid deceleration of the cranium and often have experienced loss of consciousness associated with frontal head trauma. Thin-section CT scans of the orbital apex and anterior clinoid process demonstrate fractures through or adjacent to the optic canal in many cases.

Management

The proper management of neurogenic visual loss after blunt head trauma is controversial. Observation alone, high-dose corticosteroids, and surgical decompression of the optic canal are all considered reasonable options. Interest in high-dose methylprednisolone (30 mg/kg loading dose and 15 mg/kg every 6 hours) in traumatic optic neuropathy is supported by the success of this regimen in the National Acute Spinal Cord Injury Study II, in which the regimen was found to produce significant improvement in patients treated within 8 hours of injury. When the steroid is given in such high doses, the therapeutic effect appears to derive from the steroid's antioxidant, rather than anti-inflammatory, properties. The success seen with methylprednisolone as therapy for spinal cord injuries may not be applicable to the treatment of traumatic optic neuropathy, however; trial data are lacking for optic nerve injuries.

For a time, interest focused on surgical decompression of the optic canal in patients who failed to improve on high-dose steroids. Decompression of the medial wall of the bony optic canal through a transethmoidal sphenoidal route undertaken within 5 days of injury was purported to return vision to patients with indirect traumatic optic neuropathy. However, the optimal management of traumatic optic neuropathy remains unresolved because no large, randomized studies have been carried out. A recent multicenter, prospective, nonrandomized study failed to demonstrate clear benefit for either corticosteroid therapy or optic canal decompression. Successful results with steroid therapy or surgical treatment remain anecdotal, and a number of traumatic optic neuropathy cases have documented significant visual improvement without therapy.

Joseph MP, Lessell S, Rizzo J, Momose KJ. Extracranial optic nerve decompression for traumatic optic neuropathy. *Arch Ophthalmol.* 1990;108(8):1091–1093.

Levin LA, Beck RW, Joseph MP, Seiff S, Kraker R. The treatment of traumatic optic neuropathy: the International Optic Nerve Trauma Study. *Ophthalmology.* 1999;106(7):1268–1277.

Levin LA, Joseph MP, Rizzo JF III, Lessell S. Optic canal decompression in indirect optic nerve trauma. *Ophthalmology.* 1994;101(3):566–569.

Steinsapir KD, Goldberg RA. Traumatic optic neuropathy. *Surv Ophthalmol.* 1994;38(6): 487–518.

CHAPTER 7

Orbital Surgery

Orbital surgery requires the delicacy of a neurosurgeon, the strength of an orthopedic surgeon, and the 3-dimensional sense of a general surgeon. Few other locations of the body have so many surgical spaces and so many vital structures within such a small area. Surgical comfort and success are based on the surgeon's knowledge of the relationships among the orbital structures and ability to approach the orbit from different directions and angles to achieve best access to the pathology.

Surgical Spaces

There are 5 surgical spaces within the orbit (Fig 7-1):

- the *subperiorbital (subperiosteal) surgical space,* which is the potential space between the bone and the periorbita
- the *extraconal surgical space* (peripheral surgical space), which lies between the periorbita and the muscle cone with its fascia

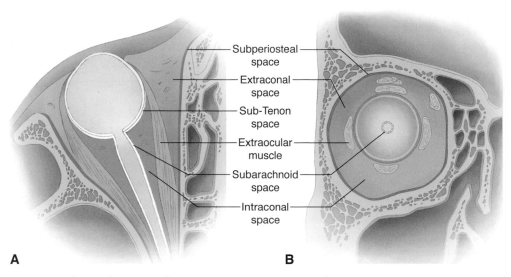

A   **B**

Figure 7-1 Surgical spaces of the orbit. **A,** Axial view. **B,** Coronal view. *(Modified from Nerad JA. Oculoplastic Surgery: The Requisites in Ophthalmology. Philadelphia: Mosby; 2001:350. Used with permission. Illustration by Cyndie C. H. Wooley.)*

- the *episcleral (sub-Tenon) surgical space,* which lies between the Tenon capsule and the globe
- the *intraconal surgical space* (central surgical space), which lies within the muscle cone
- the *subarachnoid surgical space,* which lies between the optic nerve and the nerve sheath

Orbital lesions may involve more than 1 space, and an orbital pathologic process may require a combination of approaches. Incisions to reach these surgical spaces via anterior or lateral orbitotomies are shown in Figure 7-2.

Orbitotomy

Superior Approach

More orbital lesions are found in the superoanterior part of the orbit than in any other location. Lesions in this area can usually be reached through a transcutaneous incision. The surgeon must take care to avoid damaging the levator and superior oblique muscles, trochlea, lacrimal gland, and sensory nerves and vessels entering or exiting the orbit along the superior orbital rim.

Transcutaneous incisions

For procedures in the superior subperiorbital space, an incision through the upper eyelid crease offers good access to the superior orbital rim and periosteum, with a well-hidden scar. Although it requires additional soft-tissue dissection, the cosmetic result is better with an eyelid crease incision than with an incision directly over the supraorbital rim. After making an upper eyelid crease incision, the surgeon obtains access to the superior

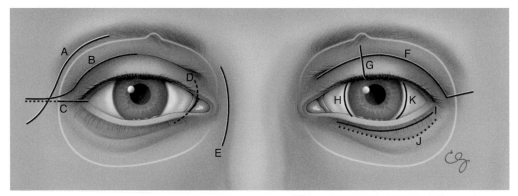

Figure 7-2 Sites of surgical entry into the orbit. *A,* Classic Stallard-Wright lateral orbitotomy. *B,* Eyelid crease lateral orbitotomy. *C,* Lateral canthotomy orbitotomy. *D,* Transcaruncular medial orbitotomy. *E,* Frontoethmoidal (Lynch) medial orbitotomy. *F,* Upper eyelid crease anterior orbitotomy. *G,* Vertical eyelid split superomedial orbitotomy. *H,* Medial bulbar conjunctival orbitotomy. *I,* Subciliary inferior orbitotomy. *J,* Transconjunctival inferior orbitotomy. *K,* Lateral bulbar conjunctival orbitotomy. *(Illustration by Christine Gralapp after a drawing by Jennifer Clemens.)*

orbital rim by dissecting superiorly in the postorbicularis fascial plane anterior to the orbital septum. After the rim is exposed, an incision is made in the arcus marginalis of the rim, and a periosteal elevator is then used to separate the periosteum from the frontal bone of the orbital roof. The periosteal dissection is facilitated by initially keeping the periorbita intact, which prevents orbital fat from obscuring the view during reflection of the periosteum.

Upper eyelid crease incisions may also be used for entry into the medial intraconal space, which requires exposure of the medial edge of the levator muscle and dissection through the intermuscular septum extending from the superior rectus to the medial rectus muscles. This approach may be used for exposure and fenestration of the retrobulbar optic nerve in cases of idiopathic intracranial hypertension.

Occasionally, a coronal scalp flap is used to expose superior orbital lesions. This route is most helpful for transcranial orbitotomies and for extensive lesions of the superior orbit and sinuses that require bone removal for access. Although the coronal incision has been used to gain access for lateral orbitotomy, this incision requires extensive elevation of the temporalis muscle, which may result in cosmetically significant temporal wasting postoperatively. Alopecia may occur at the site of the scalp incision.

Paolini S, Santoro A, Missori P, Pichierri A, Esposito V, Ciappetta P. Surgical exposure of lateral orbital lesions using a coronal scalp flap and lateral orbitozygomatic approach: clinical experience. *Acta Neurochir (Wien)*. 2006;148(9):959–963.

Stewart WB, Levin PS, Toth BA. Orbital surgery. The technique of coronal scalp flap approach to the lateral orbitotomy. *Arch Ophthalmol*. 1988;106(12):1724–1726.

Transconjunctival incision

Incisions in the superior conjunctiva can be used to reach the superonasal, episcleral, intraconal, or extraconal surgical spaces; but dissection must be performed medial to the levator muscle to prevent postoperative ptosis.

Vertical eyelid splitting

Vertical splitting of the upper eyelid at the junction of the medial and central thirds allows extended transconjunctival exposure for the removal of superomedial intraconal tumors. The surgeon incises the eyelid and levator aponeurosis vertically to expose the superomedial intraconal space. Realignment of the tarsal plate and aponeurosis with vertical closure prevents postoperative ptosis and eyelid retraction, which are likely to occur if the levator muscle is transected horizontally.

Kersten RC, Kulwin DR. Vertical lid split orbitotomy revisited. *Ophthal Plast Reconstr Surg*. 1999;15(6):425–428.

Inferior Approach

The inferior approach is suitable for masses that are visible or palpable in the inferior conjunctival fornix of the lower eyelid, as well as for deeper inferior extraconal orbital masses. The surgeon can also gain access to intraconal lesions by dissecting between the inferior rectus and lateral rectus muscles. The inferior oblique muscle inserts over the macula and may be identified and retracted while intraconal lesions are accessed. This route is also used to approach the orbital floor for fracture repair or decompression.

Transcutaneous incisions

Visible scarring can be minimized by the use of an infraciliary blepharoplasty incision in the lower eyelid and dissection beneath the orbicularis muscle to expose the inferior orbital septum and inferior orbital rim. An incision in the lower eyelid crease can provide the same exposure, but it leaves a slightly more obvious scar. The surgeon can then incise the septum to expose the extraconal surgical space.

For access to the inferior subperiorbital space, an extended subciliary incision or an incision in the lower eyelid crease with downward reflection of the skin and orbicularis muscle allows exposure of the rim. At the arcus marginalis of the inferior rim, the periosteum is incised and elevated to expose the floor of the orbit. Fractures of the orbital floor are reached by the subperiosteal route. Transcutaneous incisions made directly over the orbital rim or in the lower eyelid crease leave a more noticeable scar (Fig 7-3).

Transconjunctival incisions

The transconjunctival approach (Fig 7-4) has largely replaced the transcutaneous route for exposure of tumors in the inferior orbit and for management of fractures of the orbital floor and medial wall. To reach the extraconal surgical space and the orbital floor, the surgeon may make an incision through the inferior conjunctiva and lower eyelid retractors. Exposure of the floor is optimized when this incision is combined with a lateral canthotomy and cantholysis. The intraconal space may be reached by opening the reflected periosteum and retracting the muscles and intraconal fat.

Working on the globe surface and using an incision of the bulbar conjunctiva and Tenon capsule allows entry to the episcleral surgical space. This technique is used to reach the extraocular muscles. If the inferior rectus is retracted, the intraconal surgical space can be accessed through this incision.

Medial Approach

When dissecting in the medial orbit, the surgeon should be careful to avoid damaging the medial canthal tendon, lacrimal canaliculi and sac, trochlea, superior oblique tendon and muscle, inferior oblique muscle, and the sensory nerves and vessels along the medial aspect of the superior orbital rim.

Transcutaneous incision

Tumors within or near the lacrimal sac, the frontal or ethmoidal sinuses, and the medial rectus muscle can be approached through a skin incision (*Lynch,* or *frontoethmoidal,*

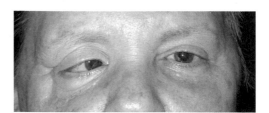

Figure 7-3 Lower eyelid retraction and visible scar following lower eyelid crease incision for fracture repair. *(Courtesy of Jill Foster, MD.)*

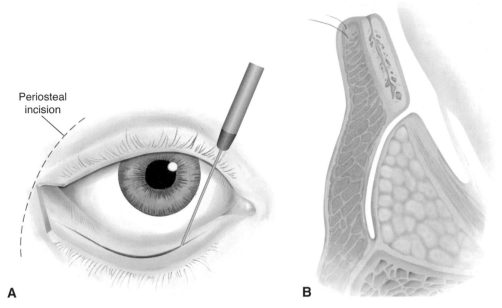

Figure 7-4   Inferior transconjunctival approach to the orbital floor. **A,** Canthotomy, cantholysis, and conjunctival incision. **B,** Plane of dissection anterior to the orbital septum. *(Modified from Nerad JA. Oculoplastic Surgery: The Requisites in Ophthalmology. Philadelphia: Mosby; 2001:335–336. Used with permission. Illustration by Cyndie C. H. Wooley.)*

incision) placed vertically just medial to the insertion of the medial canthal tendon (approximately 9–10 mm medial to the medial canthal angle). This route is generally used to enter the subperiorbital space. The medial canthal tendon can be reflected with the periosteum and, therefore, does not need to be incised.

Superomedial intraconal lesions can be approached through a medial upper eyelid crease incision. The superior oblique tendon must be identified, and dissection is then carried out medial to the medial horn of the levator muscle, providing access to the intraconal space.

> Pelton RW, Patel BC. Superomedial lid crease approach to the medial intraconal space: a new technique for access to the optic nerve and central space. *Ophthal Plast Reconstr Surg.* 2001;17(4):241–253.

Transconjunctival incision

An incision in the bulbar conjunctiva allows entry into the extraconal or episcleral surgical space. If the medial rectus is detached, the surgeon can then enter the intraconal surgical space to expose the region of the anterior optic nerve for examination, biopsy, or sheath fenestration. If the posterior optic nerve or muscle cone needs to be seen well, a combined lateral/medial orbitotomy can be performed. A lateral orbitotomy with removal of the lateral orbital wall allows the globe to be displaced temporally, thus maximizing medial access to the deeper orbit.

Transcaruncular incision

An incision through the posterior third of the caruncle or the conjunctiva immediately lateral to the caruncle allows excellent exposure of the medial periosteum. Dissection carried medially, just posterior to the lacrimal sac, allows access to the subperiorbital space along the medial wall. Incision and elevation of the medial periorbita allow exposure of the medial orbital wall. This incision has the advantage of providing better cosmetic results than the traditional frontoethmoidal, or Lynch, incision, but the surgeon must be careful to protect the lacrimal canaliculi and to remain posterior to the lacrimal apparatus. The combination of the transcaruncular route with an inferior transconjunctival incision allows extensive exposure of the inferior and medial orbit. This approach provides access for repair of medial wall fractures, for medial orbital bone decompression, and for drainage of medial subperiosteal abscesses.

Goldberg RA, Mancini R, Demer JL. The transcaruncular approach: surgical anatomy and technique. *Arch Facial Plast Surg.* 2007;9(6):443–447.

Graham SM, Thomas RD, Carter KD, Nerad JA. The transcaruncular approach to the medial orbital wall. *Laryngoscope.* 2002;112(6):986–989.

Tsirbas A, Kazim M, Close L. Endoscopic approach to orbital apex lesions. *Ophthal Plast Reconstr Surg.* 2005;21(4):271–275.

Lateral Approach

A lateral orbitotomy approach is used when a lesion is located within the lateral intraconal space, behind the equator of the globe, or in the lacrimal gland fossa. As the orbits are relatively shallower in children than in adults, extensive exposure of the orbits without the need for bone removal may be possible in children. The traditional S-shaped Stallard-Wright skin incision, extending from beneath the eyebrow laterally and curving down along the zygomatic arch, allowed good exposure of the lateral rim but left a noticeable scar. It has largely been replaced by newer approaches for lateral orbital exposure, through either an upper eyelid crease incision or a lateral canthotomy incision. Both of these approaches allow exposure of the lateral orbital rim and anterior portion of the zygomatic arch with reflection of the temporalis muscle and the periosteum of the orbit. Dissecting through the periorbita and then intermuscular septum either above or below the lateral rectus muscle and posterior to the equator of the globe provides access to the retrobulbar space. The retrobulbar optic nerve may be reached this way and fenestrated in cases of idiopathic intracranial hypertension.

If a lesion cannot be adequately exposed through a soft-tissue lateral incision, an oscillating saw is used to remove the bone of the lateral rim to expose the underlying periorbita, which is then opened. An operating microscope is often useful during intraorbital surgery, especially if dissection proceeds inside the muscle cone. Good exposure of the intraconal surgical space can be achieved with retraction of the lateral rectus muscle. Tumors can occasionally be prolapsed into the incision by application of gentle pressure over the eyelids. A cryosurgical probe or Allis forceps can be used to provide firm traction on encapsulated tumors. In cavernous hemangiomas, a suture through the lesion allows not only traction but also slow decompression of the tumor to facilitate its removal.

Complete hemostasis should be accomplished before closure. To help prevent postoperative intraorbital hemorrhage, an external drain may be placed through the skin to reach the deep orbital tissues. The lateral orbital rim is usually replaced and may be sutured back into place through predrilled tunnels in the rim. Alternatively, the surgeon may use rigid fixation with plating systems. The overlying tissues are then returned to their normal positions and sutured. The use of steel wire is avoided because it can cause artifacts on follow-up CT scans. The surgeon closes the periosteum loosely to allow postoperative hemorrhage to decompress.

Goldberg RA, Shorr N, Arnold AC, Garcia GH. Deep transorbital approach to the apex and cavernous sinus. *Ophthal Plast Reconstr Surg.* 1998;14(5):336–341.

Kersten RC, Kulwin DR. Optic nerve sheath fenestration through a lateral canthotomy incision. *Arch Ophthalmol.* 1993;111(6):870–874.

Orbital Decompression

Orbital decompression is a surgical procedure used to improve the volume-to-space discrepancy that occurs primarily in thyroid eye disease (TED). The goal of orbital decompression is to allow the enlarged muscles and orbital fat to expand into periorbital spaces. This expansion relieves pressure on the optic nerve and its blood supply and reduces proptosis.

Decompression historically involved removal of the medial orbital wall and much of the orbital floor to allow orbital tissues to expand into the ethmoid and maxillary sinuses. The approach was made through the maxillary sinus (Caldwell-Luc) or transcutaneous anterior orbitotomy incision. However, when used in patients with inflammatory eye disease featuring enlarged, restricted inferior rectus muscles, this type of decompression with removal of the medial orbital strut may exacerbate globe ptosis, upper eyelid retraction, and vertical globe excursion due to prolapse of the muscles into the maxillary sinus and downward displacement of the orbital contents. Also, limitation of lateral excursion may occur because of prolapse of a tight medial rectus muscle into the ethmoid sinus.

The approach currently used by many orbital surgeons is a transconjunctival incision combined with a lateral cantholysis to disinsert and evert the lower eyelid for exposure of the inferior and lateral orbital rims (Fig 7-5). Extension of this incision superonasally with a transcaruncular approach allows excellent access to the medial orbital wall for bone removal and decompression. (A transnasal endoscopic approach to the medial orbit via

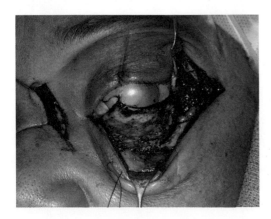

Figure 7-5 Surgical approach to the orbit combining lateral canthotomy, inferior transconjunctival incision, and medial Lynch incision. Lateral orbital rim bone removed. *(Courtesy of Jill Foster, MD.)*

the ethmoid sinus may also be useful for the medial wall.) To allow further decompression into the infratemporal fossa, the surgeon may remove the lateral orbital rim and reposition it anteriorly at the time of closure. Burring down the medial surface of the lateral wall and the sphenoid wing results in additional decompression. This type of procedure maximizes volume expansion and "balances" the decompression (Fig 7-6).

Removal of retrobulbar fat at the time of decompression further reduces proptosis and has also been shown to be beneficial in compressive optic neuropathy. Decompression through the orbital roof into the anterior cranial fossa is rarely advisable.

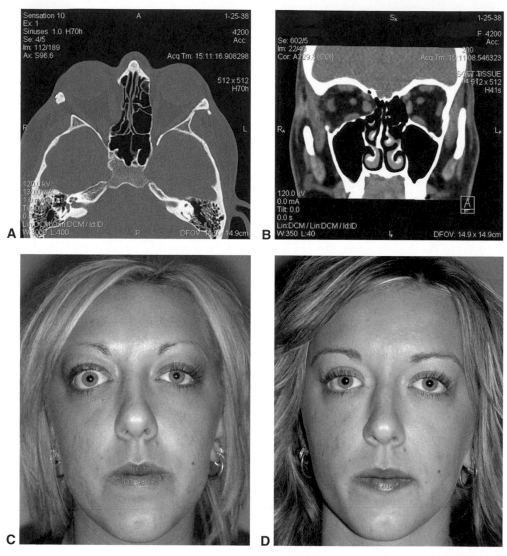

Figure 7-6 "Balanced" orbital decompression. **A,** Axial view CT scan showing surgical removal of areas of the lateral and medial walls on the right side. **B,** Coronal CT of same patient with views of medial, lateral, and inferior medial bone removal. **C,** Clinical photograph of this patient prior to surgery. **D,** Clinical photo of same patient following surgery. *(Courtesy of Jill Foster, MD.)*

Garrity JA, Fatourechi V, Bergstralh EJ, et al. Results of transantral orbital decompression in 428 patients with severe Graves' ophthalmopathy. *Am J Ophthalmol.* 1993;116(5):533–547.

Goldberg RA. The evolving paradigm of orbital decompression surgery [editorial]. *Arch Ophthalmol.* 1998;116(5):95–96.

Kacker A, Kazim M, Murphy M, Trokel S, Close LG. "Balanced" orbital decompression for severe Graves' orbitopathy: technique with treatment algorithm. *Otolaryngol Head Neck Surg.* 2003;128(2):228–235.

Perry JD, Kadakia A, Foster JA. Transcaruncular orbital decompression for dysthyroid optic neuropathy. *Ophthal Plast Reconstr Surg.* 2003;19(5):353–358.

Richter DF, Stoff A, Olivari N. Transpalpebral decompression of endocrine ophthalmopathy by intraorbital fat removal (Olivari technique): experience and progression after more than 3000 operations over 20 years. *Plast Reconstr Surg.* 2007;120(1):109–123.

Trokel S, Kazim M, Moore S. Orbital fat removal. Decompression for Graves orbitopathy. *Ophthalmology.* 1993;100(5):674–682.

White WA, White WL, Shapiro PE. Combined endoscopic medial and inferior orbital decompression with transcutaneous lateral orbital decompression in Graves' orbitopathy. *Ophthalmology.* 2003;110(9):1827–1832.

Postoperative Care for Orbital Surgery

Measures used to reduce postoperative edema are elevation of the head, iced compresses on the eyelids, administration of systemic steroids, and placement of a drain (if used, the drain is removed in 24–36 hours). Visual acuity should be checked at frequent intervals in the first 12 hours after surgery. Systemic antibiotics may be given. Patching of the operative site should be discouraged because it can delay diagnosis of a postoperative hemorrhage. Ice packs minimize swelling and still allow frequent observation of the operative site and vision monitoring.

Special Surgical Techniques in the Orbit

Fine-needle aspiration biopsy (FNAB) may have value in selected cases of lymphoid lesions, secondary tumors invading the orbit from the sinuses, suspected metastatic tumors, and blind eyes with optic nerve tumors. The technique is not very effective for obtaining tissue from fibrous lesions, from which it is difficult to aspirate cells. Although FNAB has not been considered a good technique for biopsy of lymphoproliferative disorders, it may assist in the diagnosis of selected cases when used with flow cytometry with monoclonal antibodies or polymerase chain reaction analysis. FNAB is performed with a 4-cm 22- or 23-gauge needle attached to a syringe in a pistol-grip syringe holder. The needle is passed through the skin or conjunctiva. If necessary, the needle can be guided into the tumor by ultrasonography or computed tomography. Cells (and occasionally a small block of tissue) are aspirated from the lesion. A skilled cytologist is required to study the specimen. See BCSC Section 4, *Ophthalmic Pathology and Intraocular Tumors,* for further discussion of FNAB.

Masses or traumatic injuries may involve the skull base, including posterior and superior aspects of the orbit. Advanced surgical techniques provide access to these areas via a frontal craniotomy or frontotemporal-orbitozygomatic approach. Such operations often require the combined efforts of the orbital surgeon, neurosurgeon, and otorhinolaryngologist. The neurosurgeon provides orbital access for the oculofacial surgeon by removing the frontal bar and the orbital roof, giving unparalleled access to superior apical lesions. These techniques allow removal of tumors such as meningiomas, fibrous dysplasia, hemangiomas, hemangiopericytomas, schwannomas, and gliomas that might not otherwise be resectable. In addition, the frontotemporal-orbitozygomatic approach provides access to the intracranial optic canal for decompression.

McDermott MW, Durity FA, Rootman J, Woodhurst WB. Combined frontotemporal-orbitozygomatic approach for tumors of the sphenoid wing and orbit. *Neurosurgery.* 1990; 26(1):107–116.

Shrivastava RK, Sen C, Costantino PD, Della Rocca R. Sphenoorbital menigiomas: surgical limitations and lessons learned in their long-term management. *J Neurosurg.* 2005;103(3): 491–497.

Complications of Orbital Surgery

The surgeon can reduce complications from orbital surgery by performing a complete preoperative evaluation with orbital imaging when indicated, choosing the appropriate surgical approach, obtaining adequate exposure, carefully manipulating the tissues, maintaining good hemostasis, and using a team approach when appropriate.

Decreased or lost vision is a serious complication of surgery that may be caused by excessive traction on the globe and optic nerve, contusion of the optic nerve, postoperative infection, or hemorrhage, which leads to increased orbital pressure and consequent ischemic injury to the optic nerve. A patient who has severe orbital pain postoperatively should be evaluated immediately for possible orbital hemorrhage. If this pain is associated with decreased visual acuity, proptosis, ecchymosis, increased intraocular pressure, and an afferent pupillary defect, the surgeon should consider opening the wound to minimize the effects of the compartment syndrome, evacuating any hematoma, and controlling active bleeding.

Hypoesthesia in the distribution of the infraorbital nerve may follow manipulation of the orbital floor after fracture repair or orbital floor decompression. Other complications of decompression such as downward displacement of the globe and postoperative exacerbation of upper eyelid retraction, were discussed previously. Motility disorders may be caused or exacerbated by orbital surgery. Actively inflamed TED may increase the risks of postoperative restrictive myopathy and enlarged muscle displacement in orbital decompression. In tumor resection in the superior orbit, the superior division of the third cranial nerve is especially susceptible to intraoperative injury. The ciliary ganglion is at risk in lateral approaches to the intraconal space. Other complications of orbital surgery include ptosis, neuroparalytic keratopathy, pupillary changes, vitreous hemorrhage, detached retina, hypoesthesia of the forehead, keratitis sicca, cerebrospinal fluid leak, and infection.

Kersten RC, Nerad JA. Orbital surgery. In: Tasman W, Jaeger EA, eds. *Duane's Clinical Ophthalmology.* Philadelphia: Lippincott-Raven; 2005.

Purgason PA, Hornblass A. Complications of surgery for orbital tumors. *Ophthal Plast Reconstr Surg.* 1992;8(2):88–93.

CHAPTER 8

The Anophthalmic Socket

It is occasionally necessary to remove an eye or the contents of an orbit to enhance patient comfort and cosmesis, to protect the vision in the fellow eye, or to safeguard life. With loss of an eye, the patient can suffer depression or a degraded self-image. The ophthalmologist can assist the patient both before and after anophthalmic surgery by providing reassurance and psychological support. Discussions of the procedure, the rehabilitation process, and expected functional changes can help the patient with adjustment. With very few exceptions, the monocular patient may resume the full range of home, vocational, and athletic activities.

When resuming full activity, however, patients should take a cautious approach to allow adjustment to the loss of some depth perception and visual field. This may result in occupational limitations. The ophthalmologist can help safeguard the remaining eye through regular follow-up examinations and the prescription of polycarbonate safety glasses for full-time wear.

The indications for anophthalmic surgery are diverse, and the procedure of choice varies. *Enucleation* involves removal of the entire globe while preserving other orbital tissues. *Evisceration* is the removal of the intraocular contents (lens, uvea, retina, vitreous, and sometimes cornea), leaving the sclera and extraocular muscles intact. *Exenteration* refers to the removal of some or all of the orbital tissues, including the globe. The cosmetic goals in anophthalmic surgery are to minimize any condition that draws attention to the anophthalmia. Surgical efforts to produce orbital and eyelid symmetry and to promote good prosthetic position and motility enhance cosmesis.

Brady FB. *A Singular View: The Art of Seeing With One Eye.* 6th ed. Vienna, VA: Michael O. Hughes; 2004.

Coday MP, Warner MA, Jahrling KV, Rubin PA. Acquired monocular vision: functional consequences from the patient's perspective. *Ophthal Plast Reconstr Surg.* 2002;18(1):56–63.

Enucleation

Enucleation allows for the complete histologic examination of the eye and optic nerve. It reduces the concern that surgery might contribute to the risk of sympathetic ophthalmia in the fellow eye. Enucleation is always the procedure of choice if the nature of the intraocular pathology is unknown or if ocular tumor is suspected.

Enucleation is indicated for primary intraocular malignancies not amenable to alternative modes of therapy such as external-beam irradiation or episcleral plaque brachytherapy. Retinoblastoma and choroidal melanoma are the ocular tumors that most commonly require enucleation. When enucleation is performed for an intraocular tumor, the surgeon must take care to avoid penetrating the globe during surgery and to handle the globe gently to minimize the risk of disseminating tumor cells. In cases of suspected retinoblastoma, the surgeon should obtain a long segment of optic nerve with the enucleation specimen to increase the chance of complete resection of the tumor. A lateral canthotomy or superomedial approach during enucleation surgery may provide the desired surgical exposure.

Blind eyes with opaque media should be suspected of harboring an occult neoplasm unless another cause of ocular disease can be surmised. Although blind or phthisical eyes are not at increased risk for malignancy, a tumor can occasionally be the cause of globe degeneration. Ultrasonography is useful in evaluating these eyes and planning proper management.

In severely traumatized eyes, early enucleation may be considered if the risk of sympathetic ophthalmia and harm to the remaining eye is judged to be greater than the likelihood of recovering useful vision in the traumatized eye. Sympathetic ophthalmia is thought to be a delayed hypersensitivity immune response to the uveal antigens. Enucleation with complete removal of the uveal pigment may be beneficial in preventing a subsequent immune response. The incidence of sympathetic ophthalmia is estimated to be 0.03 in 100,000 per year. The condition has been reported to occur from 9 days to 50 years after corneoscleral perforation. The infrequency of sympathetic ophthalmia, coupled with improved medical therapy for uveitis, has made early enucleation strictly for prophylaxis a debatable practice. (See BCSC Section 9, *Intraocular Inflammation and Uveitis,* Chapter 6, for additional detailed information.)

Painful eyes without useful vision can be managed with enucleation or evisceration. Patients with end-stage neovascular glaucoma, chronic uveitis, or previously traumatized blind eyes can obtain dramatic relief from discomfort and improved cosmesis with either procedure. For debilitated patients unable to undergo surgery and rehabilitation, retrobulbar injection of ethanol may provide adequate pain relief. Retrobulbar injection of chlorpromazine has also been reported to reduce pain. Serious complications of retrobulbar injections of ethanol and chlorpromazine include chronic orbital inflammation, fibrosis, and pain. In nonpainful, disfigured eyes, it is generally advisable to consider a trial of a cosmetic scleral shell at first. If tolerated, scleral shells can give excellent cosmesis and motility.

Galor A, Davis JL, Flynn HW Jr, et al. Sympathetic ophthalmia: incidence of ocular complications and vision loss in the sympathizing eye. *Am J Ophthalmol.* 2009;148(5):704–710.e2.

Guidelines for Enucleation

A functionally and aesthetically acceptable anophthalmic socket must have the following components:

- an orbital implant of sufficient volume centered within the orbit
- a socket lined with conjunctiva or mucous membrane with fornices deep enough to hold a prosthesis

- eyelids with normal appearance and adequate tone to support a prosthesis
- good transmission of motility from the implant to the overlying prosthesis
- a comfortable ocular prosthesis that looks similar to the normal eye

Enucleation can be performed satisfactorily under local or general anesthesia; however, most patients prefer general anesthesia or sedation when an eye is removed.

Enucleation in Childhood

Enucleation in early childhood, as well as congenital anophthalmia or microphthalmia, may lead to underdevelopment of the involved bony orbit with secondary facial asymmetry. Orbital soft-tissue volume is a critical determinant of orbital bone growth. When enucleation is necessary in childhood, a large implant should be used to replace orbital volume. An adult-sized implant should be placed as soon as possible to encourage symmetrical orbital bone growth. Volume loss in the adult anophthalmic socket may be adequately replaced by a 20–22-mm sphere implant. Rarely should an implant smaller than 18 mm be used, even in the very young.

Autogenous dermis-fat grafts are used successfully as anophthalmic implants in children. These grafts may grow along with the expanding orbit. The opposite effect has been observed in adults, in whom a loss of volume generally occurs when dermis-fat grafts are used as primary anophthalmic implants.

Heher KL, Katowitz JA, Low JE. Unilateral dermis-fat graft implantation in the pediatric orbit. *Ophthal Plast Reconstr Surg.* 1998;14(2):81–88.

Intraoperative Complications of Enucleation

Removal of the wrong eye

This is one of the most feared complications in ophthalmology. Taking a "time out" to reexamine the chart, the operative permit, and the patient with ophthalmoscopy in the operating room immediately before enucleation is of critical importance. Marking the skin near the eye to be enucleated and having the patient and family point to the involved eye give further assurance.

Recommendations of American Academy of Ophthalmology Wrong-Site Task Force. November 2008. Available at: http://one.aao.org/CE/PracticeGuidelines/Patient_Content.aspx?cid=d0db838c-2847-4535-baca-aebab3011217. Accessed July 1, 2010.

Ptosis and extraocular muscle damage

Avoiding excessive dissection, especially near the orbital roof and apex, reduces the chance of damaging the extraocular muscles, the levator muscle, or their innervation.

Evisceration

Evisceration involves the removal of the contents of the globe, leaving the sclera, extraocular muscles, and optic nerve intact. Evisceration should be considered *only* if the presence of an intraocular malignancy has been ruled out.

Advantages of Evisceration

- *Less disruption of orbital anatomy.* Thus, the chance of injury to extraocular muscles and nerves and atrophy of fat is reduced with less dissection within the orbit. The relationships between the muscles, globe, eyelids, and fornices remain undisturbed.
- *Good motility of the prosthesis.* The extraocular muscles remain attached to the sclera.
- *Treatment of endophthalmitis.* Evisceration is preferred by some surgeons in cases of endophthalmitis because extirpation and drainage of the ocular contents can occur without invasion of the orbit. The chance of contamination of the orbit with possible subsequent orbital cellulitis or intracranial extension is therefore theoretically reduced.
- *A technically simpler procedure.* Performing this less invasive procedure may be important when general anesthesia is contraindicated or when bleeding disorders increase the risk of orbital dissection.
- *Lower rate of migration, extrusion, and reoperation.*

Disadvantages of Evisceration

- *Not every patient is a candidate.* Evisceration should never be performed if an ocular tumor is suspected. Severe phthisis bulbi is a contraindication to evisceration.
- *Theoretical increased risk of sympathetic ophthalmia.* Initial report of 4 cases more than 25 years ago has not been subsequently confirmed by additional case reports.
- *Evisceration affords a less complete specimen for pathologic examinations.*

Levine MR, Pou CR, Lash RH. Evisceration: is sympathetic ophthalmia a concern in the new millennium? The 1998 Wendell Hughes Lecture. *Ophthal Plast Reconstr Surg.* 1999;15(1):4–8.

Techniques of Evisceration

Evisceration can be performed with either retention or excision of the cornea. The cornea can be retained if it is of normal thickness and shows no active corneal disease. The corneal epithelium and endothelium should be removed at the time of surgery. If there is mild thinning of the cornea, a bridge flap of conjunctiva and Tenon capsule can be brought down from the bulbar area just above the cornea and sutured over the cornea. This technique has the advantage of allowing placement of a larger implant, thus enhancing orbital volume. The disadvantage is that the cornea may erode eventually, with possible extrusion of the implant. Regardless of the technique used for evisceration, all visible pigmented uvea should be removed before the implant is placed.

If there is active disease in the cornea, the cornea should be excised and the implant sutured within the sclera. Posterior relaxing incisions of the sclera (radially in each quadrant or concentric to the optic nerve) may be used to allow placement of a larger implant.

Lucarelli MJ, Kaltreider SA. Advances in evisceration and enucleation. *Focal Points: Clinical Modules for Ophthalmologists.* San Francisco: American Academy of Ophthalmology; 2004, module 6.

Massry GG, Holds JB. Evisceration with scleral modification. *Ophthal Plast Reconstr Surg.* 2001;1(1)7:42–47.

Orbital Implants

The implant's function is to replace lost orbital volume, maintain the structure of the orbit, and impart motility to the overlying ocular prosthesis. Modern implants are usually either spheres or buried implants with anterior surface projections to which the extraocular muscles can be attached. Spherical implants may be grouped according to the materials from which they are manufactured: *inert materials,* such as glass, silicone, or methylmethacrylate; and *biointegrated materials,* such as hydroxyapatite or porous polyethylene (Fig 8-1). The latter are designed to be incorporated by soft-tissue ingrowth into the socket.

Inert spherical implants provide comfort and low rates of extrusion. They are considered an appropriate cost-effective choice in patients not requiring implant integration. Disadvantages of nonporous implants include decreased motility and implant migration. Inert implants transfer motility to the prosthesis only through passive movement of the socket. Buried motility implants with anterior surface projections push the overlying prosthesis with direct force and can improve prosthetic motility. The anterior surface projections, however, may pinch the conjunctiva between the implant and the prosthesis, leading to a painful socket or implant erosion.

Hydroxyapatite and porous polyethylene implants allow for drilling and placement of a peg to integrate the prosthesis directly with the moving implant. Pegging is usually carried out 6–12 months after enucleation. Although pegged porous implants offer excellent motility, they also have a higher rate of postoperative complications, including inflammation and exposure. It should be noted that the majority of porous implants are never pegged and are able to achieve adequate motility.

Locations for implants are either within the Tenon capsule or behind the posterior Tenon capsule in the muscle cone. Spheres may be covered with other materials such as sclera (homologous or cadaveric) or autogenous fascia, which serve as further barriers to migration and extrusion. Secure closure of Tenon fascia over the anterior surface of an anophthalmic implant is an important barrier to later extrusion.

Extraocular muscles should not be crossed over the front surface of a sphere implant or purse-stringed anteriorly because the implant migrates when the muscles slip off the anterior surface. Muscles sutured into the normal anatomical locations, either directly to the implant or to sclera or autogenous fascia surrounding the implant, allow superior motility and prevent migration.

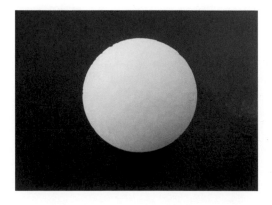

Figure 8-1 Porous polyethylene orbital implant. *(Courtesy of Vikram D. Durairaj, MD.)*

Following enucleation surgery, an acrylic or silicone conformer is placed in the conjunctival fornices to maintain the conjunctival space that will eventually accommodate the prosthesis.

Prostheses

An ocular prosthesis is fitted within 4–8 weeks after enucleation or evisceration. The ideal prosthesis is custom fitted to the exact dimensions of the orbit after postoperative edema has subsided. Premade or stock eyes are less satisfactory cosmetically, and they limit prosthetic motility. In addition, they may trap secretions between the prosthesis and the socket.

The American Society of Ocularists is an international nonprofit professional and educational organization founded by technicians specializing in the fabrication and fitting of custom ocular prosthetics.

Custer PL, Kennedy RH, Woog JJ, Kaltreider SA, Meyer DR. Orbital implants in enucleation surgery: a report by the American Academy of Ophthalmology. *Ophthalmology.* 2003;110(10):2054–2061.

Custer PL, Trinkaus KM, Fornoff J. Comparative motility of hydroxyapatite and alloplastic enucleation implants. *Ophthalmology.* 1999;106(3):513–516.

Edelstein C, Shields CL, De Potter P, Shields JA. Complications of motility peg placement for the hydroxyapatite orbital implant. *Ophthalmology.* 1997;104(10):1616–1621.

Anophthalmic Socket Complications and Treatment

Deep Superior Sulcus

Deep superior sulcus deformity is caused by decreased orbital volume (Fig 8-2). The surgeon can correct this deformity by increasing the orbital volume through placement of a subperiosteal secondary implant on the orbital floor. This implant pushes the initial implant and superior orbital fat upward to fill out the superior sulcus. Dermis-fat grafts may be implanted in the upper eyelid to fill out the sulcus, but eyelid contour and function may be damaged and the graft may undergo resorption. Superior sulcus deformity can also be corrected with replacement of the original implant with a larger secondary implant. Alternatively, modification of the ocular prosthesis may be used to correct a deep superior sulcus.

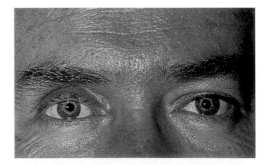

Figure 8-2 Superior sulcus deformity following enucleation of right eye.

Contracture of Fornices

Preventing contracted fornices includes preserving as much conjunctiva as possible and limiting dissection in the fornices. Placing extraocular muscles in their normal anatomical positions also minimizes shortening of the fornices. It is recommended that the patient wear a conformer as much as possible postoperatively to minimize conjunctival shortening. Conformers and prostheses should not be removed for periods greater than 24 hours. The prosthesis can be removed frequently and cleaned in the presence of infection but should be replaced promptly after irrigation of the socket.

Exposure and Extrusion of Implant

Implants may extrude if placed too far forward or if closure of anterior Tenon fascia is not satisfactory. Postoperative infection, poor wound healing, poorly fitting prostheses or conformers, and pressure points between the implant and prosthesis may also contribute to extrusion of the implant. Exposed implants are subject to infection. Although small defects over porous implants may rarely close spontaneously, most exposures should be covered with scleral patch grafts or autogenous tissue grafts to promote conjunctival healing (Fig 8-3).

A dermis-fat graft may be used when a limited amount of conjunctiva remains in the socket. This graft increases the net amount of conjunctiva available as the conjunctiva reepithelializes over the front surface of the dermis. Unpredictable fat resorption is a serious drawback to the dermis-fat graft technique in adults. However, as stated earlier, dermis-fat grafts in children appear to continue to grow along with the surrounding orbit and may help stimulate orbital development if enucleation is required during infancy or childhood.

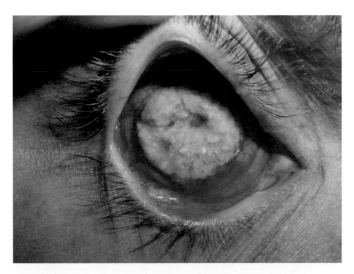

Figure 8-3 Large exposure of the porous polyethylene orbital implant in a patient who had undergone evisceration for trauma. *(Courtesy of Martín Devoto, MD.)*

Contracted Sockets

Causes of contracted sockets include

- radiation treatment (usually as treatment of the tumor that necessitated removal of the eye)
- extrusion of an enucleation implant
- severe initial injury (alkali burns or extensive lacerations)
- poor surgical techniques (excessive sacrifice or destruction of conjunctiva and Tenon capsule; traumatic dissection within the socket causing excessive scar tissue formation)
- multiple socket operations
- removal of the conformer or prosthesis for prolonged periods

Sockets are considered to be contracted when the fornices are too small to retain a prosthesis (Fig 8-4). Socket reconstruction procedures involve incision or excision of the scarred tissues and placement of a graft to enlarge the fornices. Full-thickness mucous membrane grafting is preferred because it allows the grafted tissue to match conjunctiva histologically. Buccal mucosal grafts may be taken from the cheeks (beware of damaging the duct to the parotid gland) or from the upper lip, lower lip, or hard palate. Goblet cells and mucus production are preserved.

Contracture of the fornices alone (more common with the inferior fornix) usually is associated with milder degrees of socket contracture. In these cases, the buccal mucosal graft is placed in the defect, and a silicone sheet is attached by sutures to the superior or inferior orbital rim, depending on which fornix is involved. In 2 weeks, the sheet may be removed and a prosthesis placed.

Anophthalmic Ectropion

Lower eyelid ectropion may result from the loosening of lower eyelid support under the weight of a prosthesis. Frequent removal of the prosthesis or use of a larger prosthesis

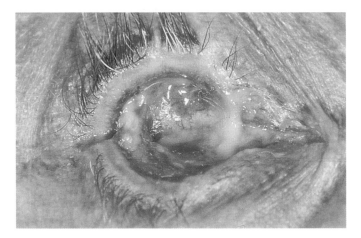

Figure 8-4 Socket contraction of right anophthalmic orbit. Note obliteration of conjunctival fornices. Patient is unable to wear an ocular prosthesis.

accelerates the development of lid laxity. Tightening the lateral or medial canthal tendon may remedy the situation. Surgeons may combine ectropion repair with correction of eyelid retraction by recessing the inferior retractor muscle layer and grafting mucous membrane tissue in the inferior fornix.

Anophthalmic Ptosis

Ptosis of the anophthalmic socket results from superotemporal migration of sphere implants, cicatricial tissue in the upper fornix, or damage to the levator muscle or nerve. Small amounts of ptosis may be managed by modification of the prosthesis. Greater amounts of ptosis require tightening of the levator aponeurosis. This procedure is best done under local anesthesia with intraoperative adjustment of eyelid height and contour because mechanical forces may cause the surgeon to underestimate true levator function. Ptosis surgery usually improves a deep sulcus by bringing the preaponeurotic fat forward. Mild ptosis may be corrected with conjunctiva/Müller muscle resection. Frontalis suspension is usually a less acceptable procedure because there is no visual drive to stimulate contracture of the frontalis muscle to elevate the eyelid.

Lash Margin Entropion

Lash margin entropion, trichiasis, and ptosis of the eyelashes are common in the anophthalmic socket. Contracture of fornices or cicatricial tissue near the lash margin contributes to these abnormalities. Horizontal tarsal incisions and rotation of the lash margin may correct the problem. In more severe cases, splitting of the eyelid margins at the gray line with mucous membrane grafting to the eyelid margin may correct the entropic lash margin.

Cosmetic Optics

The style of frames and tinted lenses chosen for spectacles can help camouflage residual defects in reconstructed sockets. Plus (convex) lenses or minus (concave) lenses may be placed in the glasses in front of the prosthesis to alter the apparent size of the prosthesis. Prisms in the glasses may be used to change the apparent vertical position of the prosthesis.

Kaltreider SA, Lucarelli MJ. A simple algorithm for selection of implant size for enucleation and evisceration: a prospective study. *Ophthal Plast Reconstr Surg.* 2002;18(5):336–341.

Neuhaus R, Hawes MJ. Inadequate inferior cul-de-sac in the anophthalmic socket. *Ophthalmology.* 1992;99(1):153–157.

Smit TJ, Koornneef L, Zonneveld FW, Groet E, Otto AJ. Computed tomography in the assessment of the postenucleation socket syndrome. *Ophthalmology.* 1990;97(10):1347–1351.

Smit TJ, Koornneef L, Zonneveld FW, Groet E, Otto AJ. Primary and secondary implants in the anophthalmic orbit: preoperative and postoperative computed tomographic appearance. *Ophthalmology.* 1991;98(1):106–110.

Exenteration

Exenteration involves the removal of the soft tissues of the orbit, including the globe.

Considerations for Exenteration

Exenteration should be considered in the following circumstances:

- *Destructive tumors extending into the orbit from the sinuses, face, eyelids, conjunctiva, or intracranial space* (Fig 8-5). However, exenteration is not indicated for all such tumors: some are responsive to radiation, and some have extended too far to be completely removed by surgical excision.
- *Intraocular melanomas or retinoblastomas that have extended outside the globe (if evidence of distant metastases is excluded).* When local control of the tumor would benefit the nursing care of the patient, exenteration is indicated.
- *Malignant epithelial tumors of the lacrimal gland.* Although the procedure is somewhat controversial, these tumors may require extended exenteration with radical bone removal of the roof, lateral wall, and floor.
- *Sarcomas and other primary orbital malignancies that do not respond to nonsurgical therapy.* Some tumors such as rhabdomyosarcomas that were previously treated by exenteration are now initially treated by radiation and chemotherapy.
- *Fungal infection.* Subtotal or total exenteration may be necessary for the management of orbital zygomycosis, which occurs most commonly in patients who are diabetic or immunosuppressed. However, attention is now being focused on achieving control through more limited debridement of involved orbital tissues.

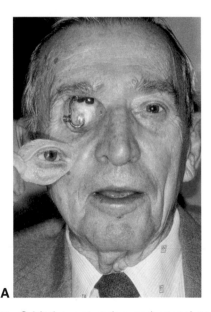
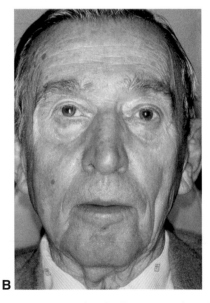

A   B

Figure 8-5 Orbital exenteration and osseointegrated prosthesis. **A,** Exenterated socket for sebaceous cell carcinoma. **B,** Prosthesis in place, retained with magnets attached to bone-anchored framework. *(Courtesy of Jeffrey A. Nerad, MD.)*

Types of Exenteration

Exenterations vary in the amount of tissue that is removed. Following are the types of exenteration:

- *Subtotal.* The eye and adjacent intraorbital tissues are removed such that the lesion is locally excised (leaving the periorbita and part or all of the eyelids). This technique is used for some locally invasive tumors, for debulking of disseminated tumors, or for partial treatment in selected patients.
- *Total.* All intraorbital soft tissues, including periorbita, are removed, with or without the skin of the eyelids.
- *Extended.* All intraorbital soft tissues are removed, together with adjacent structures (usually bony walls and sinuses).

The technique selected depends on the pathologic process. The goal is to remove all lesions along with appropriate margins of adjacent tissue while retaining as much healthy tissue as possible. Following removal of the orbital contents, the bony socket may be allowed to spontaneously granulate and epithelialize or may be covered by a split-thickness skin graft, which may be placed onto bare bone or over a temporalis muscle or temporoparietal fascial flap.

Bartley GB, Garrity JA, Waller RR, Henderson JW, Ilstrup DM. Orbital exenteration at the Mayo Clinic: 1967–1986. *Ophthalmology.* 1989;96(4):468–474.

Goldberg RA, Kim JW, Shorr N. Orbital exenteration: results of an individualized approach. *Ophthal Plast Reconstr Surg.* 2003;19(3):229–236.

Levin PS, Dutton JJ. A 20-year series of orbital exenteration. *Am J Ophthalmol.* 1991;112(5): 496–501.

Yeatts RP, Marion JR, Weaver RG, Orkubi GA. Removal of the eye with socket ablation: a limited subtotal exenteration. *Arch Ophthalmol.* 1991;109(9):1306–1309.

PART II

Periocular Soft Tissues

CHAPTER 9

Facial and Eyelid Anatomy

Face

The surgeon who undertakes surgical manipulation of the face should understand its anatomy. The structural planes of the face include skin; subcutaneous tissue; the *superficial musculoaponeurotic system (SMAS)* and mimetic muscles; the deep facial fascia; and the plane containing the facial nerve, parotid duct, and buccal fat pad.

The superficial facial fascia, an extension of the superficial cervical fascia in the neck, invests the facial mimetic muscles (platysma, zygomaticus major, zygomaticus minor, and orbicularis oculi), making up the SMAS (Fig 9-1). The SMAS distributes facial muscle contractions, facilitating facial expression. These muscle actions are transmitted to the skin by ligamentous attachments located between the SMAS and the dermis. The SMAS is also connected to the underlying bone by a network of fibrous septa and ligaments. Thus, facial support is transmitted from the deep fixed structures of the face to the overlying dermis. Two major components of this system are the osteocutaneous ligaments (orbito-malar, zygomatic, and mandibular) and the ligaments formed by a condensation of superficial and deep facial fasciae (parotidocutaneous and masseteric). As these ligaments become attenuated in conjunction with facial dermal elastosis, facial aging becomes apparent. Dissection and repositioning of the SMAS have important implications for facial cosmetic surgery.

As the SMAS continues superiorly over the zygomatic arch, it becomes continuous with the *temporoparietal fascia* (also called the *superficial temporal fascia*); more superiorly, the SMAS becomes continuous with the galea aponeurotica. Interior to the loose areolar tissue and the temporoparietal fascia, the deep temporal fascia of the temporal muscle splits and envelops the temporal fat pad, creating deep and superficial layers of the deep temporal fascia (see Fig 9-1B).

The mimetic muscles (Fig 9-2) can be grouped into those of the upper face and those of the lower face. In the upper face, the frontalis, corrugator, and procerus muscles animate the forehead and glabella. The orbicularis oculi depresses the eyebrows and closes the eyelids. The frontalis elevates the eyebrows, and contraction of the muscle causes transverse forehead rhytids.

In the lower face, mimetic muscles can be further categorized as superficial or deep. The *superficial mimetic muscles,* which receive their neurovascular supply on the posterior surfaces, include the platysma, zygomaticus major, zygomaticus minor, and risorius. The *deep mimetic muscles* receive their neurovascular supply anteriorly and include the

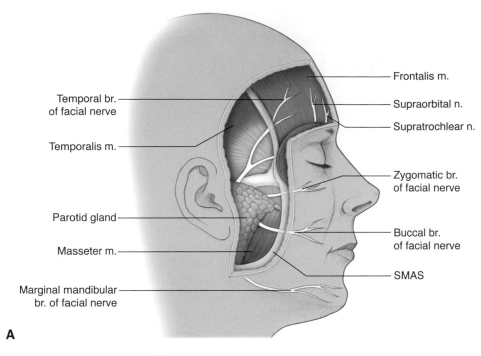

Frontalis m.

Temporal br.
of facial nerve

Supraorbital n.

Supratrochlear n.

Temporalis m.

Zygomatic br.
of facial nerve

Parotid gland

Buccal br.
of facial nerve

Masseter m.

SMAS

Marginal mandibular
br. of facial nerve

A

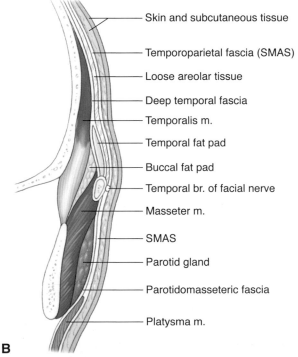

Skin and subcutaneous tissue

Temporoparietal fascia (SMAS)

Loose areolar tissue

Deep temporal fascia

Temporalis m.

Temporal fat pad

Buccal fat pad

Temporal br. of facial nerve

Masseter m.

SMAS

Parotid gland

Parotidomasseteric fascia

Platysma m.

B

Figure 9-1 **A,** Superficial musculoaponeurotic system (SMAS). Note that the facial nerve branches inferior to the zygomatic arch are deep to the SMAS. **B,** Coronal section of face. The temporal branch of the facial nerve is found within the superficial portion of the temporoparietal fascia (extension of the SMAS). *(Illustration by Christine Gralapp.)*

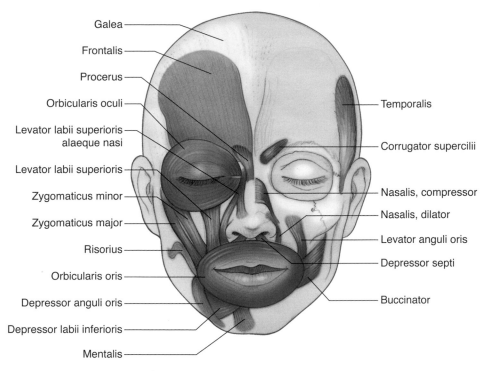

Galea
Frontalis
Procerus
Orbicularis oculi
Levator labii superioris alaeque nasi
Levator labii superioris
Zygomaticus minor
Zygomaticus major
Risorius
Orbicularis oris
Depressor anguli oris
Depressor labii inferioris
Mentalis

Temporalis
Corrugator supercilii
Nasalis, compressor
Nasalis, dilator
Levator anguli oris
Depressor septi
Buccinator

Figure 9-2 Facial mimetic muscles. *(Illustration by Christine Gralapp.)*

buccinator, mentalis, and levator anguli oris. Other facial muscles include the orbicularis oris, the levator labii superioris, the levator labii superioris alaeque nasi, the depressor anguli oris and the depressor labii inferioris, the masseter, and the temporalis.

In the neck, the superficial cervical fascia and platysma are continuous with the SMAS, and the deep cervical fascia is found on the superficial surface of the strap muscles, superior to the hyoid bone. The deep cervical fascia overlies the myelohyoid muscle and extends superiorly over the body of the mandible. The parotidomasseteric fascia is a continuation of the deep cervical fascia of the neck. The facial nerve lies deep to this thin layer in the lower face. In the temporal region, above the zygomatic arch, this layer is continuous with the deep temporal fascia, and the facial nerve (frontal branch) lies superficial to this fascial layer.

The facial nerve, cranial nerve VII (CN VII), which innervates the mimetic muscles, divides into 5 major branches within or deep to the parotid gland (Fig 9-3): temporal (frontal), zygomatic, buccal, marginal mandibular, and cervical. Landmarks identifying the depth of the nerve have special significance. In general, dissection deep to the SMAS and deep to CN VII (on top of the deep temporalis fascia) in the upper face and temporal region avoids the frontal nerve, whereas dissection superficial to the SMAS and superficial to the plane of the facial nerve (especially anterior to the parotid gland) avoids the facial nerve branches in the lower face.

In the temporal area, the frontal branch of CN VII (see Fig 9-3) crosses the zygomatic arch and courses superomedially in the deep layers of the temporoparietal fascia. The temporoparietal fascia bridges the SMAS of the lower face to the galea aponeurosis of the

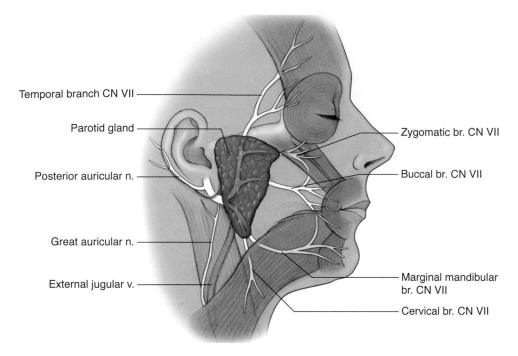

Figure 9-3 Five major branches of the facial nerve. *(Illustration by Christine Gralapp.)*

upper face. Deep to the temporoparietal fascia, a dense, immobile fascia called the *deep temporal fascia* overlies the temporalis muscle (see Fig 9-1B). Dissection along this fascia allows mobilization of the temporal forehead while avoiding the overlying frontal branch of the facial nerve. This is an important anatomical principle in brow- and forehead-lifting procedures.

In the lower face, the facial nerve branches, sensory nerves, vascular networks, and parotid gland and duct are deep to the SMAS (see Fig 9-1). Dissection just superficial to the SMAS, parotid gland, and parotidomasseteric fascia in the lower face avoids injury to these structures.

The face receives its sensory innervation from the 3 branches of CN V: V_1, ophthalmic; V_2, maxillary; and V_3, mandibular. Damage to these nerves causes numbness and paresthesia. Fortunately, overlapping of the distal branches makes permanent sensation loss unusual unless injury occurs at the proximal neurovascular bundles or with extensive distal disruption, as can be seen with a bicoronal incision.

Eyelids

For discussion purposes, the eyelids can be conveniently divided into the following 7 structural layers:

- skin and subcutaneous tissue
- muscles of protraction

- orbital septum
- orbital fat
- muscles of retraction
- tarsus
- conjunctiva

Figures 9-4 through 9-8 detail the anatomy of the eyelids.

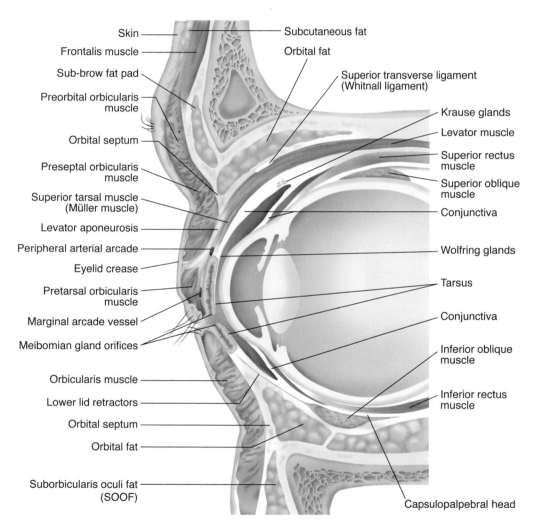

Figure 9-4 Upper and lower eyelid anatomy. *(Modified from Stewart WB*. Surgery of the Eyelid, Orbit, and Lacrimal System. *Ophthalmology Monograph 8, vol 2. San Francisco: American Academy of Ophthalmology; 1994:23, 85. Illustration by Cyndie C. H. Wooley.)*

Skin and Subcutaneous Tissue

Eyelid skin is the thinnest of the body and is unique in having no subcutaneous fat layer. Because the thin skin of the eyelids is subjected to constant movement with each blink, the laxity that often occurs with age is not surprising. In both the upper and the lower eyelids, the pretarsal tissues are normally firmly attached to the underlying tissues, whereas the preseptal tissues are more loosely attached, creating potential spaces for fluid accumulation. The contours of the eyelid skin are defined by the *eyelid crease* and the *eyelid fold*. The upper eyelid crease approximates the attachments of the levator aponeurosis to the pretarsal orbicularis bundles and skin. This site is near or at the level of the superior border of the tarsus. The upper eyelid fold consists of the loose preseptal skin and subcutaneous tissues above the confluence of the levator aponeurosis and the septum.

Racial variation can be noted in the location of the eyelid crease and eyelid fold. The Asian eyelid normally has a relatively low upper lid crease because, in contrast to the supratarsal fusion, the orbital septum in the Asian eyelid fuses with the levator aponeurosis between the eyelid margin and the superior border of the tarsus. This also allows preaponeurotic fat to occupy a position more inferior and anterior in the eyelid. Although the lower eyelid crease is less well defined than the upper eyelid crease, these racial differences are apparent in the lower eyelid as well.

Protractors

The orbicularis oculi muscle is the main protractor of the eyelid. Contraction of this muscle, which is innervated by CN VII, narrows the palpebral fissure. Specific portions of this muscle also constitute the lacrimal pump.

The orbicularis muscle is divided into *pretarsal, preseptal,* and *orbital* parts (see Fig 9-5). The palpebral (pretarsal and preseptal) parts are integral to involuntary eyelid movements (blinking), whereas the orbital portion is primarily involved in forced eyelid closure. The pretarsal parts of the upper and lower eyelid orbicularis arise from deep origins at the posterior lacrimal crest and superficial origins at the anterior limb of the medial canthal tendon. Near the common canaliculus, the deep heads of the pretarsal orbicularis fuse to form a prominent bundle of fibers known as the *Horner muscle,* which runs just behind the posterior arm of the canthal tendon. The Horner muscle continues posteriorly to the posterior lacrimal crest, just behind the posterior arm of the medial canthal tendon. The upper and lower eyelid segments of the pretarsal orbicularis fuse in the lateral canthal area to become the lateral canthal tendon.

The preseptal orbicularis arises from the upper and lower borders of the medial canthal tendon. The inferior preseptal muscle arises as a single head from the common tendon. In the upper eyelid, the preseptal muscle has an anterior head from the common tendon and a posterior head from both the superior and posterior arms of the tendon. Laterally, the preseptal muscles form the lateral palpebral raphe.

The orbital portions of the orbicularis muscle arise from the anterior limb of the medial canthal tendon, the orbital process of the frontal bone, and the frontal process of the maxillary bone in front of the anterior lacrimal crest. Its fibers form a continuous ellipse

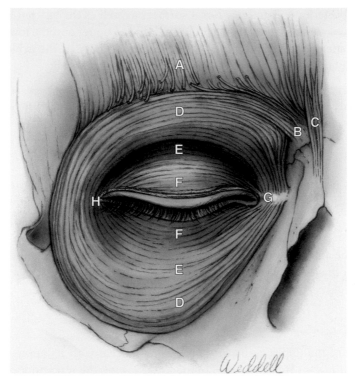

Figure 9-5 Orbicularis muscle and related musculature. *A,* Frontalis muscles; *B,* corrugator supercilii muscle; *C,* procerus muscle; *D,* orbicularis muscle (orbital portion); *E,* orbicularis muscle (preseptal portion); *F,* orbicularis muscle (pretarsal portion); *G,* medial canthal tendon; *H,* lateral canthal tendon. *(Adapted from Beard C. Ptosis. 3rd ed. St Louis: Mosby; 1981. Used with permission. Modified by Cyndie C. H. Wooley.)*

and insert just below the point of origin. Near the eyelid margin, a specialized bundle of striated muscle, the *muscle of Riolan,* lies more posterior than the main portion of the orbicularis and creates the gray line (see Fig 9-8). The muscle of Riolan may play a role in meibomian glandular discharge, blinking, and the position of the eyelashes.

Dutton JJ. *Atlas of Clinical and Surgical Orbital Anatomy.* Philadelphia: Saunders; 1994.

Muzaffar AR, Mendelson BC, Adams WP Jr. Surgical anatomy of the ligamentous attachments of the lower lid and lateral canthus. *Plast Reconstr Surg.* 2002;110(3):873–884; discussion 897–911.

Orbital Septum

The orbital septum, a thin, multilayered sheet of fibrous tissue, arises from the periosteum over the superior and inferior orbital rims at the arcus marginalis. In the upper eyelid, the orbital septum fuses with the levator aponeurosis 2–5 mm above the superior tarsal border in non-Asians. In the lower eyelid, the orbital septum fuses with the capsulopalpebral fascia at or just below the inferior tarsal border. The fused capsulopalpebral orbital septum complex, along with a small contribution from the inferior tarsal smooth muscle, inserts on the posterior and anterior tarsal surfaces as well as the tapered inferior border of the tarsus. As a result of aging, the septum in both the upper and the lower eyelids may become quite attenuated. Thinning of the septum and laxity of the orbicularis muscle contribute to anterior herniation of the orbital fat in the aging eyelid.

Meyer DR, Linberg JV, Wobig JL, McCormick SA. Anatomy of the orbital septum and associated eyelid connective tissues. Implications for ptosis surgery. *Ophthal Plast Reconstr Surg.* 1991;7(2):104–113.

Orbital Fat

Orbital fat lies posterior to the orbital septum and anterior to the levator aponeurosis (upper lid) or the capsulopalpebral fascia (lower lid). In the upper eyelid, there are 2 fat pockets: nasal and central. In the lower eyelid, there are 3 fat pockets: nasal, central, and temporal. These pockets are surrounded by thin fibrous sheaths that are forward continuations of the anterior orbitoseptal system. The central orbital fat pad is an important landmark in both elective eyelid surgery and lid laceration repair because it lies directly behind the orbital septum and in front of the levator aponeurosis.

Retractors

The retractors of the upper eyelid are the levator muscle with its aponeurosis and the superior tarsal muscle *(Müller muscle)*. In the lower eyelid, the retractors are the capsulopalpebral fascia and the inferior tarsal muscle.

Upper eyelid retractors

The levator muscle originates in the apex of the orbit, arising from the periorbita of the lesser wing of the sphenoid, just above the annulus of Zinn. The muscular portion of the levator is approximately 40 mm long; the aponeurosis is 14–20 mm in length. The superior transverse ligament *(Whitnall ligament)* is a sleeve of elastic fibers around the levator muscle located in the area of transition from levator muscle to levator aponeurosis (see Fig 9-6).

The Whitnall ligament functions primarily as a suspensory support for the upper eyelid and the superior orbital tissues. The ligament also acts as a fulcrum for the levator, transferring its vector force from an anterior–posterior to a superior–inferior direction. Its analogue in the lower eyelid is the *Lockwood ligament.* Medially, the Whitnall ligament attaches to connective tissue around the trochlea and superior oblique tendon. Laterally, it forms septa through the stroma of the lacrimal gland, then arches upward to attach to the inner aspect of the lateral orbital wall approximately 10 mm above the lateral orbital tubercle, with a small group of fibers extending inferiorly to insert onto the lateral retinaculum. The Whitnall ligament has sometimes been confused with the horns of the levator aponeurosis. However, the horns of the levator aponeurosis lie more inferior and toward the canthi. The lateral horn inserts onto the lateral orbital tubercle; the medial horn inserts onto the posterior lacrimal crest. The lateral horn of the levator aponeurosis is strong, and it divides the lacrimal gland into orbital and palpebral lobes, attaching firmly to the orbital tubercle. The medial horn of the aponeurosis is more delicate and

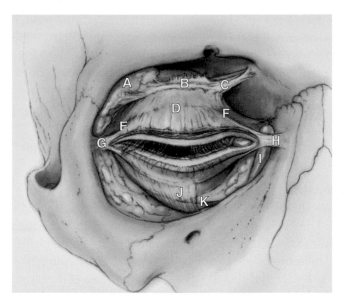

Figure 9-6 Deeper eyelid and anterior orbital structures from anterior view. *A,* Lacrimal gland; *B,* superior transverse ligament (Whitnall ligament); *C,* superior oblique tendon sheath; *D,* levator aponeurosis; *E,* lateral horn; *F,* medial horn; *G,* lateral canthal tendon; *H,* medial canthal tendon; *I,* lacrimal sac; *J,* lower eyelid retractors; *K,* inferior oblique muscle. *(Adapted from Beard C. Ptosis. 3rd ed. St Louis: Mosby; 1981. Used with permission. Modified by Cyndie C. H. Wooley.)*

forms loose connective attachments to the posterior aspect of the medial canthal tendon and to the posterior lacrimal crest.

As the levator aponeurosis continues toward the tarsus, it divides into an anterior and posterior portion a variable distance above the superior tarsal border. The anterior portion is composed of fine strands of aponeurosis that insert into the septa between the pretarsal orbicularis muscle bundles and skin. These fine attachments are responsible for the close apposition of the pretarsal skin and orbicularis muscle to the underlying tarsus. The upper eyelid crease is formed by the most superior of these attachments and by contraction of the underlying levator complex. The upper eyelid fold is created by the overhanging skin, fat, and orbicularis muscle superior to the crease.

The levator muscle is innervated by the superior division of CN III, which also supplies the superior rectus muscle. A superior division palsy, resulting in ptosis and decreased upgaze, implies an intraorbital disruption of CN III.

The posterior portion of the levator aponeurosis inserts firmly onto the anterior surface of the lower half of the tarsus. It is most firmly attached approximately 3 mm above the eyelid margin and is only very loosely attached to the superior 2–3 mm of the tarsus. Disinsertion, dehiscence, or rarefaction of the aponeurosis following ocular surgery or due to intraocular inflammation, eyelid trauma, or senescence may give rise to ptosis.

The Müller muscle originates in the undersurface of the levator aponeurosis approximately at the level of the Whitnall ligament, 12–14 mm above the upper tarsal margin. This sympathetically innervated smooth muscle extends inferiorly to insert along the upper eyelid superior tarsal margin. This muscle provides approximately 2 mm of elevation of the upper eyelid; if it is interrupted (as in Horner syndrome), mild ptosis results. The Müller muscle is firmly attached to the adjacent conjunctiva posteriorly, especially just above the superior tarsal border. The peripheral arterial arcade is found between the levator aponeurosis and the Müller muscle, just above the superior tarsal border. This vascular arcade serves as a useful surgical landmark to identify the Müller muscle.

Codère F, Tucker NA, Renaldi B. The anatomy of Whitnall ligament. *Ophthalmology.* 1995; 102(12):2016–2019.

Stasior GO, Lemke BN, Wallow IH, Dortzbach RK. Levator aponeurosis elastic fiber network. *Ophthal Plast Reconstr Surg.* 1993;9(1):1–10.

Lower eyelid retractors

The capsulopalpebral fascia in the lower eyelid is analogous to the levator aponeurosis in the upper eyelid. The fascia originates as the capsulopalpebral head from attachments to the terminal muscle fibers of the inferior rectus muscle. The capsulopalpebral head divides as it encircles the inferior oblique muscle and fuses with the sheath of the inferior oblique muscle. Anterior to the inferior oblique muscle, the 2 portions of the capsulopalpebral head join to form the Lockwood suspensory ligament. The capsulopalpebral fascia extends anteriorly from this point, sending strands to the inferior conjunctival fornix. The capsulopalpebral fascia inserts onto the inferior tarsal border, just after it fuses with the orbital septum.

The inferior tarsal muscle in the lower eyelid is analogous to the Müller muscle. The poorly developed inferior tarsal muscle runs posterior to the capsulopalpebral fascia. The smooth muscle fibers are most abundant in the area of the inferior fornix.

Tarsus

The tarsi are firm, dense plates of connective tissue that serve as the structural support of the eyelids (see Fig 9-7). The upper eyelid tarsal plates measure 10–12 mm vertically in

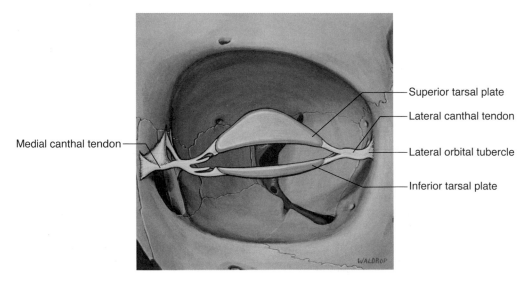

Figure 9-7 Eyelids, deep dissection of structural elements. *(Reproduced with permission from Dutton JJ. Atlas of Clinical and Surgical Orbital Anatomy. Philadelphia: Saunders; 1994:126.)*

the center of the eyelid; the maximum lower eyelid tarsal plate measurement is 4 mm. The tarsal plates have rigid attachments to the periosteum through the canthal tendons medially and laterally. The tarsal plates may become horizontally displaced with age as a result of stretching of the medial and lateral supporting tendons. Both tarsal plates are usually 1 mm thick and taper at the medial and lateral ends as they approach the canthal tendons. Located within the tarsus, the meibomian glands are holocrine sebaceous glands.

Conjunctiva

The conjunctiva is composed of nonkeratinizing squamous epithelium. It forms the posterior layer of the eyelids and contains the mucin-secreting goblet cells and the accessory lacrimal glands of Wolfring and Krause. The accessory lacrimal glands are found in the subconjunctival tissue mainly in the upper and lower eyelids. The glands of Wolfring are found primarily along the nonmarginal tarsal borders, and the glands of Krause are found in the fornices.

Additional Anatomical Considerations

Connective tissue

Suborbicularis fat pads Deep to the orbicularis muscle overlying the maxillary and zygomatic periosteum is a plane of nonseptate fat called the *suborbicularis oculi fat (SOOF)*. This fat is analogous to the superiorly located *retro-orbicularis oculi fat (ROOF)*, which is situated deep to the eyebrow and extends into the eyelid, where it merges with postorbicularis fascia in the upper eyelid.

The SOOF plays an important role in the aging process of gradual gravitational descent of the midfacial soft tissues. Studies and surgical procedures suggest that elevation of the SOOF into its previous anatomical position restores more youthful contours in the lower eyelid and midfacial soft tissues.

Similarly, the *sub-brow fat pad* undergoes gravitational descent, compounding a redundant upper eyelid skin fold. The displaced sub-brow fat pad can be confused with a coexisting redundant upper eyelid fold and prominent prolapsed upper eyelid preaponeurotic fat pad. To achieve an adequate functional and aesthetic result, the surgeon must address the descended sub-brow fat pad, in addition to skin and eyelid fat adjustment, during blepharoplasty.

Lucarelli MJ, Khwarg SI, Lemke BN, Kozel JS, Dortzbach RK. The anatomy of midfacial ptosis. *Ophthal Plast Reconstr Surg.* 2000;16(1):7–22.

Mendelson BC, Muzaffar AR, Adams WP Jr. Surgical anatomy of the midcheek and malar mounds. *Plast Reconstr Surg.* 2002;110(3):885–896; discussion 897–911.

Canthal tendons The configuration of the palpebral fissure is maintained by the medial and lateral canthal tendons in conjunction with the attached tarsal plates. The 2 origins of the medial canthal tendon from the anterior and posterior lacrimal crests fuse just temporal to the lacrimal sac and then again split into an upper limb and a lower limb that attach to the upper and lower tarsal plates. The attachment of the tendon to the periosteum overlying the anterior lacrimal crest is diffuse and strong; the attachment to the posterior lacrimal crest is more delicate but important in maintaining apposition of the eyelids to the globe, allowing the puncta to lie in the tear lake.

The lateral canthal tendon attaches at the lateral orbital tubercle on the inner aspect of the orbital rim. It splits into superior and inferior branches that attach to the respective tarsal plates. Cutting, stretching, or disinsertion of either of the canthal tendons usually causes cosmetic or functional problems such as telecanthus and horizontal eyelid laxity. Horizontal eyelid instability is frequently the result of lateral canthal lengthening. Therefore, surgical correction should be directed at shortening the lateral canthus, rather than resecting the normal eyelid in the palpebral fissure. The lateral canthal tendon usually inserts 2 mm higher than does the medial canthal tendon, giving the normal horizontal palpebral fissure an upward slope medial to lateral. Insertion of the lateral canthal tendon inferior to the medial canthal tendon causes a downward (antimongoloid) slant.

Eyelid margin

The eyelid margin is the confluence of the mucosal surface of the conjunctiva, the edge of the orbicularis, and the cutaneous epithelium. Along the margin are eyelashes and glands, which provide protection for the ocular surface. The mucocutaneous junction of the eyelid margin is often erroneously referred to as the *gray line.* The gray line is an isolated section of pretarsal orbicularis muscle (Riolan) just anterior to the tarsus. The mucocutaneous junction is located posterior to the meibomian gland orifices on the eyelid margin (see Fig 9-8). The horizontal palpebral fissure is approximately 30 mm long. The main portion of the margin, called the *ciliary margin,* has a rather well-defined anterior and posterior edge. Medial to the punctum, the eyelid is thinner.

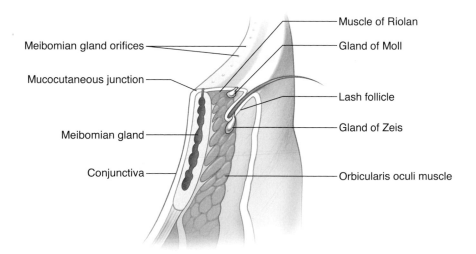

Meibomian gland orifices
Mucocutaneous junction
Meibomian gland
Conjunctiva

Muscle of Riolan
Gland of Moll
Lash follicle
Gland of Zeis
Orbicularis oculi muscle

Figure 9-8 Eyelid margin anatomy. *(Illustration by Christine Gralapp.)*

Eyelashes

There are approximately 100 eyelashes, or cilia, in the upper eyelid and 50 in the lower eyelid. The lashes usually originate in the anterior aspect of the eyelid margin just anterior to the tarsal plate and form 2 or 3 irregular rows. A few cilia may be found in the caruncle.

Meibomian glands

The meibomian glands originate in the tarsus and number approximately 25 in the upper eyelid and 20 in the lower eyelid. During the second month of gestation, both the eyelashes and the meibomian glands differentiate from a common pilosebaceous unit. This dual potentiality explains why, following trauma or chronic irritation, a lash follicle may develop from a meibomian gland *(acquired distichiasis)*. Similarly, an extra row of lashes arising from the meibomian orifices may be present from birth *(congenital distichiasis)*.

Vascular and lymphatic supply

The extensive vascularity of the eyelids promotes healing and helps defend against infection. The arterial supply of the eyelids comes from 2 main sources: (1) the internal carotid artery by way of the ophthalmic artery and its branches (supraorbital and lacrimal) and (2) the external carotid artery by way of the arteries of the face (angular and temporal). Collateral circulation between these 2 systems is extensive, anastomosing throughout the upper and lower eyelids and forming the marginal and peripheral arcades.

The marginal arterial arcade should not be confused with the peripheral arterial arcade. In the upper eyelid, the marginal arcade lies 2 mm superior to the margin, near the follicles of the cilia and anterior to the tarsal plate. The peripheral arcade lies superior to the tarsus, between the levator aponeurosis and the Müller muscle (see Fig 9-4). The lower eyelid often has only 1 arterial arcade, located at the inferior tarsal border.

Eyelid venous drainage may be divided into pretarsal and posttarsal. The *pretarsal* tissues drain into the angular vein medially and into the superficial temporal vein laterally. *Posttarsal* drainage is into the orbital veins and the deeper branches of the anterior facial vein and pterygoid plexus. Lymphatic vessels serving the medial portion of the eyelids drain into the submandibular lymph nodes. Lymph channels serving the lateral portions of the eyelids drain first into the superficial preauricular nodes and then into the deeper cervical nodes.

CHAPTER 10

Classification and Management of Eyelid Disorders

Like the orbit, the eyelids can be affected by a variety of congenital, acquired, infectious, inflammatory, neoplastic, and traumatic conditions. These disorders and their management are discussed in this chapter. In addition, the eyelids are subject to various positional abnormalities and involutional changes; these disorders are discussed in Chapter 11.

Congenital Anomalies

Congenital anomalies of the eyelid may be isolated or associated with other eyelid, facial, or systemic anomalies. Careful evaluation of patients in cases of hereditary syndromes is helpful before proceeding with treatment. Most congenital anomalies of the eyelids occur during the second month of gestation as the result of a failure of fusion or an arrest of development. The majority of the defects described in this section are rare. (See also BCSC Section 6, *Pediatric Ophthalmology and Strabismus*.)

Blepharophimosis Syndrome

This eyelid syndrome is an autosomal dominantly inherited blepharophimosis, usually presenting with telecanthus, epicanthus inversus (fold of skin extending from the lower to upper eyelid), and severe ptosis. Additional findings may include lateral lower eyelid ectropion secondary to vertical lid deficiency, a poorly developed nasal bridge, hypoplasia of the superior orbital rims, lop ears, and hypertelorism (Fig 10-1).

Surgical modification may require multiple surgeries. Timing of the repair is based first on eyelid function and then on eyelid appearance. Visually disruptive ptosis should be addressed promptly. Whether performed simultaneously with the ptosis repair or separately, the medial canthal repositioning will place traction on the upper eyelid and potentially exacerbate the ptosis. Repair of the ptosis usually requires frontalis suspension for adequate lift. Multiple Z-plasties or Y–V-plasties, sometimes combined with transnasal wiring of the elongated medial canthal tendons, are used to modify the telecanthus and epicanthus. Additional procedures may be needed to correct associated problems such as ectropion or hypoplasia of the orbital rims.

Allen CE, Rubin PA. Blepharophimosis-ptosis-epicanthus inversus syndrome (BPES): clinical manifestation and treatment. *Int Ophthalmol Clin.* 2008;48(2):15–23.

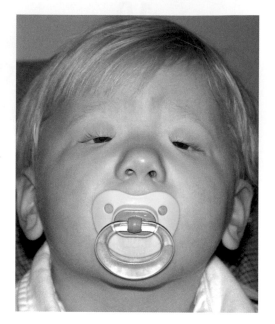

Figure 10-1 Blepharophimosis syndrome. *(Courtesy of Jill Foster, MD.)*

Anderson RL, Nowinski TS. The five-flap technique for blepharophimosis. *Arch Ophthalmol.* 1989;107(3):448–452.

Congenital Ptosis of the Upper Eyelid

Congenital ptosis of the upper eyelid is discussed in Chapter 11.

Congenital Ectropion

In rare cases, congenital ectropion occurs as an isolated finding. It is more often associated with blepharophimosis syndrome, Down syndrome, or ichthyosis. Congenital ectropion is caused by a vertical insufficiency of the anterior lamella of the eyelid and may give rise to chronic epiphora and exposure keratitis. Mild congenital ectropion usually requires no treatment. If it is severe and symptomatic, congenital ectropion is treated like a cicatricial ectropion, with horizontal tightening of the lateral canthal tendon and vertical lengthening of the anterior lamella by means of a full-thickness skin graft.

A complete eversion of the upper eyelids occasionally occurs in newborns (Fig 10-2). Possible causes include inclusion conjunctivitis, anterior lamellar inflammation or shortage, or Down syndrome. Topical lubrication and short-term patching of both eyes may be curative. Full-thickness sutures or a temporary tarsorrhaphy are used when necessary.

Euryblepharon

Euryblepharon is a unilateral or bilateral horizontal widening of the palpebral fissure sometimes associated with blepharophimosis syndrome. Euryblepharon usually involves the lateral portion of the lower eyelids and is associated with both vertical shortening

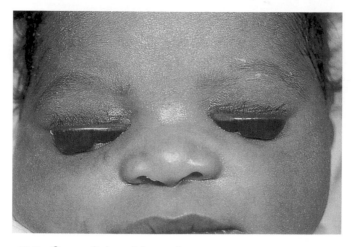

Figure 10-2 Congenital eyelid eversion. *(Courtesy of Thaddeus S. Nowinski, MD.)*

and horizontal lengthening of the involved eyelids (Figs 10-3, 10-4). The palpebral fissure often has a downward (antimongoloid) slant because of the inferiorly displaced lateral canthal tendon. Impaired blinking, poor closure, and lagophthalmos may result in exposure keratitis. If the condition is symptomatic, reconstruction may include lateral canthal repositioning along with suspension of the suborbicularis oculi fat to the lateral orbital rim so that the lower eyelid is supported. If excess horizontal length is still apparent, a lateral tarsal strip or eyelid margin resection may be added. Skin grafts may occasionally be necessary.

Ankyloblepharon

Ankyloblepharon is partial or complete fusion of the eyelids by webs of skin (see Fig 10-3). These webs can usually be opened with scissors after being clamped for a few seconds with a hemostat.

Epicanthus

Epicanthus is a medial canthal fold that may result from immature midfacial bones or a fold of skin and subcutaneous tissue (Fig 10-5; also see Fig 10-3). The condition is usually bilateral. An affected child may appear esotropic because of decreased scleral exposure nasally *(pseudostrabismus)*. Traditionally, 4 types of epicanthus are described:

- *epicanthus tarsalis* if the fold is most prominent in the upper eyelid
- *epicanthus inversus* if the fold is most prominent in the lower eyelid
- *epicanthus palpebralis* if the fold is equally distributed in the upper and lower eyelids
- *epicanthus supraciliaris* if the fold arises from the eyebrow region running to the lacrimal sac

Epicanthus tarsalis can be a normal variation of the Asian eyelid, whereas epicanthus inversus is frequently associated with blepharophimosis syndrome.

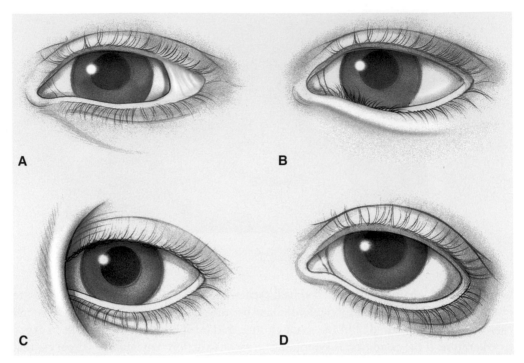

Figure 10-3 Congenital eyelid deformities. **A,** Ankyloblepharon. **B,** Epiblepharon. **C,** Epicanthus. **D,** Euryblepharon. *(Illustration by Christine Gralapp.)*

Most forms of epicanthus resolve with normal growth of the facial bones. If no associated eyelid anomalies are present, observation is recommended until the face achieves maturity. Epicanthus inversus, however, rarely resolves with facial growth. Most cases of isolated epicanthus requiring treatment respond well to linear revisions such as Z-plasty or Y–V-plasty. Epicanthus tarsalis in the Asian patient may be eliminated by a Y–V-plasty with or without construction of an upper eyelid crease.

Epiblepharon

In epiblepharon, the lower eyelid pretarsal muscle and skin ride above the lower eyelid margin to form a horizontal fold of tissue that causes the cilia to assume a vertical position (Fig 10-6; also see Fig 10-3). The eyelid margin, therefore, is in normal position with respect to the globe. Epiblepharon is most common in Asian children.

The cilia often do not touch the cornea except in downgaze, and this rarely causes corneal staining. Epiblepharon may not require surgical treatment because it tends to diminish with the maturation of the facial bones. However, epiblepharon occasionally results in keratitis; in that case, the excess skin and muscle fold should be excised just inferior to the eyelid margin (in the case of the lower eyelid) and the skin edges approximated.

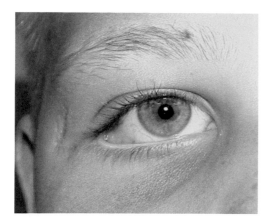

Figure 10-4   Euryblepharon. *(Courtesy of Jill Foster, MD.)*

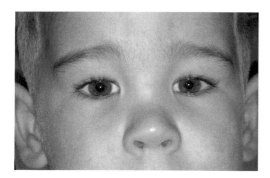

Figure 10-5   Epicanthal folds. *(Courtesy of Jill Foster, MD.)*

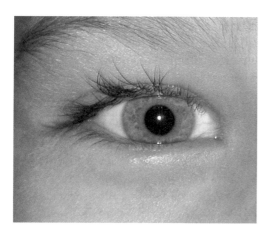

Figure 10-6   Epiblepharon. *(Courtesy of Jill Foster, MD.)*

Congenital Entropion

In contrast to epiblepharon, eyelid margin inversion is present in congenital entropion (Fig 10-7). Developmental factors that lead to this rare condition include lower eyelid retractor dysgenesis, structural defects in the tarsal plate, and relative shortening of the posterior lamella. Congenital entropion often does not improve spontaneously and may

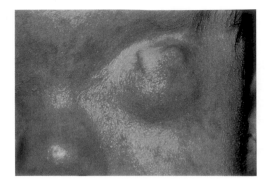

Figure 10-10 Cryptophthalmos.

following even a single injection. Treatment with systemic steroids eliminates the risks attributed to the injection delivery but increases the dosage and risk of systemic side effects. Topical treatment with clobetasol propionate has also been reported to successfully shrink eyelid hemangiomas. However, topical treatment does not eliminate the risks of systemic steroid exposure. Interferon-α is usually reserved for life-threatening or sight-threatening lesions because of the risk of serious adverse effects. Surgical excision may be used on well-circumscribed lesions. Use of the carbon-dioxide laser as an incisional device is helpful for controlling bleeding. Topical lasers may be used on the superficial (1–2 mm) layers of the skin to diminish the redness of a lesion. However, cutaneous lasers do not penetrate deeply enough to shrink a visually disabling lesion.

Cryptophthalmos

Cryptophthalmos is a rare condition that presents with partial or complete absence of the eyebrow, palpebral fissure, eyelashes, and conjunctiva (Fig 10-10). The partially developed adnexa are fused to the anterior segment of the globe. Cryptophthalmos may be unilateral or bilateral. Histologically, the levator, orbicularis, tarsus, conjunctiva, and meibomian glands are attenuated or absent; thus, attempts at reconstruction are difficult. Severe ocular defects are present in the underlying eye.

Acquired Eyelid Disorders

Chalazion

Chalazion is a focal inflammation of the eyelids that results from an obstruction of the meibomian glands (an internal posterior hordeolum). This disorder is often associated with rosacea and chronic blepharitis. This common disorder may occasionally be confused with a malignant neoplasm.

The *meibomian glands* are oil-producing sebaceous glands located in the tarsal plates of both upper and lower eyelids. If the gland orifices on the eyelid margin become plugged, the contents of the glands (sebum) are released into the tarsus and the surrounding eyelid soft tissue. This elicits an acute inflammatory response accompanied by pain and erythema of the skin. The exact role of bacterial agents (most commonly *Staphylo-*

coccus aureus) in the production of chalazia is not clear. Histologically, these lesions are characterized by chronic lipogranulomatous inflammation.

Treatment

In the acute inflammatory phase, treatment consists of warm compresses and appropriate eyelid hygiene. Although topical antibiotic or anti-inflammatory ocular medications can be used, they may have minimal effect in resolving a chalazion. Acute secondary infection may be treated with an antibiotic directed at skin flora. Doxycycline or tetracycline given for systemic effect may be appropriate when a case requires long-term suppression of meibomian gland inflammation associated with ocular rosacea. Patients should be counseled about the possible side effects of systemically administered antibiotics.

Occasionally, chalazia become chronic, requiring surgical management to facilitate clearing of the inflammatory mass. In most cases, the greatest inflammatory response is on the posterior eyelid margin, and an incision through tarsus and conjunctiva is appropriate for drainage. Sharp dissection and excision of all necrotic material, including the posterior wall, are indicated. This results in a posterior marsupialization of the chalazion (Fig 10-11). Caution is needed in the removal of inflammatory tissue at the eyelid margin or adjacent to the punctum. Rarely, the greatest inflammatory response is anterior; in such cases, incision through the skin and orbicularis muscle, with appropriate removal of granulomatous tissue, is possible. Pathologic examination is appropriate for atypical or recurrent chalazia. Local injection of corticosteroids in chalazia resistant to conservative

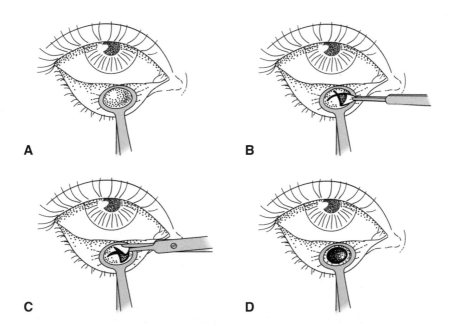

Figure 10-11 Excision of chalazion. **A,** After a clamp is placed around the chalazion, a blade is used to make a vertical incision into the tarsus. **B,** Cruciate incision of conjunctiva and cyst wall. **C,** Flaps are excised with a scissors. **D,** Defect is allowed to heal by secondary intention. *(Illustration by Jeanne C. Koelling.)*

management can cause depigmentation of the overlying skin and is not as effective as surgical treatment. Combining excision with steroid injection into the excisional bed results in a 95% resolution rate.

Epstein GA, Putterman AM. Combined excision and drainage with intralesional corticosteroid injection in the treatment of chronic chalazia. *Arch Ophthalmol.* 1988;106(4):514–516.

Hordeolum

An acute infection (usually staphylococcal) can involve the sebaceous secretions in the glands of Zeis *(external hordeolum,* or *stye)* or the meibomian glands *(internal hordeolum).* In the case of external hordeola, the infection often appears to center around an eyelash follicle, and the eyelash can be plucked to promote drainage. Spontaneous resolution often occurs. If needed, diligent application of hot compresses and topical antibiotic ointment is usually curative. Rarely, hordeola may progress to true superficial cellulitis, or even abscesses, of the eyelid. In such cases, systemic antibiotic therapy and possible surgical incision and drainage may be required.

Eyelid Edema

Swelling of the eyelids may be caused by local conditions such as insect bites or allergy or by systemic conditions such as cardiovascular disease, renal disease, certain collagen vascular diseases, or thyroid eye disease. Cerebrospinal fluid leakage into the orbit or eyelids following trauma may mimic eyelid edema. Lymphedema may be present if the lymphatic drainage system from the eyelid is interrupted.

Floppy Eyelid Syndrome

Floppy eyelid syndrome is characterized by ocular irritation and mild mucus discharge that is frequently worse on awakening. Patients have a chronic papillary conjunctivitis. The superior tarsal plate is soft, rubbery, flaccid, and easily everted (Fig 10-12). During examination, if the clinician pulls the skin of the upper eyelid up toward the forehead, the upper eyelid will evert spontaneously, especially in the temporal area. Associations have been reported with obesity, keratoconus, eyelid rubbing, mechanical pressure, hyperglycemia, and sleep apnea. A marked decrease in the number of elastin fibers in the tarsus plate has been reported from histologic examination. Often, patients have a history of sleeping prone; this can cause mechanical upper eyelid eversion, allowing the superior

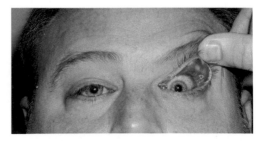

Figure 10-12 Easy eversion of loose eyelid, characteristic of floppy eyelid syndrome. *(Courtesy of Morris Hartstein, MD.)*

palpebral conjunctiva to rub against the pillow or bedding. Initial conservative treatment using viscous lubrication and a patch or eyelid shield at night is helpful. Frequently, surgical correction by horizontal tightening of the eyelid is indicated. Sleep studies are recommended to rule out sleep apnea.

Eyelid imbrication syndrome occurs when a lax upper eyelid with normal tarsal plate overrides the lower eyelid margin during closure. This results in chronic conjunctivitis. Management consists of topical lubrication in mild cases. In more severe cases, horizontal tightening of the upper eyelid is indicated.

Ezra DG, Beaconsfield M, Sira M, et al. Long-term outcomes of surgical approaches to the treatment of floppy eyelid syndrome. *Ophthalmology.* 2010;117(4):839–846.

Karesh JW, Nirankari VS, Hameroff SB. Eyelid imbrication: an unrecognized cause of chronic ocular irritation. *Ophthalmology.* 1993;100(6):883–889.

Trichotillomania

Trichotillomania is an impulse control disorder most commonly seen in preteen or teenage girls. It is characterized by the repeated desire to pull out hairs, frequently eyebrows or eyelashes. Diagnosis may be elusive, as affected patients usually deny the cause. Characteristically, multiple hairs are broken off and regrowing at different lengths. Applying ophthalmic ointment to the affected area sometimes helps diagnosis and treatment by allowing hairs to regrow. Habit reversal therapy or oral treatment with selective serotonin reuptake inhibitors may be effective, as employed in the treatment of obsessive-compulsive behavior.

Eyelid Neoplasms

Numerous benign and malignant cutaneous neoplasms can develop in the periocular skin, arising from the epidermis, dermis, or eyelid adnexal structures. Most lesions, whether benign or malignant, develop from the epidermis, the rapidly growing superficial layer of the skin. Although many of these lesions may occur elsewhere on the body, their appearance and behavior in the eyelids may be unique owing to the particular characteristics of eyelid skin and the specialized adnexal elements. The malignant lesions most frequently affecting the eyelids are basal cell carcinoma, squamous cell carcinoma, sebaceous cell carcinoma, and melanoma. Because clinical judgment is not as exact as pathologic diagnosis, histologic examination of suspected cutaneous malignancies is generally recommended.

Clinical Evaluation of Eyelid Tumors

The history and physical examination of eyelid lesions offer important clues regarding the likelihood of malignancy. Predisposing factors in the development of skin cancer include

- a history of prior skin cancer
- excessive sun exposure, especially blistering sunburn during adolescence
- previous radiation therapy

- history of smoking
- Celtic or Scandinavian ancestry, with fair skin, red hair, blue eyes
- immunosuppression

Signs suggesting eyelid malignancy are

- slow, painless growth of a lesion
- ulceration, with intermittent drainage, bleeding, and crusting
- irregular pigmentary changes
- destruction of normal eyelid margin architecture (especially meibomian orifices) and loss of cilia
- heaped-up, pearly, translucent margins with central ulceration
- fine telangiectasias
- loss of fine cutaneous wrinkles

Palpable induration extending well beyond visibly apparent margins suggests tumor infiltration into the dermis and subcutaneous tissue.

Lesions near the puncta should be evaluated for punctal or canalicular involvement. Probing and irrigation may be required to exclude lacrimal system involvement or to prepare for surgical resection.

Large lesions should be palpated for evidence of fixation to deeper tissues or bone. In addition, regional lymph nodes should be palpated for evidence of metastases in cases of suspected squamous cell carcinoma, sebaceous carcinoma, melanoma, or Merkel cell carcinoma. Lymphatic tumor spread may produce rubbery swelling along the line of the jaw or in front of the ear. Restriction of ocular motility and proptosis suggest orbital extension of an eyelid malignancy. The function of cranial nerves VII and V is assessed so that any deficiencies possibly indicating perineural tumor spread can be detected. Perineural invasion is a feature of squamous cell carcinoma. Systemic evidence of liver, pulmonary, bone, or neurological involvement should be sought in cases of sebaceous adenocarcinoma or melanoma of the eyelid.

It is important to obtain photographs prior to treatment of the lesion. If photographs cannot be obtained, drawings and measurements are recorded for future comparison.

The following discussions of eyelid neoplasms are intended to provide a brief overview of the most prevalent lesions. For more extensive coverage and additional clinical and pathologic photographs, see BCSC Section 4, *Ophthalmic Pathology and Intraocular Tumors.*

Cook BE Jr, Bartley GB. Epidemiologic characteristics and clinical course of patients with malignant eyelid tumors in an incidence cohort in Olmsted County, Minnesota. *Ophthalmology.* 1999;106(4):746–750.

de la Garza AG, Kersten RC, Carter KD. Evaluation and treatment of benign eyelid lesions. *Focal Points: Clinical Modules for Ophthalmologists.* San Francisco: American Academy of Ophthalmology; 2010, module 5.

Benign Eyelid Lesions

Epithelial hyperplasias

The terminology used by dermatopathologists to describe various benign epithelial proliferations continues to evolve. It is helpful to group the various benign epithelial proliferations under the clinical heading of *papillomas*. (This designation does not necessarily imply any association with the papillomavirus.) Clinical and histologic characterizations of the various benign epithelial proliferations overlap considerably. Included within this group are seborrheic keratosis; pseudoepitheliomatous hyperplasia; verruca; acrochordon (skin tag, fibroepithelial polyp, squamous papilloma; Fig 10-13); basosquamous acanthoma; squamous acanthoma; and many others. These benign epithelial proliferations can all be managed with shave excision at the dermal–epidermal junction.

Seborrheic keratosis is an example of acquired benign eyelid papillomas (Fig 10-14). It tends to affect middle-aged and elderly patients. Its clinical appearance varies; it may be

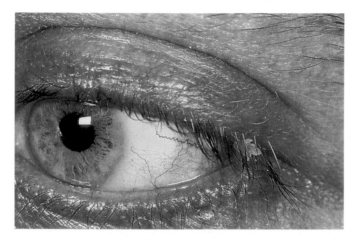

Figure 10-13 Acrochordon (also called *skin tag* or *squamous papilloma*).

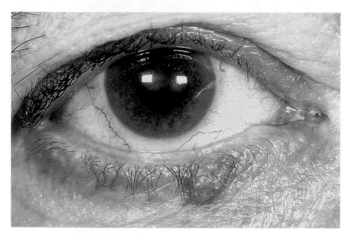

Figure 10-14 Seborrheic keratosis.

sessile or pedunculated and have varying degrees of pigmentation and hyperkeratosis. On facial skin, seborrheic keratosis typically appears as a smooth, greasy, stuck-on lesion. On the thinner eyelid skin, this lesion can be more lobulated, papillary, or pedunculated with visible excrescences on its surface. Even large lesions of this type remain superficial. They can be managed by shave excision at the dermal–epidermal junction.

Pseudoepitheliomatous hyperplasia is not a discrete lesion but rather refers to a pattern of reactive changes in the epidermis that may develop over areas of inflammation or neoplasia.

Verruca vulgaris, caused by epidermal infection with the human papillomavirus (type 6 or 11), rarely occurs in thin eyelid skin (Fig 10-15). Cryotherapy may eradicate the lesion and minimizes the risk of viral spread.

Cutaneous horn is a descriptive, nondiagnostic term referring to *exuberant hyperkeratosis.* This lesion may be associated with a variety of benign or malignant histologic processes, including seborrheic keratosis, verruca vulgaris, and squamous or basal cell carcinoma. Biopsy of the base of the cutaneous horn is required to establish a definitive diagnosis.

Benign epithelial lesions

Cysts of the epidermis are the second most common type of benign periocular cutaneous lesions, accounting for approximately 18% of excised benign lesions. Most of these are *epidermal inclusion cysts,* which arise from the infundibulum of the hair follicle, either spontaneously or following traumatic implantation of epidermal tissue into the dermis (Fig 10-16). The lesions are slow-growing, elevated, round, and smooth. They often have a central pore, indicating the remaining pilar duct. Although these cysts are often called *sebaceous cysts,* they are actually filled with keratin. Rupture of the cyst wall may cause an inflammatory foreign-body reaction. The cysts may also become secondarily infected. Recommended treatment for small cysts is marsupialization, excising around the periphery of the cyst but leaving the base of the cyst wall to serve as the new surface epithelium.

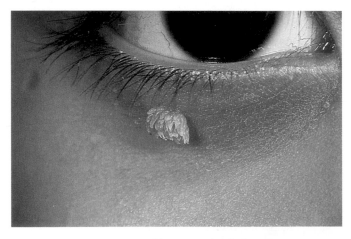

Figure 10-15 Verruca vulgaris (wart).

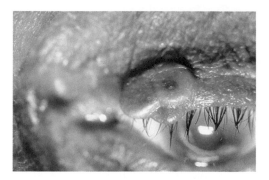

Figure 10-16 Epidermal inclusion cyst. *(Courtesy of Robert C. Kersten, MD.)*

Larger or deeper cysts may require a complete excision, in which case the cyst wall should be removed intact to reduce the possibility of recurrence.

Multiple tiny epidermal inclusion cysts are called *milia*. Milia may appear spontaneously, following trauma, or during the healing phase of a bullous disease process. They are particularly common in newborn infants. Generally, milia resolve spontaneously, but they may be marsupialized with a sharp blade or needle. Multiple confluent milia may be treated with topical retinoic acid cream.

A less common epidermal cyst is the *pilar,* or *trichilemmal, cyst.* These cysts are clinically indistinguishable from epidermal inclusion cysts, but they tend to occur in areas containing large and numerous hair follicles. Approximately 90% of pilar cysts occur on the scalp; in the periocular region, they are generally found in the eyebrows. The cysts are filled with desquamated epithelium, and calcification occurs in approximately 25%.

Molluscum contagiosum is a viral infection of the epidermis that often involves the eyelid in children (Fig 10-17). Occasionally, multiple exuberant lesions appear in adult patients with acquired immunodeficiency syndrome (AIDS). The lesions are characteristically waxy and nodular, with a central umbilication. They may produce an associated

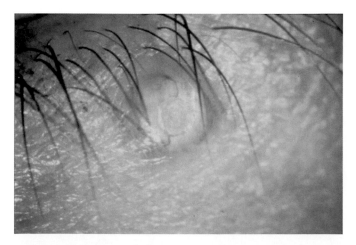

Figure 10-17 Molluscum lesion of eyelid. *(Courtesy of Jill Foster, MD.)*

follicular conjunctivitis. Treatment is observation, excision, controlled cryotherapy, or curettage.

Xanthelasmas are yellowish plaques that occur commonly in the medial canthal areas of the upper and lower eyelids (Fig 10-18). They represent lipid-laden macrophages in the superficial dermis and subdermal tissues. Although xanthelasmas usually occur in patients with normal serum cholesterol levels, they are sometimes associated with hyper-cholesterolemia or congenital disorders of lipid metabolism. When excising these lesions, the surgeon must be careful to avoid removing too much of the anterior lamella of the eyelids, because doing so can lead to cicatricial ectropion. Xanthelasmas may recur. Other treatment options include serial excision, CO_2 laser ablation, or topical 100% trichloro-acetic acid. Deep extension into the orbicularis muscle can occur, in which case the lesion may not be amenable to surface ablative therapies.

Benign Adnexal Lesions

The term *adnexa* refers to skin appendages that are located within the dermis but communicate through the epidermis to the surface. They include oil glands, sweat glands, and hair follicles. The eyelids contain both the specialized eyelashes and the normal vellus hairs found on skin throughout the body. Periocular adnexal oil glands include the *meibomian glands* within the tarsal plate, the *glands of Zeis* associated with eyelash follicles, and normal *sebaceous glands* that are present as part of the pilosebaceous units in the skin hair. Sweat glands in the periocular region include the *eccrine sweat glands,* which have a general distribution throughout the body and are responsible for thermal regulation, and the eccrine glands with apocrine secretion (the *glands of Moll*) associated with the eyelid margin.

Lesions of oil gland origin

Chalazion and hordeolum These common eyelid lesions are discussed earlier in this chapter under Acquired Eyelid Disorders.

Sebaceous hyperplasia Sebaceous gland hyperplasia presents as multiple small yellow papules that may have central umbilication. They tend to occur on the forehead and cheeks and are common in patients older than 40 years. These lesions may sometimes

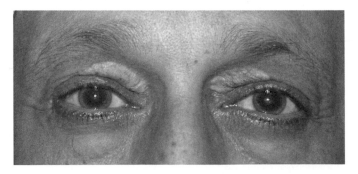

Figure 10-18 Xanthelasma. *(Courtesy of Jill Foster, MD.)*

be mistaken for basal cell carcinoma because of their tendency for central umbilication and fine telangiectasias. However, they are cream colored and are soft on palpation. They may result from chronic dermatitis and can also be seen in patients with rosacea. Patients with multiple acquired sebaceous gland adenomas, adenomatoid sebaceous hyperplasia, or basal cell carcinomas with sebaceous differentiation have an increased incidence of visceral malignancy *(Muir-Torre syndrome)* and should be evaluated accordingly.

When sebaceous gland hyperplasia occurs in the meibomian glands in the tarsal plate, the eyelids may become thickened and ectropic. This condition may coexist with chronic blepharitis, and the possibility of sebaceous gland carcinoma must be considered.

Sebaceous adenoma This rare tumor appears as a yellowish papule on the face, scalp, or trunk and may mimic a basal cell carcinoma or seborrheic keratosis.

Tumors of eccrine sweat gland origin

Eccrine hidrocystoma Eccrine hidrocystomas are common cystic lesions 1–3 mm in diameter that occur in groups and tend to cluster around the lower eyelids and canthi and the face. They are considered to be ductal retention cysts, and they often enlarge in conditions such as heat and increased humidity, which stimulate perspiration. Treatment consists of surgical excision.

Syringoma Benign eccrine sweat gland tumors found commonly in young females, syringomas present as multiple small, waxy, pale yellow nodules 1–2 mm in diameter on the lower eyelids (Fig 10-19). Syringomas can also be found in the axilla and sternal region. They become more apparent at the time of puberty. Because the eccrine glands are located within the dermis, these lesions lie too deep to allow shave excision. Removal requires complete surgical excision, which is often best accomplished in a staged fashion.

Eccrine spiradenoma This uncommon benign tumor appears as a solitary nodule 1–2 cm in diameter that may be tender and painful. It tends to occur in early adulthood, and eyelid involvement is rare. Treatment is surgical excision.

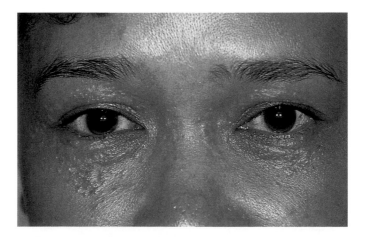

Figure 10-19 Syringomas. *(Courtesy of Robert C. Kersten, MD.)*

a role in ultimate resolution. At present, incisional biopsy followed by complete surgical excision is recommended.

Grossniklaus HE, Wojno TH, Yanoff M, Font RL. Invasive keratoacanthoma of the eyelid and ocular adnexa. *Ophthalmology.* 1996;103(6):937–941.

Premalignant Melanocytic Lesions

Lentigo maligna

Also known as *Hutchinson melanotic freckle* or *precancerous melanosis,* lentigo maligna is a flat, irregularly shaped, unevenly pigmented, slowly enlarging lesion that typically oc- curs on the malar regions in older white persons. Unlike senile or solar lentigo, character- istics of lentigo maligna include significant pigmentary variation, irregular borders, and progressive enlargement. These characteristics reflect a radial, intraepidermal, uncon- trolled growth phase of melanocytes, which in 30%–50% of patients eventually progresses to nodules of vertically invasive melanoma.

The area of histologic abnormality frequently extends beyond the visible pigmented borders of the lesion; in the periocular region, cutaneous lentigo maligna of the eyelid may extend onto the conjunctival surface, where the lesion appears identical to primary acquired melanosis. Excision with adequate surgical margins is recommended, with per- manent sections for final monitoring. Close observation for recurrence is warranted.

Malignant Eyelid Tumors

Basal cell carcinoma

Basal cell carcinoma, the most common eyelid malignancy, accounts for approximately 90%–95% of malignant eyelid tumors. Basal cell carcinomas are often located on the lower eyelid margin (50%–60%) and near the medial canthus (25%–30%). Less commonly, they may occur on the upper eyelid (15%) and lateral canthus (5%). Basal cell carcinoma may have many different clinical manifestations in the eyelid (Fig 10-27).

Patients at highest risk for basal cell carcinoma are fair-skinned, blue-eyed, red-haired or blond, middle-aged and older people with English, Irish, Scottish, or Scandinavian an- cestry. They may have a history of prolonged sun exposure during the first 2 decades of life. A history of cigarette smoking also increases the risk of basal cell carcinoma. Patients with prior basal cell carcinomas have a higher probability of developing additional skin cancers.

Basal cell carcinoma is being seen with increasing frequency in younger patients, and discovery of malignant eyelid lesions in these patients or those with a positive family his- tory should prompt inquiry into possible systemic associations such as basal cell nevus syndrome or xeroderma pigmentosum. *Basal cell nevus syndrome (Gorlin syndrome)* is an uncommon autosomal dominant, multisystem disorder characterized by multiple nevoid basal cell carcinomas, which appear early in life and are associated with skeletal anoma- lies, especially of the mandible, maxilla, and vertebrae. *Xeroderma pigmentosum* is a rare autosomal recessive disorder characterized by extreme sun sensitivity and a defective re- pair mechanism for ultraviolet light–induced DNA damage in skin cells.

Library and eLearning Centre
Gartnavel General Hospital
CHAPTER 10: Classification and Management of Eyelid Disorders • 169

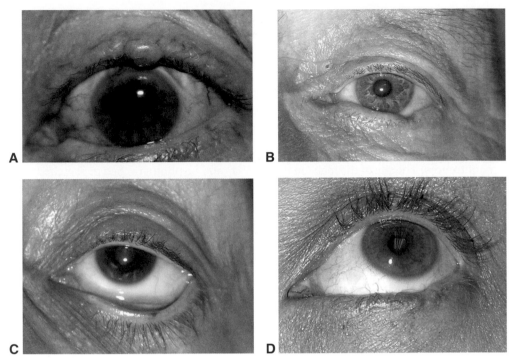

Figure 10-27 Basal cell carcinoma. **A,** Nodular. **B,** Ulcerative. **C,** Pigmented. **D,** Morpheaform. *(Courtesy of Jill Foster, MD.)*

Nodular basal cell carcinoma, the most common clinical appearance of basal cell carcinoma, is a firm, raised, pearly nodule that may be associated with telangiectasia and central ulceration. Histologically, tumors of this form demonstrate nests of basal cells that originate from the basal cell layer of the epithelium and may show peripheral palisading. As the nests of atypical cells break through to the surface of the epithelium, central necrosis and ulceration may occur.

The *morpheaform* tumor type is less common, and behaves more aggressively, than the nodular form of basal cell carcinoma. Morpheaform lesions may be firm and slightly elevated, with margins that may be indeterminate on clinical examination. Histologically, these lesions do not show peripheral palisading but rather occur in thin cords that radiate peripherally. The surrounding stroma may show proliferation of connective tissue into a pattern of fibrosis.

Basal cell carcinoma may simulate chronic inflammation of the eyelid margin and is frequently associated with loss of eyelashes (madarosis). *Multicentric* or *superficial* basal cell carcinoma may be mistaken for chronic blepharitis and can silently extend along the eyelid margin.

Carneiro RC, de Macedo EM, Matayoshi S. Imiquimod 5% cream for the treatment of periocular basal cell carcinoma. *Ophthal Plast Reconstr Surg.* 2010;26(2):100–102.

Margo CE, Waltz K. Basal cell carcinoma of the eyelid and periocular skin. *Surv Ophthalmol.* 1993;38(2):169–192.

Management A biopsy is necessary to confirm any clinical suspicion of basal cell carcinoma (Fig 10-28). The most accurate diagnosis can be ensured if every incisional biopsy provides tissue that

- is representative of the clinically evident lesion
- is of adequate size for histologic processing
- is not excessively traumatized or crushed
- contains normal tissue at the margin to show the transitional area

An *incisional biopsy* can be used as a confirmatory office procedure for suspected malignant tumors. The site of the incisional biopsy should be photographed or sketched with measurements because the site may heal so well that the original location of the tumor becomes difficult to find for subsequent tumor removal.

An *excisional biopsy* is reasonable when eyelid lesions are small and do not involve the eyelid margin or when eyelid margin lesions are centrally located, away from the lateral canthus or lacrimal punctum. However, histologic monitoring of tumor borders to ensure complete excision is mandatory. The borders of any excisional biopsy should be marked in case the excision is incomplete and further resection is necessary. Excisional biopsies should be oriented vertically so that closure does not put vertical traction on the eyelid. If the margins of the excised portion of the eyelid are positive for residual tumor cells, the involved area of the eyelid should be reexcised, with surgical monitoring of the margins by Mohs micrographic technique or by frozen-section technique.

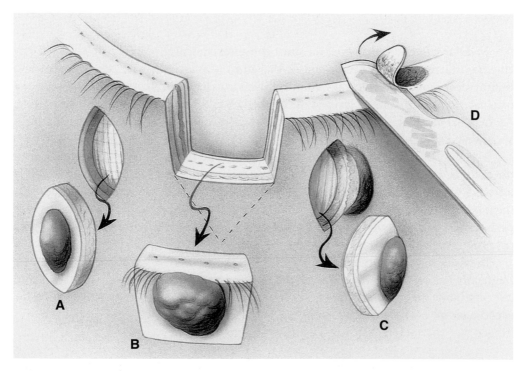

Figure 10-28 Techniques of eyelid biopsy. **A,** Excisional biopsy. **B,** Full-thickness eyelid biopsy. **C,** Incisional or punch biopsy including normal skin. **D,** Shave biopsy of eyelid margin lesion. *(Illustration by Christine Gralapp.)*

Surgery is the treatment of choice for all basal cell carcinomas of the eyelid. Surgical excision affords the advantages of complete tumor removal with histologic control of the margins. The recurrence rate is lower with excision than with any other treatment modality. It also offers superior cosmetic results in most cases.

When basal cell carcinomas involve the medial canthal area, the lacrimal drainage system may have to be removed in order to completely eradicate the tumor. If the lacrimal drainage system has been removed for tumor eradication, reconstruction of the lacrimal outflow system should not be undertaken until it is established that the patient is tumor free.

Orbital invasion of basal cell carcinoma is particularly common in cases that have been inadequately treated, in clinically neglected tumors, or in morpheaform tumors. Orbital exenteration may be required in such cases. Retrospective studies show that the mortality rate from ocular adnexal basal cell carcinoma is 3%. The vast majority of patients who died from basal cell carcinoma had disease that started in the canthal areas, had undergone prior radiation therapy, or had clinically neglected tumors.

Histological examination of the margins of an excised malignant tumor should be performed to check for complete tumor excision. Frozen-section techniques permit such examination during the course of surgery. The surgeon excises the clinically apparent tumor along with 1–2 mm of clinically uninvolved tissue, and then sends the entire specimen, oriented on a drawing, to the pathologist. The pathologist then samples the margins with frozen-section technique.

Reconstruction is undertaken when all margins are found to be free of tumor. Some tumors have subcutaneous extensions that are not recognized preoperatively. Consequently, the surgeon must always be prepared to do a much larger reconstruction than originally anticipated from the clinical appearance of the tumor.

To ensure complete removal of recurrent, deeply infiltrated, or morpheaform tumors and tumors in the medial canthal region, dermatologists with special training often use *Mohs micrographic surgery*. Tissue may be removed in thin layers that provide a 3-dimensional mapping of the tumor excision. Mohs micrographic tumor resection is most commonly used in the excision of morpheaform basal cell carcinoma and squamous cell carcinoma.

Micrographic excision preserves the maximal amount of healthy tissue while providing the best assurance of complete cancer removal. Preoperative planning between the micrographic surgeon and oculoplastic reconstructive surgeon allows for most efficient patient care. In some cases, micrographic excision may allow the preservation of a globe, whereas conventional surgical techniques might indicate the need for exenteration. However, a major limitation of Mohs micrographic surgery is in identifying margins of the tumor when the tumor has invaded orbital fat.

Following Mohs tumor resection, the eyelid should be reconstructed by standard oculoplastic procedures. Urgent reconstruction is not critical, but surgery should be performed expeditiously. Early surgery affords maximum protection for the globe and allows reconstruction to take place while the remaining eyelid margins are still fresh. If immediate reconstruction is not possible, the cornea should be protected by patching or temporarily suturing the remaining eyelids closed over the globe. If defects are small, spontaneous granulation may be a treatment alternative.

The recurrence rate following *cryotherapy* is higher than that following surgical therapy for well-circumscribed nodular lesions. When cryotherapy is used to treat more diffuse sclerosing lesions, the recurrence rate is unacceptably high. In addition, histologic margins cannot be evaluated with cryotherapy. Consequently, this treatment modality is avoided for canthal lesions, recurrent lesions, lesions greater than 1 cm in diameter, and morpheaform lesions. Further, because cryotherapy may lead to depigmentation and tissue atrophy, it should not be used when final cosmesis is important. Accordingly, cryotherapy for eyelid basal cell carcinoma is generally reserved for patients who are otherwise unable to tolerate surgery, such as elderly patients confined to bed or those with serious medical conditions that prevent surgical intervention.

Radiation therapy also should be considered only a palliative treatment that should generally be avoided for periorbital lesions. In particular, it should not be used for canthal lesions because of the risk of orbital recurrence. As with cryotherapy, histologic margins cannot be evaluated with radiation treatment. The recurrence rate following radiation treatment is higher than that following surgical treatment. Moreover, recurrence after radiation is more difficult to detect, occurs at a longer interval after initial treatment, and is more difficult to manage surgically because of the altered healing of previously irradiated tissues.

Complications of radiation therapy include cicatricial changes in the eyelids, lacrimal drainage scarring with obstruction, keratitis sicca, and radiation-induced malignancy. Radiation-induced injury to the globe may also occur if the globe is not shielded during treatment. See also BCSC Section 4, *Ophthalmic Pathology and Intraocular Tumors.*

Howard GR, Nerad JA, Carter KD, Whitaker DC. Clinical characteristics associated with orbital invasion of cutaneous basal cell and squamous cell tumors of the eyelid. *Am J Ophthalmol.* 1992;113(2):123–133.

Leshin B, Yeatts P. Management of periocular basal cell carcinoma. I, Mohs' micrographic surgery. *Surv Ophthalmol.* 1993;38(2):193–203.

Mohs FE. Micrographic surgery for the microscopically controlled excision of eyelid cancers. *Arch Ophthalmol.* 1986;104(6):901–909.

Waltz K, Margo CE. Mohs' micrographic surgery. *Ophthalmol Clin North Am.* 1991;4:153–163.

Squamous cell carcinoma

Squamous cell carcinoma of the eyelid is 40 times less common than basal cell carcinoma, but it is biologically more aggressive. Tumors can arise spontaneously or from areas of solar injury and actinic keratosis, and they may be potentiated by immunodeficiency (Fig 10-29). The treatment modalities available for squamous cell carcinoma are similar to those for basal cell carcinoma. Mohs micrographic resection or surgical excision with wide margins and frozen sections is preferred because of the potentially lethal nature of this tumor. Squamous cell carcinoma may metastasize through lymphatic transmission, blood-borne transmission, or direct extension, often along nerves. Recurrences of squamous cell carcinoma should be treated with wide surgical resection, possibly including orbital exenteration, and may require collaboration with a head and neck cancer surgeon.

Reifler DM, Hornblass A. Squamous cell carcinoma of the eyelid. *Surv Ophthalmol.* 1986; 30(6):349–365.

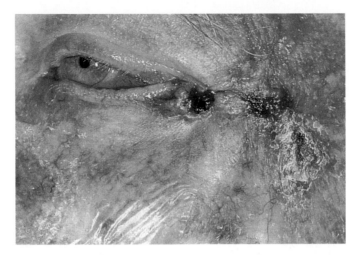

Figure 10-29 Squamous cell carcinoma of the eyelid. *(Courtesy of Jeffrey A. Nerad, MD.)*

Sebaceous adenocarcinoma

Carcinoma of the sebaceous glands is a highly malignant and potentially lethal tumor that arises from the meibomian glands of the tarsal plate; from the glands of Zeis associated with the eyelashes; or from the sebaceous glands of the caruncle, eyebrow, or facial skin. Unlike basal cell or squamous cell carcinoma, sebaceous gland carcinoma occurs more frequently in females and originates twice as often in the upper than in the lower eyelid, reflecting the greater numbers of meibomian and Zeis glands in the upper lid. Multicentric origin is common, and separate upper and lower eyelid tumors occur in 6%–8% of patients. The tumor often exhibits a yellow coloration as a result of lipid material within the neoplastic cells. Patients are commonly older than 50 years, but these tumors have been reported in younger patients as well.

These tumors often masquerade as benign eyelid diseases. Clinically, they may simulate chalazia, chronic blepharitis, basal cell or squamous cell carcinoma, ocular cicatricial pemphigoid, superior limbic keratoconjunctivitis, or pannus associated with adult inclusion conjunctivitis. Typically, effacement of the meibomian gland orifices with destruction of follicles of the cilia occurs, leading to loss of lashes (Fig 10-30).

In sebaceous carcinoma, there is a tendency for the tumor within the tarsal plate to progress to an intraepidermal growth phase, which may extend over the palpebral and bulbar conjunctiva. A fine papillary elevation of the tarsal conjunctiva may indicate pagetoid spread of tumor cells; intraepithelial growth may replace corneal epithelium as well. Sebaceous secretions from the intraepithelial cancer cells may cause marked conjunctival inflammation and injection.

A nodule that initially simulates a chalazion but later causes loss of eyelashes and destruction of the meibomian gland orifices warrants a biopsy, as this presentation is characteristic of sebaceous gland carcinoma. Solid material from a chalazion that has been surgically excised more than once should be submitted for histologic examination. Because the rate of histologic misdiagnosis is high among general pathologists, the clinician

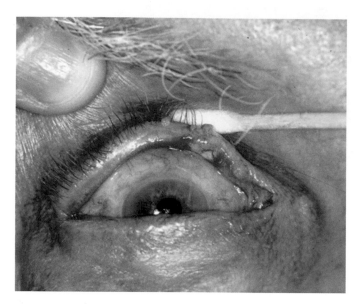

Figure 10-30 Sebaceous gland carcinoma. *(Courtesy of John B. Holds, MD.)*

should maintain suspicion based on clinical findings and request special stains (lipid) or outside consultation. Any chronic unilateral blepharitis could also raise the possibility of sebaceous gland carcinoma.

Because eyelid margin sebaceous carcinomas originate in the tarsal plate or the eyelash margin, superficial shave biopsies may reveal chronic inflammation but miss the underlying tumor. A full-thickness eyelid biopsy with permanent sections may be required to assist in the correct diagnosis. Alternatively, full-thickness punch biopsy of the tarsal plate may be diagnostic.

Wide surgical excision is mandatory for adequate treatment of sebaceous adenocarcinoma. Mohs micrographic surgery has been used in some cases; however, considerable caution is required because of the skip areas, pagetoid spread, and polycentricity characteristic of these tumors. Map biopsies of the conjunctiva are helpful to eliminate the potential of pagetoid spread. If pagetoid spread is present, cryotherapy may be used. Orbital exenteration may be considered for recurrent or large tumors invading through the orbital septum (see Chapter 8). These tumors usually metastasize to regional lymph nodes but may rarely spread hematogenously or through direct extension. Radiation therapy is usually not appropriate, as sebaceous carcinomas are relatively radioresistant.

Sentinel lymph node (SLN) biopsy is considered for patients with eyelid sebaceous cell carcinoma with high-risk features (recurrent lesions or extensive involvement of the eyelid or orbit); conjunctival or eyelid melanoma with a Breslow thickness greater than 1 mm; or Merkel cell carcinoma of the eyelid. With the exception of basal cell carcinoma, cancers of the eyelid and conjunctiva typically metastasize to the regional lymph nodes, and regional metastasis commonly occurs before metastasis to distant sites. SLN biopsy has evolved as a technique for identifying early subclinical, microscopic regional lymph node metastasis for many solid tumors throughout the body. The identification of microscopic regional nodal metastases may indicate that more extensive therapy is warranted. It can also provide prognostic information to the physician and patient.

Ho VH, Ross MI, Prieto VG, Khaleeq A, Kim S, Esmaeli B. Sentinel lymph node biopsy for sebaceous cell carcinoma and melanoma of the ocular adnexa. *Arch Otolaryngol Head Neck Surg.* 2007;133(8):820–826.

Khan JA, Doane JF, Grove AS Jr. Sebaceous and meibomian carcinomas of the eyelid: recognition, diagnosis, and management. *Ophthal Plast Reconstr Surg.* 1991;7(1):61–66.

Nijhawan N, Ross MI, Diba R, Ahmadi MA, Esmaeli B. Experience with sentinel lymph node biopsy for eyelid and conjunctival malignancies at a cancer center. *Ophthal Plast Reconstr Surg.* 2004;20(4):291–295.

Shields JA, Demirci H, Marr BP, Eagle RC Jr, Shields CL. Sebaceous carcinoma of the eyelids: personal experience with 60 cases. *Ophthalmology.* 2004;111(12):2151–2157.

Melanoma

Melanoma accounts for approximately 5% of cutaneous cancers. The incidence of melanoma has been steadily increasing over the last half century. Multiple factors, including sunlight exposure, genetic predisposition, and environmental mutagens, have been implicated in this increase. Cutaneous melanomas may develop de novo or from preexisting melanocytic nevi or lentigo maligna. Although melanoma accounts for about 5% of all skin cancers, primary cutaneous melanoma of the eyelid skin is rare (<0.1% of eyelid malignancies). Melanomas should be suspected in any patient with an acquired pigmented lesion beyond the first 2 decades of life. Melanomas typically have variable pigmentation, with darker and lighter hues within the lesion. They usually have irregular borders and may also ulcerate and bleed.

There are 4 clinicopathologic forms of cutaneous melanoma:

- lentigo maligna melanoma
- nodular melanoma
- superficial spreading melanoma
- acrolentiginous melanoma

The eyelid is most often involved by either lentigo maligna melanoma or nodular melanoma.

Lentigo maligna melanoma represents the invasive vertical malignant growth phase that occurs in 10%–20% of patients with lentigo maligna. It accounts for 90% of head and neck melanomas. Clinically, the invasive areas are marked by nodule formation within the broader, flat, tan to brown irregular macule. The eyelid is usually involved by secondary extension from the malar region, and pigmentation may progress over the eyelid margin and onto the conjunctival surface. Surgical excision is recommended for a premalignant lentigo maligna and is mandatory in patients with lentigo maligna melanoma.

Nodular melanoma (Fig 10-31) accounts for approximately 10% of cutaneous melanomas but is extremely rare on the eyelids. These tumors may be amelanotic. The vertical invasive growth phase is the initial presentation of these lesions; thus, they are likely to have extended deeply by the time of the diagnosis.

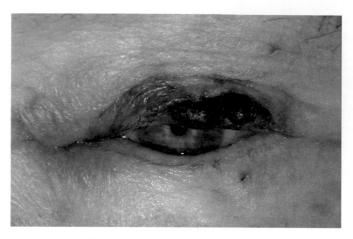

Figure 10-31 Upper eyelid melanoma. *(Courtesy of Jill Foster, MD.)*

Treatment for cutaneous melanoma includes wide surgical excision with histologic assurance (by means of permanent sections) of complete tumor removal. Randomized trials have so far provided insufficient information to address optimal excision margins for primary cutaneous melanoma. In the periocular regions, margins less than 1 cm are often used to help preserve tissue needed for reconstruction and protection of the eye. Regional lymph node dissection or SLN biopsy may be performed in patients with melanomas that show microscopic evidence of vascular or lymphatic involvement or Breslow thickness greater than 1 mm. Complete preoperative metastatic workup is indicated for tumors with thickness greater than 1.5 mm. Thin lesions (<0.75 mm) confer a 5-year survival rate of 98%; thicker lesions (>4 mm) with ulceration confer a survival rate of less than 50%. Because tumor thickness has strong prognostic implications, a biopsy should be performed on these lesions, specifically, a biopsy with a disposable punch that allows a core to be taken through the full depth of the tumor. Biopsy of these lesions does not increase the risk of metastatic spread. Although cryotherapy may have a role in the treatment of acquired melanomas in the conjunctiva, it should not be considered for treatment of cutaneous melanoma.

Boulos PR, Rubin PA. Cutaneous melanomas of the eyelid. *Semin Ophthalmol.* 2006;21(3): 195–206.

Sladden MJ, Balch C, Barzilai DA, Berg D, et al. Surgical excision margins for primary cutaneous melanoma. *Cochrane Database Syst Rev.* 2009;4:CD004835.

Sober AJ, Chuang TY, Duvic M, et al; Guidelines/Outcome Committee. Guidelines of care for primary cutaneous melanoma. *J Am Acad Dermatol.* 2001;45(4):579–586.

Kaposi sarcoma

This previously rare tumor presents as a chronic reddish dermal mass and is a frequent manifestation of AIDS (Fig 10-32). The conjunctival lesions can be mistaken for foreign-body granuloma or cavernous hemangioma. The lesion is composed of spindle cells of probable endothelial origin. It may be treated with cryotherapy, excision, radiation, or intralesional chemotherapeutic agents. Kaposi sarcoma may regress with adequate antiviral treatment of the HIV infection.

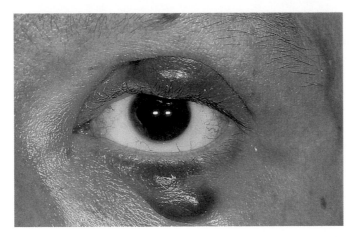

Figure 10-32 Kaposi sarcoma.

Shuler JD, Holland GN, Miles SA, Miller BJ, Grossman I. Kaposi sarcoma of the conjunctiva and eyelids associated with the acquired immunodeficiency syndrome. *Arch Ophthalmol.* 1989;107(6):858–862.

Merkel cell carcinoma

The Merkel cell is part of the dendritic (neuroendocrine) cell population of the skin. Studies suggest that, as a slowly adapting mechanoreceptor, it has a role in mediating the sense of touch. Merkel cells can give rise to malignant neoplasms, 10% of which occur in the eyelid and periocular area and manifest as painless, erythematous nodules with overlying telangiectatic blood vessels. Merkel cell carcinoma can mimic other malignant lesions; thus, the diagnosis can be difficult. One-third of the tumors recur after excision, and there is a high rate of metastasis. The estimated 5-year survival rate is 38%. Initial treatment should be aggressive and include surgical resection, with consideration of postoperative radiation and/or chemotherapy.

Peters GB 3rd, Meyer DR, Shields JA, et al. Management and prognosis of Merkel cell carcinoma of the eyelid. *Ophthalmology.* 2001;108(9):1575–1579.

Eyelid Trauma

Injury of the eyelid may be divided into blunt and penetrating trauma. Cardinal rules in the management of eyelid trauma include the following:

- Take a careful history.
- Record the best acuity for each eye.
- Thoroughly evaluate the globe and orbit.
- Obtain appropriate radiologic studies.
- Have a detailed knowledge of eyelid and orbital anatomy.
- Ensure the best possible primary repair.

Blunt Trauma

Ecchymosis and edema are the most common presenting signs of blunt trauma. Patients should be evaluated for intraocular injury with a thorough biomicroscopic evaluation and a dilated fundus examination. Computed tomography, both axial and direct coronal, may be necessary to determine whether an orbital fracture is present. See Chapter 6 for further discussion of orbital fractures.

Penetrating Trauma

A detailed knowledge of eyelid anatomy helps the surgeon in repairing a penetrating eyelid injury and often reduces the need for secondary repairs. Generally, the treatment of eyelid lacerations depends on the depth and location of the injury.

Lacerations not involving the eyelid margin

Superficial eyelid lacerations involving just the skin and orbicularis muscle usually require only skin sutures. Unnecessary scarring can be avoided by following the basic principles of plastic repair. These include conservative debridement of the wound, use of small-caliber sutures, eversion of the wound edges, and early suture removal.

The presence of orbital fat in the wound means that the orbital septum has been violated. Superficial or deep foreign bodies should be searched for meticulously before these deeper eyelid lacerations are repaired. Copious irrigation washes away contaminated material in the wound. Orbital fat prolapse in an upper eyelid wound is an indication for levator exploration. A lacerated levator muscle or aponeurosis must be carefully repaired to enable the levator to function as normally as possible. Upper eyelid lagophthalmos and tethering to the superior orbital rim are common if the orbital septum is inadvertently incorporated into the laceration repair. Orbital septum lacerations should not be sutured. Meticulous closure of overlying eyelid skin and orbicularis muscle is adequate in all cases and avoids possible vertical shortening of the sutured orbital septum.

Lacerations involving the eyelid margin

Repair of eyelid margin lacerations requires precise suture placement and critical suture tension to minimize notching of the eyelid margin. Many techniques have been described, but the most important principle is that tarsal approximation must be made in a meticulous, direct manner (Fig 10-33). Eyelid margin closure may be accomplished by placing 2 or 3 sutures for alignment through the lash line, the meibomian gland plane, and (optionally) the gray line. Surgeons differ as to whether they place the tarsal or the eyelid margin sutures first. Precise anatomical alignment of the margin and secure tarsal closure are the goals, and many variations of techniques are acceptable. To avoid corneal epithelial disruption, the tarsal sutures should not extend through the conjunctival surface. The eyelid margin closure should result in a moderate eversion of the well-approximated wound edges. Resorbable buried sutures may be used in the margin as an alternative to the permanent externally tied sutures.

Trauma involving the canthal soft tissue

Trauma to the medial or lateral canthal areas is usually the result of horizontal traction on the eyelid, which causes an avulsion of the eyelid at its weakest points, the medial or

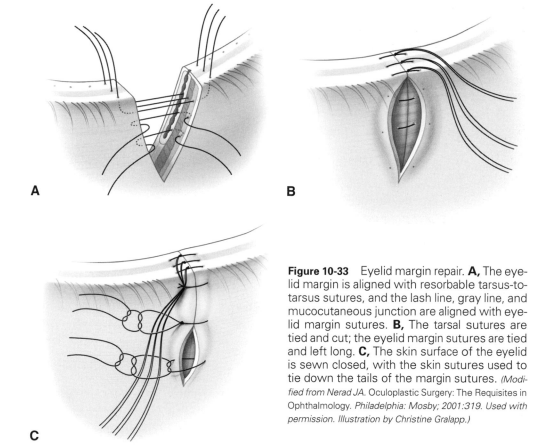

Figure 10-33 Eyelid margin repair. **A,** The eyelid margin is aligned with resorbable tarsus-to-tarsus sutures, and the lash line, gray line, and mucocutaneous junction are aligned with eyelid margin sutures. **B,** The tarsal sutures are tied and cut; the eyelid margin sutures are tied and left long. **C,** The skin surface of the eyelid is sewn closed, with the skin sutures used to tie down the tails of the margin sutures. *(Modified from Nerad JA.* Oculoplastic Surgery: The Requisites in Ophthalmology. *Philadelphia: Mosby; 2001:319. Used with permission. Illustration by Christine Gralapp.)*

lateral canthal tendon. Careful review of the patient's history often confirms that an object or finger engaged the eyelid soft tissue in the central aspect of the eyelid, with subsequent horizontal traction of the eyelid. Hence, lacerations in the medial canthal area demand evaluation of the lacrimal drainage apparatus, which is often involved in an avulsion injury. Canalicular involvement is usually confirmed by inspection and gentle probing. The examiner can assess the integrity of the inferior and superior limbs of medial or lateral canthal tendons by grasping each lid with a toothed forceps and tugging away from the injury while palpating the insertion of the tendon. Even trivial medial canthal injuries can result in canalicular lacerations.

Medial canthal tendon avulsion should be suspected when there is rounding of the medial canthal angle and acquired telecanthus. Attention to the posterior portion of the tendon's attachment to the posterior lacrimal crest is critical.

Treatment of medial canthal tendon avulsions depends on the nature of the avulsion. If the upper or lower limb is avulsed but the posterior attachment of the tendon is intact, the avulsed limb may be sutured to its stump or to the periosteum overlying the anterior lacrimal crest. If the entire tendon, including the posterior portion, is avulsed but there is no naso-orbital fracture, the avulsed tendon should be wired through small drill holes in the ipsilateral posterior lacrimal crest. If the entire tendon is avulsed and there is a naso-orbital fracture, transnasal wiring or plating is necessary after reduction of the fracture. A Y-shaped miniplate may be fixed anteriorly on the nasal bone, with posterior extension into the orbit. The suture is sewn through the severed tendons and passed through the holes in the miniplate. This technique is particularly helpful when the bone of the posterior lacrimal crest is missing.

A 3-dimensional perspective is crucial in the evaluation and repair of canthal lacerations; that is, to ensure optimal functional and cosmetic repair, the surgeon must always keep in mind the horizontal, vertical, and anteroposterior position of the canthal angle and medial canthal tendon. The different configurations of the medial and lateral canthal angles must also be considered. Whereas the lateral canthal angle is sharp, the medial canthal angle is slightly rounded. Failure to appreciate this difference gives rise to postoperative cosmetic and functional problems.

Devoto MH, Kersten RC, Teske SA, Kulwin DR. Simplified technique for eyelid margin repair. *Arch Ophthalmol.* 1997;115(4):566–567.

Goldenberg DC, Bastos EO, Alonso N, Friedhofer J, Ferreira MC. The role of micro-anchor devises in medial canthoplexy. *Ann Plast Surg.* 2008;61(1):47–51.

Howard GR, Nerad JA, Kersten RC. Medial canthoplasty with microplate fixation. *Arch Ophthalmol.* 1992;110(12):1793–1797.

Secondary Repair

Secondary repair of eyelid trauma usually requires treatment of cicatricial changes that resulted from either the initial trauma or the subsequent surgical repair. Revision of scars may require simple fusiform excision with primary closure or a more complex rearrangement of tissue. The location of a particular scar in relation to the relaxed skin tension lines (which correspond to the facial wrinkles in most cases) determines the best technique or combination of techniques to use. An elliptical excision of the scar is most useful for revision of scars that follow the relaxed skin tension lines. Single Z-plasty or multiple Z-plasty reconstructive techniques can be used for the revision of scars that do not conform to relaxed skin tension lines.

Free skin grafts alone or in combination with various flaps are used when tissue has been lost. Although any non–hair-bearing skin can be used, full-thickness postauricular or preauricular skin is the most commonly used donor site for lower and upper eyelid reconstruction. Ipsilateral or contralateral upper eyelid, supraclavicular or subclavicular areas, and even brachial or inner thigh areas are all potential donor sites for eyelid reconstruction.

Tarsoconjunctival grafts are good substitutes for posterior lamella eyelid defects when both the tarsal plate and the conjunctiva are deficient. Buccal mucosa may be used when only the conjunctiva is insufficient. Hard palate composite grafts have also become increasingly popular for posterior lamella defects in the lower eyelid. However, they should be avoided as a tarsal replacement in the upper eyelid because of the presence of keratinized epithelium, which can irritate the cornea.

Before treatment is considered for traumatic ptosis, the patient should be observed for 6 months or until no further spontaneous return of function occurs. An exception to this rule may be in a young child, in whom the possibility of deprivation amblyopia may necessitate early surgery to clear the visual axis.

Dog and Human Bites

Tearing and crushing injuries occur secondary to dog or human bites. Partial-thickness and full-thickness eyelid lacerations, canthal avulsions, and canalicular lacerations are common. Serious facial and intracranial injury is possible, especially in infants, as bites generate hundreds of pounds of force per square inch. Irrigation and early wound repair are mandatory, and tetanus and rabies protocols should be observed. Systemic antibiotics are recommended.

Bartley GB. Periorbital animal bites. *Focal Points: Clinical Modules for Ophthalmologists.* San Francisco: American Academy of Ophthalmology; 1992, module 3.

Burns

Burns of the eyelid are rare and generally are seen in patients who have sustained significant burns over large areas of the body. Often, these patients are semiconscious or heavily sedated and require ocular surface protection to prevent corneal exposure, ulceration, and infection. Lubricating antibiotic eyedrops and ointments, moisture chambers, and frequent evaluation of both the globes and the eyelids are part of the early treatment of these patients. Once cicatricial changes begin in the eyelids, a relentless and rapid deterioration of the patient's ocular status often ensues secondary to cicatricial eyelid retraction, lagophthalmos, and corneal exposure. If tarsorrhaphies are used, they should always be more extensive than seems to be immediately necessary. Unfortunately, with progression of the cicatricial traction, even the most aggressive eyelid adhesions may dehisce. In the past, skin grafting was usually delayed until the cicatricial changes stabilized, but the early use of full-thickness skin grafts, amniotic membrane, and various types of flaps can effectively reduce ocular morbidity in selected patients.

Eyelid and Canthal Reconstruction

The following discussion of eyelid reconstruction applies to defects resulting from tumor resection as well as congenital and traumatic defects. Several methods may be appropriate for reconstruction of a particular eyelid defect. The surgeon's choice of procedure depends on the age of the patient, the condition of the eyelids, the size and position of the defect, and personal experience and preference. Priorities in eyelid reconstruction are

- development of a stable eyelid margin
- provision of adequate vertical eyelid height
- adequate eyelid closure

involved, advancement of adjacent tissue or grafting of distant tissue may be required. The surgeon can cut the superior limb of the lateral canthal tendon to allow 3–5 mm of medial mobilization of the remaining lateral eyelid margin, taking care to avoid the lacrimal ductules in the lateral third of the upper eyelid. Removal or destruction of these ductules may lead to dry-eye problems. Postoperatively, the eyelid appears tight and ptotic because of traction, but it relaxes over several weeks.

Moderate upper eyelid defects

Moderate defects of the upper eyelid margin (33%–50% involvement) can be repaired by advancement of the lateral segment of the eyelid. The lateral canthal tendon is incised, and a semicircular skin flap is made below the lateral portion of the eyebrow and canthus to allow for further mobilization of the eyelid. Tarsal-sharing procedures in the upper eyelid may also be employed.

Large upper eyelid defects

Upper eyelid defects involving more than 50% of the upper eyelid margin require advancement of adjacent tissues. With an incision below the lower eyelid tarsus, a full-thickness lower eyelid flap is moved into the defect of the upper eyelid by advancement of the flap behind the remaining lower eyelid margin *(Cutler-Beard procedure)*. This procedure, however, results in a thick and relatively immobile upper eyelid. Alternatively, a free tarsoconjunctival graft taken from the contralateral upper eyelid can be positioned and covered with a skin-muscle flap if adequate redundant upper eyelid skin is present.

Small lower eyelid defects

Small defects of the lower eyelid (<33% involvement) can be repaired by primary closure (Fig 10-35). In addition, the inferior crus of the lateral canthal tendon can be released so that there is an additional 3–5 mm of medial mobilization of the remaining lateral eyelid margin.

Moderate lower eyelid defects

Semicircular advancement or rotation flaps, which have been described for upper eyelid repair, can be used for reconstruction of moderate defects in the lower eyelid as well. The flap most commonly used in such cases is a modification of the Tenzel semicircular rotation flap. Tarsoconjunctival autografts harvested from the underside of the upper eyelid may be transplanted into the lower eyelid defect for reconstruction of the posterior lamella of the eyelid. When tarsal grafts are being harvested, the marginal 4–5 mm height of tarsus is preserved to prevent distortion of the donor eyelid margin. Tarsoconjunctival autografts may be covered with skin flaps of various types. Cheek elevation may also be required so that vertical traction on the lid and ectropion can be avoided. Alternatively, a tarsoconjunctival flap developed from the upper eyelid and a full-thickness skin graft can also be used.

Large lower eyelid defects

Defects involving more than 50% of the lower eyelid margin can be repaired by advancement of a tarsoconjunctival flap from the upper eyelid into the posterior lamellar defect of the lower eyelid. The anterior lamella of the reconstructed eyelid is then created with an

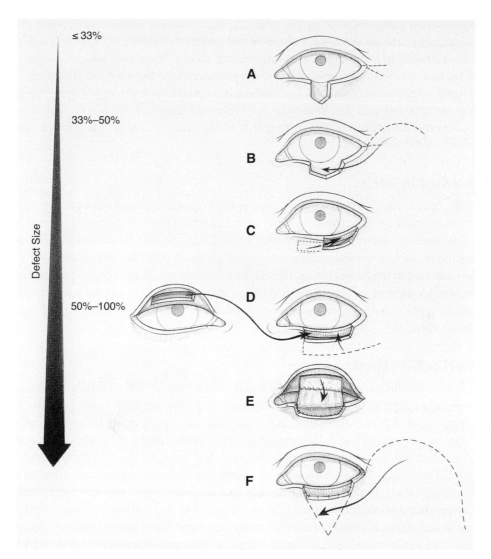

Figure 10-35 Reconstructive ladder for lower eyelid defect. **A,** Primary closure with or without lateral canthotomy or superior cantholysis. **B,** Semicircular flap. **C,** Adjacent tarsoconjunctival flap and full-thickness skin graft. **D,** Free tarsoconjunctival graft and skin flap. **E,** Tarsoconjunctival flap from upper eyelid and skin graft (Hughes procedure). **F,** Composite graft with cheek advancement flap (Mustardé flap). *(Illustration by Christine Gralapp.)*

advancement skin flap or, in most cases, a free skin graft taken from the preauricular or postauricular area *(modified Hughes procedure)*. The modified Hughes procedure therefore results in placement of a bridge of conjunctiva from the upper eyelid across the pupil for several weeks. The vascularized pedicle of conjunctiva is then released in a staged, second procedure once the lower eyelid flap is revascularized. Eyelid-sharing techniques should be avoided in children, as these patients may develop deprivation amblyopia. Large rotating cheek flaps *(Mustardé procedure)* can work well for repair of large anterior lamellar defects, but they require some tarsal substitute such as a free tarsoconjunctival autograft, hard palate mucosa, or a Hughes flap for posterior lamella replacement. Both the Mustardé cheek rotation flap and the Tenzel semicircular rotation flap frequently result in a rounded lateral canthus. The surgeon can reduce this problem by creating a very high incision toward the lateral end of the eyebrow where the incision emanates from the lateral commissure. Free tarsoconjunctival autografts from the upper eyelid covered with a vascularized skin flap have been used to repair large defects as well. This type of procedure has the advantage of requiring only 1 surgical stage and avoids even temporary occlusion of the visual axis.

Lateral Canthal Defects

Laterally based transposition flaps of upper eyelid tarsus and conjunctiva can be used for large lower eyelid defects extending to the lateral canthus. These flaps can be covered with free skin grafts. Semicircular advancement flaps of skin can also be used to repair defects extending to the lateral canthal area. Sometimes, strips of periosteum and temporalis fascia left attached at the lateral orbital rim can be swung over and attached to the remaining lateral eyelid margins for reconstruction of the entire lateral canthal posterior lamella. A Y-shaped pedicle flap of periosteum is optimal to reconstruct the entire lateral canthal posterior lamella.

Medial Canthal Defects

The medial canthal area lends itself to a variety of reconstructive methods. Spontaneous granulation of anterior lamellar defects has been used with varying success. Full-thickness skin grafting or flap reconstructions are more widely accepted repair techniques for medial canthal defects. When full-thickness medial eyelid defects are present, the medial canthal attachments of the remaining eyelid margin must be fixed to firm periosteum or bone. This fixation may be accomplished with heavy permanent suture, wire, or titanium miniplates. Defects involving the lacrimal drainage apparatus are more complex and require simultaneous microsurgical reconstruction and possible silicone intubation or marsupialization. If extensive sacrifice of the canaliculi has occurred in the resection of a tumor, the patient may have to tolerate epiphora until recurrence of the tumor is no longer a risk. Until tumor recurrence is ruled out, it is critical to avoid lacrimal surgery that could create a pathway for tumor to spread into the nose or sinuses. After a recurrence-free period of up to 5 years (based on clinical judgment), the patient may undergo a conjunctivodacryocystorhinostomy with a Jones tube to eliminate the epiphora.

Full-thickness skin grafts offer an excellent method of reconstruction of the medial canthus compared with the cicatrix resulting from spontaneous granulation. The full-thickness grafts are thin enough to allow for early detection of tumor recurrence. However, every effort should be made at the time of tumor resection to minimize the risk of recurrent medial canthal tumors. Frozen sections and wide margins or Mohs micrographic resection techniques minimize the risk of recurrent medial canthal tumors and the risk of orbital or lacrimal extension of these tumors. Large medial canthal defects of anterior lamellar structures may be reconstructed through the transposition of forehead or glabellar flaps. However, such flaps have the disadvantage of being thick, thereby making early detection of recurrences difficult. In addition, they often require second-stage thinning in order to achieve the best cosmetic result. Mohs micrographic resection of tumors offers the highest cure rates for eradication of medial canthal epithelial malignancies.

Lowry JC, Bartley GB, Garrity JA. The role of second-intention healing in periocular reconstruction. *Ophthal Plast Reconstr Surg.* 1997;13(3):174–188.

Spinelli HM, Jelks GW. Periocular reconstruction: a systematic approach. *Plast Reconstr Surg.* 1993;91(6):1017–1024; discussion 1025–1026.

CHAPTER 11

Periocular Malpositions and Involutional Changes

History and Examination

Whether young or old, presenting for medical (functional) or cosmetic complaints, all patients with eyelid malpositions require careful evaluation. A history of the presenting complaints, as well as a general medical history, is essential. The presenting morphology must be compared with normal, and any deviations noted. A basic eye examination should be performed, including visual acuity, ocular motility, corneal assessment (slit-lamp examination), and tests of tearing and protective mechanisms. Photography to document the preoperative state is generally indicated, with specialized testing of visual function, visual field, and other parameters as appropriate.

Preoperative Considerations

Preoperatively, careful attention to the patient's history and general medical problems helps to minimize unexpected complications, whether or not such conditions are related to the planned surgery. Pregnant women should wait until after delivery before proceeding with elective surgery. All patients should be asked about any history of bleeding diatheses or use of anticoagulants (such as warfarin sodium) or antiplatelet agents, including aspirin, clopidogrel, or nonsteroidal anti-inflammatory drugs (NSAIDs), any of which can lead to severe intraoperative or postoperative bleeding and adverse cosmetic and functional sequelae. Accordingly, anticoagulants such as warfarin are usually discontinued 2–5 days before elective surgery, if approved by the patient's primary care physician. Aspirin, because of its irreversible platelet inhibitory function, is generally stopped at least 5 days before elective surgery. NSAIDs, which are reversible platelet inhibitors, should be stopped at least 72 hours before surgery. Prothrombin time and partial thromboplastin time may be useful tests if coagulation status is a concern. Patients with a more complicated history of poor clotting should receive a preoperative hematologic consultation. The risks and benefits of stopping medications should be carefully discussed with the patient and his or her primary care physician.

Patients should also be asked about their use of over-the-counter preparations (eg, ginkgo biloba, vitamin E). As the popularity of alternative medicine has increased, so has the number of patients who use herbal and supplemental products. The lay population generally considers such products to be "natural" and therefore harmless or even

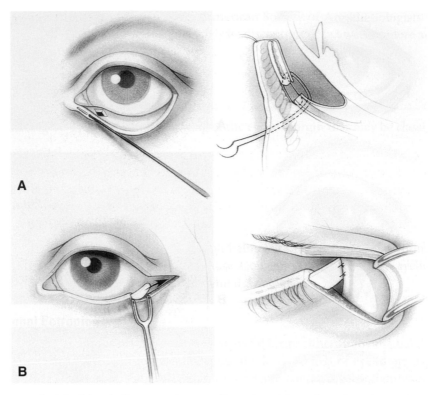

Figure 11-2 **A,** Medial spindle procedure: outline of excision of conjunctiva and retractors. **B,** Lateral tarsal strip procedure: anchoring of tarsal strip to periosteum inside lateral orbital rim. *(Illustration by Christine Gralapp.)*

Horizontal eyelid shortening

Horizontal eyelid laxity may be treated by direct shortening of the lateral canthal tendon or the lateral edge of the tarsal plate. The lateral tarsus is reattached to the lateral orbital rim periosteum (tarsal strip procedure). This procedure does not compromise the horizontal dimension of the palpebral fissure and maintains a sharp, correctly positioned lateral canthal angle.

Horizontal tightening can be achieved by means of a full-thickness excision of the eyelid just medial to the lateral canthal angle *(Bick procedure)*. Resection of the eyelid in this location may cause rounding and medial displacement of the lateral canthal angle. Repair of the eyelid defect following full-thickness resection is similar to that described in Chapter 10 for a full-thickness eyelid margin laceration (see Fig 10-35).

Laxity of the lower limb of the medial canthal tendon can be diagnosed by demonstration of excessive lateral movement of the lower punctum with lateral eyelid traction. Lateral canthal tendon laxity or disinsertion can be similarly detected. Repair of medial canthal laxity is difficult at best. Techniques can often be complicated by a kinking of the canaliculus or distraction of the punctum away from the globe, with resultant epiphora. A time-tested alternative to tighten and reposition the medial eyelid is the *lazy-T procedure,* which entails a medial wedge resection and spindle-type resection of the conjunctiva to tighten the eyelid and invert the lower punctum. This may correct medial ectropion with less lateralization of the punctum than a lateral tarsal strip procedure.

Fante RG, Elner VM. Transcaruncular approach to medial canthal tendon plication for lower eyelid laxity. *Ophthal Plast Reconstr Surg.* 2001;17(1):16–27.

Repair of lower eyelid retractors

Retractor laxity, disinsertion, or dehiscence may be associated with ectropion, especially when the eyelid is completely everted, a condition known as *tarsal ectropion*. Attenuation or disinsertion of the inferior retractors may occur as an isolated defect or may accompany horizontal laxity in involutional ectropion. When both defects are present, repair of the retractors is combined with a horizontal tightening of the eyelid. Reattachment of the retractors is performed directly through a conjunctival approach to advance the lower eyelid retractors to the inferior border of tarsus. These sutures exit more inferiorly through the skin to invert the lid margin (see Fig 11-2A).

Long-standing involutional ectropion with contraction of the anterior lamella (skin) usually requires horizontal tightening of the eyelid combined with midface lifting or full-thickness skin grafting. See discussion under Cicatricial Ectropion.

Jordan DR, Anderson RL. The lateral tarsal strip revisited. The enhanced tarsal strip. *Arch Ophthalmol.* 1989;107(4):604–606.

Nowinski TS, Anderson RL. The medial spindle procedure for involutional medial ectropion. *Arch Ophthalmol.* 1985;103(10):1750–1753.

Tse DT, Kronish JW, Buus D. Surgical correction of lower-eyelid tarsal ectropion by reinsertion of the retractors. *Arch Ophthalmol.* 1991;109(3):427–431.

Paralytic Ectropion

See discussion under Facial Paralysis later in this chapter.

Cicatricial Ectropion

Cicatricial ectropion of the upper or lower eyelid occurs following loss of skin secondary to thermal or chemical burns, mechanical trauma, surgical trauma, or chronic actinic skin damage. Cicatricial ectropion can also be caused by chronic inflammation of the eyelid from dermatologic conditions such as rosacea, atopic dermatitis, eczematoid dermatitis, or herpes zoster infections. Treatment of the underlying cause, along with conservative medical protection of the cornea, is essential as primary management. Cicatricial ectropion of the lower eyelid is usually treated in a 3-step procedure:

1. Vertical cicatricial traction is surgically released.
2. The eyelid is horizontally tightened with a lateral tarsal strip operation.
3. The anterior lamella is vertically lengthened via a midface lift or full-thickness skin graft.

Treatment of cicatricial ectropion or retraction of the upper eyelid usually requires only release of traction and augmentation of the vertically shortened anterior lamella with a full-thickness skin graft.

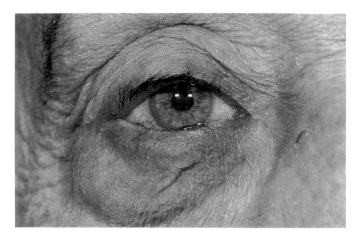

Figure 11-4 Involutional entropion.

Temporizing measures for acute intervention

Lubrication and a bandage contact lens may be used to protect the cornea from mechanical abrasion by the eyelashes. Suture techniques (Quickert sutures; see Fig 11-3) are occasionally helpful as temporizing measures in involutional entropion; but, when used as an isolated intervention, these techniques are associated with high recurrence rates. Similarly, thermal cautery is rarely successful in permanently stabilizing the eyelid, but it may be a valuable tool for in-office modification of the lid position to protect the cornea. Horizontal tightening of the eyelid at the lateral canthus, as in the lateral tarsal strip operation, stabilizes the eyelid and often corrects the entropion (see Fig 11-2B).

Repair of lower eyelid retractors

The Quickert suture procedure, a fast but usually temporary means of reinserting the retractors, can be combined with horizontal shortening techniques to increase the success rate and duration of the repair. Direct exploration and repair of lower eyelid retractor defects through a skin incision (Fig 11-5) or transconjunctival approach (Fig 11-6) can be performed to stabilize the inferior border of the tarsus. The retractor reinsertion operation is usually combined with a lateral canthal tightening of the eyelid. When retractor reinsertion is performed using an incision through the skin and orbicularis muscle at or near the inferior tarsal border, the incisional scar helps prevent postoperative orbicularis override. A small amount of preseptal orbicularis muscle can also be removed in selected patients who have a large amount of override. Reinsertion of the eyelid retractors and modification of the orbicularis in conjunction with a lateral tarsal strip operation corrects all 3 etiologic factors in involutional entropion.

Barnes JA, Bunce C, Olver JM. Simple effective surgery for involutional entropion suitable for the general ophthalmologist. *Ophthalmology.* 2006;113(1):92–96.

Ben Simon GJ, Molina M, Schwarcz RM, McCann JD, Goldberg RA. External (subciliary) vs internal (transconjunctival) involutional entropion repair. *Am J Ophthalmol.* 2005;139(3): 482–487.

Erb MH, Uzcategui N, Dresner SC. Efficacy and complications of the transconjunctival entropion repair for lower eyelid involutional entropion. *Ophthalmology.* 2006;113(12):2351–2356.

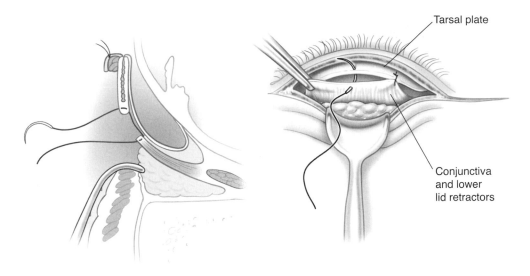

Figure 11-5 Retractor repair of involutional entropion. *(Illustration by Christine Gralapp.)*

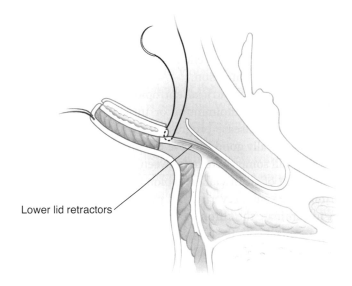

Figure 11-6 Retractor repair (transconjunctival approach). *(Illustration by Christine Gralapp.)*

Cicatricial Entropion

Cicatricial entropion is caused by vertical tarsoconjunctival contracture and internal rotation of the eyelid margin, with resulting irritation of the globe from inturned cilia or the keratinized eyelid margin (Fig 11-7). A variety of conditions may lead to cicatricial entropion, including *autoimmune* (cicatricial pemphigoid), *inflammatory* (Stevens-Johnson syndrome), *infectious* (trachoma, herpes zoster), *surgical* (enucleation, posterior-approach ptosis correction), and *traumatic* (thermal or chemical burns, scarring) conditions. The long-term use of topical glaucoma medications, especially miotics, a full-thickness conjunctival graft or flap, a partial-thickness buccal mucous membrane graft, or amniotic membrane graft.

Trichiasis

Trichiasis is an acquired misdirection of the eyelashes. The method used for treating trichiasis is usually dictated by the pattern (segmental or diffuse) of the misdirected lashes and the quality of the posterior lamella of the involved eyelid. Inturned lashes not associated with involutional entropion are usually seen in cases of posterior lamellar scarring (marginal cicatricial entropion). If the eyelid margin is misdirected, treatment should be directed at correcting the entropion.

Management

Trichiasis may be initially treated using *mechanical epilation,* removing misdirected lashes with forceps at the slit lamp. Because of eyelash regrowth, recurrence can be expected 3–8 weeks after epilation. Broken cilia are often more irritating to the cornea than mature longer lashes.

Standard *electrolysis* is still used for the treatment of trichiasis. However, the recurrence rate is high, adjacent normal lashes may be damaged, and scarring of the adjacent eyelid margin tissue can worsen the problem.

The *radiofrequency* unit allows treatment of each misdirected eyelash using a partially insulated needle tip inserted along the shaft of the cilia to the cilia's base. The radiofrequency signal is delivered for approximately 1 second on cut mode at a very low power setting to destroy the hair follicle. When the needle tip is removed, the lash is easily extracted.

Segmental trichiasis can be treated with *cryotherapy* in an office procedure that requires only local infiltrative anesthesia. The involved area is frozen for approximately 25 seconds, allowed to thaw, and then refrozen for 20 seconds *(double freeze–thaw technique).* The lashes are mechanically removed with a forceps after treatment. Edema lasting several days, loss of skin pigmentation, notching of the eyelid margin, and possible interference with goblet cell function are disadvantages of cryotherapy. This method may be combined with various surgical techniques and repeated if offending lashes persist or recur.

Argon laser treatment of trichiasis is not as effective as cryotherapy but can be useful when only a few scattered eyelashes require ablation or when the stimulation of larger areas of inflammation is undesirable. Some pigment is required in the base of the lash to absorb the laser energy and ablate the lash, making this technique sensitive to hair color.

In all these procedures, success rates vary, and additional treatment sessions are commonly necessary. *Full-thickness pentagonal resection* with primary closure may be considered when trichiasis is confined to a segment of the eyelid. Techniques for repair of entropion may be employed when extensive involvement is seen.

Dutton JJ, Tawfik HA, DeBacker CM, Lipham WJ. Direct internal eyelash bulb extirpation for trichiasis. *Ophthal Plast Reconstr Surg.* 2000;16(2):142–145.

Rosner M, Bourla N, Rosen N. Eyelid splitting and extirpation of hair follicles using a radiosurgical technique for treatment of trichiasis. *Ophthalmic Surg Lasers Imaging.* 2004;35(2):116–122.

Wilcsek GA, Francis IC. Argon laser and trichiasis. *Br J Ophthalmol.* 2003;87(3):375.

Blepharoptosis

The shortened form, *ptosis,* is frequently used in place of the more accurate term, *blepharoptosis,* to describe drooping or inferodisplacement of the upper eyelid. Ptosis is a common cause of reversible peripheral visual loss. Although the superior visual field is most often involved, central vision can also be affected. Many patients with ptosis complain of difficulty with reading because the ptosis worsens in downgaze. Ptosis has also been shown to decrease the overall amount of light reaching the macula and, therefore, can reduce visual acuity, especially at night.

Two classification systems are used to describe upper eyelid ptosis. It may be categorized by onset: congenital or acquired. In addition, it may be classified by the cause: myogenic, aponeurotic, neurogenic, mechanical, or traumatic. The most common type of *congenital* ptosis results from a poorly developed levator muscle (myogenic cause); the most common type of *acquired* ptosis is caused by stretching or disinsertion of the levator aponeurosis (aponeurotic cause).

Federici TJ, Meyer DR, Lininger LL. Correlation of the vision-related functional impairment associated with blepharoptosis and the impact of blepharoptosis surgery. *Ophthalmology.* 1999;106(9):1705–1712.

Evaluation

The patient's history usually distinguishes congenital from acquired ptosis. Patients with congenital or acquired blepharoptosis may be aware of a family history of the condition. Marked variability in the degree of ptosis during the day and complaints of diplopia should suggest ocular myasthenia gravis (MG). Complaints of dysphonia, dyspnea, dysphagia, or proximal muscle weakness suggest systemic MG.

Physical Examination

Physical examination of the ptosis patient begins with 5 clinical measurements:

- margin–reflex distance
- vertical palpebral fissure height
- upper eyelid crease position
- levator function (upper eyelid excursion)
- presence of lagophthalmos

The physician can record these data by using a drawing showing the cornea, the pupil size, and the position of the upper and lower eyelids in relation to these structures (Fig 11-9).

The *margin–reflex distance 1 (MRD$_1$),* which is the distance from the upper eyelid margin to the corneal light reflex in primary position, is probably the single most important measurement in describing the amount of ptosis. In severe ptosis, the light reflex may be obstructed by the eyelid and therefore have a zero or negative value. If the patient complains of visual obstruction while reading, the MRD$_1$ is also checked in the reading position. Lower eyelid retraction (or scleral show) should be noted separately as the *margin–reflex distance 2 (MRD$_2$).* The MRD$_2$ is the distance from the corneal light reflex

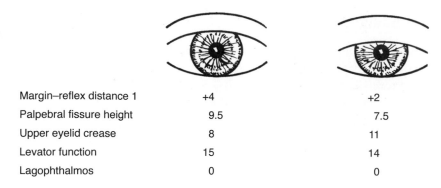

Margin–reflex distance 1	+4	+2
Palpebral fissure height	9.5	7.5
Upper eyelid crease	8	11
Levator function	15	14
Lagophthalmos	0	0

Figure 11-9 Example of ptosis data sheet.

to the lower eyelid margin. The sum of the MRD_1 and the MRD_2 should equal the vertical interpalpebral fissure height.

The *vertical interpalpebral fissure* is measured at the widest point between the lower eyelid and the upper eyelid. This measurement is taken with the patient fixating on a distant object in primary gaze.

The distance from the *upper eyelid crease* to the eyelid margin is measured. Because the insertion of fibers from the levator muscle into the skin contributes to formation of the upper eyelid crease, high, duplicated, or asymmetric creases may indicate an abnormal position of the levator aponeurosis. In the typical Caucasian eyelid, the upper eyelid crease is 8–9 mm in males and 9–11 mm in females. The crease is usually elevated in patients with involutional ptosis and is often shallow or absent in patients with congenital ptosis. The upper eyelid crease is typically lower or obscured in the Asian eyelid, with or without ptosis.

Levator function is estimated by measuring the upper eyelid excursion, or ULE, from downgaze to upgaze with frontalis muscle function negated (Fig 11-10). Fixating the brow with digital pressure minimizes contributions from accessory elevators of the eyelids such as the frontalis muscle. Failure to negate the influence of the frontalis muscle results in overestimation of levator function, which may affect the diagnosis and treatment plan.

Finally, the patient should be assessed for *lagophthalmos;* and if it is present, the degree should be noted.

Baroody M, Holds JB, Vick VL. Advances in the diagnosis and treatment of ptosis. *Curr Opin Ophthalmol.* 2005;16(6):351–355.

Other

Physical examination also includes checking head position, chin elevation, brow position, and brow action in attempted upgaze. These features help to show the patient how ptosis affects function. Quantity and quality of the tear film is documented in the initial examination. Lagophthalmos and poor tear-film quantity or quality may predispose a patient to complications of ptosis repair such as dryness and exposure keratitis. The exam-

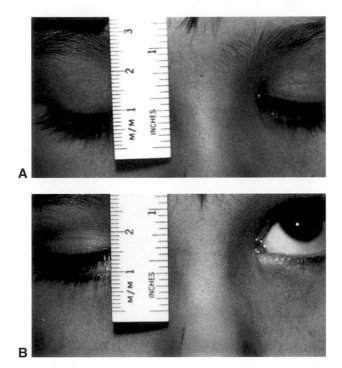

Figure 11-10 Measurement of levator excursion. **A,** Downgaze. **B,** Upgaze.

iner should also note the presence or absence of a normal Bell phenomenon and assess whether corneal sensation is normal; these factors may also affect the treatment plan.

Variation in the amount of ptosis with extraocular muscle or jaw muscle movements *(synkinesis)* is assessed. Synkinesis may be seen in Marcus Gunn jaw-winking ptosis, aberrant regeneration of the oculomotor nerve or the facial nerve, and some types of Duane syndrome. The examiner should attempt to elicit synkinesis as part of the evaluation of patients with congenital blepharoptosis or those with possible aberrant regeneration.

The *position of the ptotic eyelid in downgaze* can help differentiate between congenital and acquired causes. The congenitally ptotic eyelid is typically higher in downgaze than the contralateral, normal eyelid, as a result of eyelid lag. The congenitally ptotic eyelid may also manifest lagophthalmos. By contrast, in acquired involutional ptosis the affected eyelid remains ptotic in all positions of gaze and may even worsen in downgaze with relaxation of the frontalis muscle.

The ophthalmologist must assess *visual function and refractive error* in all cases of congenital or childhood ptosis in order to identify and treat the child with concomitant amblyopia resulting from anisometropia, high astigmatism, strabismus, or occlusion of the pupil. Amblyopia occurs in approximately 20% of patients with congenital ptosis. *Extraocular muscle function* should also be assessed because extraocular muscle dysfunction associated with ptosis occurs in various congenital conditions (combined superior rectus/levator muscle maldevelopment, congenital oculomotor palsy) and acquired conditions (ocular or systemic MG, chronic progressive external ophthalmoplegia, oculopharyngeal dystrophy, and oculomotor palsy with or without aberrant regeneration).

In addition, *pupillary examination* is important in the evaluation of ptosis. Pupil abnormalities are present in some acquired and congenital conditions associated with ptosis (eg, Horner syndrome, cranial nerve III palsy). Miosis that is most apparent in dim illumination is 1 finding in Horner syndrome; mydriasis is seen in some cases of oculomotor nerve palsy.

External examination may reveal other abnormalities as well. For example, severe bilateral congenital ptosis may be associated with telecanthus, epicanthus inversus, flattening of the superior orbital rim, horizontal shortening of the eyelids, and hypoplasia of the nasal bridge. These findings characterize an autosomal dominant condition known as *blepharophimosis syndrome* (discussed in Chapter 10, in the section Congenital Anomalies).

Ancillary Tests

Visual field testing with the eyelids untaped (in the natural, ptotic state) and taped (artificially elevated) helps determine the patient's level of functional visual impairment. Comparison of the taped and untaped visual fields gives an estimate of the superior visual field improvement that can be anticipated following surgery. Visual field testing and external full-face photography are required by third-party payers as a part of the initial evaluation in order to distinguish *functional* from *cosmetic* blepharoptosis repair.

Pharmacologic testing may be helpful in confirming the clinical diagnosis of *Horner syndrome* (Fig 11-11) and in localizing the causative lesion (see BCSC Section 5, *Neuro-Ophthalmology*). Although the differentiation among first-, second-, and third-order neuron dysfunction in the cause of Horner syndrome is important in the patient's general medical assessment, this information seldom alters treatment for the ptosis. Third-order neuron dysfunction resulting in Horner syndrome is typically benign. However, neuron dysfunction of the first or second order is sometimes associated with malignant neoplasms such as an apical lung (Pancoast) tumor, aneurysm, or dissection of the carotid artery.

Pharmacological testing may also be used in the diagnosis of myasthenia gravis (MG), a disease in which ptosis is the most common presenting sign. Fluctuating ptosis that seems to worsen with fatigue or prolonged upgaze, especially when accompanied by diplopia or other clinical signs of systemic MG, is an indication for further diagnostic

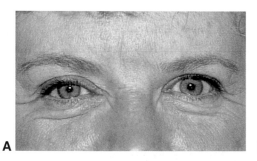 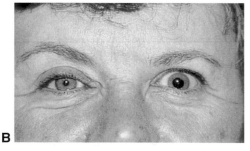

A **B**

Figure 11-11 Horner syndrome. **A,** Before instillation of topical cocaine. **B,** Pupil of normal left eye dilates after instillation of cocaine, but right pupil does not respond. *(Courtesy of Robert C. Kersten, MD.)*

evaluation with the edrophonium chloride, ice-pack, or acetylcholine receptor antibody tests. These tests are discussed later in this chapter under Neurogenic ptosis.

Classification

Myogenic ptosis

The patient's history usually distinguishes congenital from acquired ptosis. Patients with congenital or acquired blepharoptosis may be aware of a family history of the condition. *Congenital myogenic ptosis* results from dysgenesis of the levator muscle. Instead of normal muscle fibers, fibrous or adipose tissue is present in the muscle belly, diminishing the ability of the levator to contract and relax. Therefore, most congenital ptosis caused by maldevelopment of the levator muscle is characterized by decreased levator function, eyelid lag, and, sometimes, lagophthalmos (Fig 11-12). The amount of levator function is an indication of the amount of normal muscle. The upper eyelid crease is often absent or poorly formed, especially in cases of more severe ptosis. Congenital myogenic ptosis associated with a poor Bell phenomenon or with vertical strabismus may indicate concomitant maldevelopment of the superior rectus muscle (*double elevator palsy*, or *monocular elevation deficiency*).

Acquired myogenic ptosis is uncommon and results from localized or diffuse muscular disease such as muscular dystrophy, chronic progressive external ophthalmoplegia, MG, or oculopharyngeal dystrophy. Because of the underlying muscle dysfunction, surgical correction may be difficult, requiring frontalis sling procedures and/or procedures to repair lower eyelid retraction and improve corneal protection.

Demartelaere SL, Blaydon SM, Shore JW. Tarsal switch levator resection for the treatment of blepharoptosis in patients with poor eye protective mechanisms. *Ophthalmology.* 2006;113(12):2357–2363.

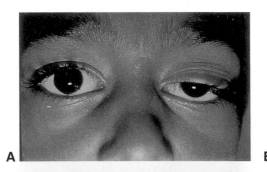
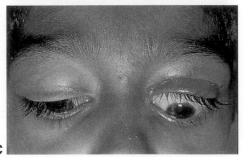
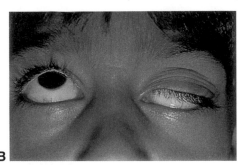

Figure 11-12 Bilateral asymmetric congenital ptosis. **A,** Note margin–reflex distance (MRD$_1$ = 5.0 mm OD, 1.0 mm OS). Normal = 4.5 mm. **B,** Upgaze accentuates ptosis. **C,** Downgaze exhibits eyelid lag. *(Courtesy of Robert C. Kersten, MD.)*

Aponeurotic ptosis

The levator aponeurosis transmits levator force to the eyelid. Thus, any disruption in its anatomy or function can lead to ptosis.

Acquired aponeurotic ptosis is the most common form of ptosis. It results from stretching or dehiscence of the levator aponeurosis or disinsertion from its normal position. Common causes are involutional attenuation or repetitive traction on the eyelid, which may occur with frequent eye rubbing or prolonged use of rigid contact lenses. Aponeurotic ptosis may also be caused or exacerbated by intraocular surgery or eyelid surgery (Fig 11-13).

Eyelids with aponeurotic defects characteristically have a high or an absent upper eyelid crease secondary to upward displacement or loss of the insertion of levator fibers into the skin. Thinning of the eyelid superior to the upper tarsal plate is often an associated finding and may allow visualization of the iris through the eyelid. Because the levator muscle itself is healthy, levator function in aponeurotic ptosis is usually normal (12–15 mm). Acquired aponeurotic ptosis may worsen in downgaze and therefore interfere with the patient's ability to read as well as limiting the superior visual field. Table 11-1 compares acquired aponeurotic ptosis with congenital myogenic ptosis.

Kersten RC, de Conciliis C, Kulwin DR. Acquired ptosis in the young and middle-aged adult population. *Ophthalmology.* 1995;102(6):924–928.

Neurogenic ptosis

Congenital conditions Congenital neurogenic ptosis is caused by innervational defects that occur during embryonic development. This condition is relatively rare and is most

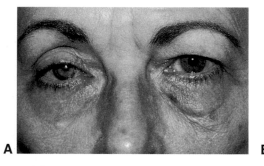

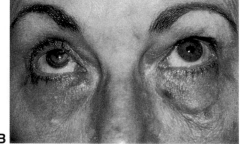

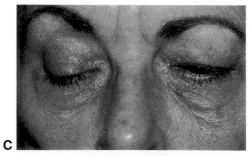

Figure 11-13 **A,** Levator aponeurosis ptosis following cataract surgery. Similar aponeurotic ptosis can occur following various other intraocular and eyelid surgical procedures as well. **B,** Excellent levator function on upgaze. **C,** Depression is greater than normal (eyelid drop) in downgaze.

Table 11-1 Blepharoptosis Comparison

	Congenital Myogenic Ptosis	Acquired Aponeurotic Ptosis
Margin–reflex distance 1	Mild to severe ptosis	Mild to severe ptosis
Upper eyelid crease	Weak or absent crease in normal position	Higher than normal crease
Levator function	Reduced	Near normal
Downgaze	Eyelid lag	Eyelid drop

commonly associated with congenital cranial nerve III (CN III) palsy, congenital Horner syndrome, or the Marcus Gunn jaw-winking syndrome.

Congenital oculomotor nerve (CN III) palsy is manifested as ptosis together with inability to elevate, depress, or adduct the globe. The pupils may also be dilated. This palsy may be partial or complete, but ptosis is very rarely an isolated finding in CN III palsy. It is uncommon to find aberrant innervation in congenital CN III palsies. Management of strabismus and amblyopia is difficult in many cases of congenital third nerve palsy. Treatment of the associated ptosis is also complicated, usually requiring a frontalis suspension procedure, which often leads to some degree of lagophthalmos. As a result of lagophthalmos, poor ocular motility, and poor postoperative eyelid excursion, postoperative management may be complicated by diplopia, exposure keratitis, and corneal ulceration.

Congenital Horner syndrome is a manifestation of an interrupted sympathetic nervous chain and may cause mild ptosis associated with miosis, anhidrosis, and decreased pigmentation of the iris on the involved side. The mild ptosis of Horner syndrome is due to an innervational deficit to the sympathetic Müller muscle, an eyelid elevator second in importance to the levator muscle. Decreased sympathetic tone to the inferior tarsal muscle in the lower lid, the analogue of the Müller muscle in the upper eyelid, results in elevation of the lower eyelid, sometimes called *lower eyelid reverse ptosis.* The combined upper and lower eyelid ptosis decreases the vertical interpalpebral fissure and may falsely suggest enophthalmos. The pupillary miosis is most apparent in dim illumination, when the contralateral pupil dilates more (see Fig 11-11).

Congenital neurogenic ptosis may also be synkinetic. *Marcus Gunn jaw-winking syndrome* is the most common form of congenital synkinetic neurogenic ptosis (Fig 11-14). In this synkinetic syndrome, the unilaterally ptotic eyelid elevates with jaw movements. The movement that most commonly causes elevation of the ptotic eyelid is lateral mandibular movement to the contralateral side. This phenomenon is usually first noticed by the mother when she is feeding or nursing the baby. This synkinesis is thought to be caused by aberrant connections between the motor division of CN V and the levator muscle. Infrequently, this syndrome is associated with abnormal connections between CN III and other cranial nerves. Some forms of Duane retraction syndrome also cause elevation of a ptotic eyelid with movement of the globe. This congenital syndrome is also thought to result from aberrant nerve connections.

Malone TJ, Nerad JA. The surgical treatment of blepharoptosis in oculomotor nerve palsy. *Am J Ophthalmol.* 1988;105(1):57–64.

Mechanical ptosis

Mechanical ptosis usually refers to the condition in which an eyelid or orbital mass weighs or pulls down the upper eyelid, resulting in inferodisplacement. It may be caused by a *congenital abnormality,* such as a plexiform neuroma or hemangioma, or by an *acquired neoplasm,* such as a large chalazion, skin carcinoma, or orbital mass. Postsurgical or post-traumatic edema may also cause temporary mechanical ptosis.

Traumatic ptosis

Trauma to the levator aponeurosis or the levator muscle may also cause ptosis through myogenic, aponeurotic, neurogenic, or mechanical defects. Eyelid lacerations exposing preaponeurotic fat indicate that the orbital septum has been transected and suggest the possibility of damage to the levator aponeurosis. Exploration of the levator muscle or apo-neurosis is indicated in these patients if levator function is diminished or ptosis is present. Orbital and neurosurgical procedures may also lead to traumatic ptosis. Because such ptosis may resolve or improve spontaneously, the ophthalmologist normally observes the patient for 6 months before considering surgical intervention.

Pseudoptosis

Pseudoptosis—apparent eyelid drooping—should be differentiated from true ptosis. An eyelid may appear to be abnormally low in various conditions, including hypertropia, en-ophthalmos, microphthalmia, anophthalmia, phthisis bulbi, or a superior sulcus defect secondary to trauma or other causes. Contralateral upper eyelid retraction may also simu-late ptosis. The term *pseudoptosis* is also sometimes used to describe *dermatochalasis,* the condition in which excess upper eyelid skin overhangs the eyelid margin, transects the pupil, and gives the appearance of a true ptosis of the eyelid margin (Fig 11-15).

Treatment of Ptosis

Ptosis repair is a challenging oculoplastic surgical procedure that requires correct diag-nosis, thoughtful planning, thorough understanding of eyelid anatomy, experience, and good surgical technique. The patient's ocular, medical, and surgical history help deter-mine whether surgical repair of ptosis is appropriate for that individual. The surgeon should be aware of any history of dry-eye syndrome and should temper blepharoptosis re-pair in the presence of significant dry-eye problems. Patients should be questioned about their coagulation status. Other pertinent historical queries should include the presence of thyroid eye disease, previous eye or eyelid surgery, and prior periorbital trauma. See also the section Preoperative Considerations earlier in this chapter.

Ptosis that causes significant superior visual field loss or difficulty with reading is considered to be a *functional* problem, and correction of this defect often improves a pa-tient's ability to perform the activities of daily living. In many instances, ptosis is consid-ered to be a *cosmetic* issue, causing a tired or sleepy appearance in the absence of a visual function deficit. Because ptosis repair is an elective surgical procedure, it is particularly important for the surgeon to have a preoperative discussion with the patient to communi-cate the alternatives, potential risks, and benefits.

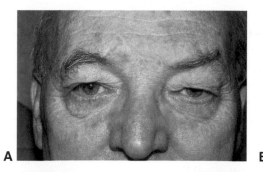
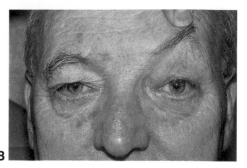
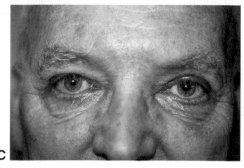

Figure 11-15 **A,** Patient with apparent ptosis of left upper eyelid. **B,** Manual elevation of dermatochalasis reveals this to be pseudoptosis; the underlying palpebral fissure is actually within normal limits. **C,** Clearance of visual axis is achieved following blepharoplasty alone. *(Courtesy of Robert C. Kersten, MD.)*

Surgical procedures designed to correct ptosis should be directed toward correction of the underlying pathologic condition. The 3 categories of surgical procedures most commonly used in ptosis repair are

- external (transcutaneous) levator advancement
- internal (transconjunctival) levator/tarsus/Müller muscle resection approaches
- frontalis muscle suspensions

The amount and type of ptosis and the degree of levator function are the most common determining factors in the choice of the surgical procedure for ptosis repair. The surgeon's comfort level and experience with various procedures is also an important factor. In patients with good levator function, surgical correction is generally directed toward the levator aponeurosis: the levator muscle is the most potent and useful elevator of the eyelid in most patients. However, if levator function is poor or absent, frontalis muscle suspension techniques are the preferred repair procedures.

External (transcutaneous) levator advancement surgery is most commonly used when levator function is normal and the upper eyelid crease is high. In this setting, the levator muscle itself is normal, but the levator aponeurosis (its tendinous attachment to the tarsal plate) is stretched or disinserted, thus requiring advancement. The levator aponeurosis is approached from the outside of the eyelid through the upper eyelid crease. This approach for acquired aponeurotic ptosis repair is particularly useful because it allows the surgeon to simultaneously remove excess eyelid skin (dermatochalasis). Reinsertion of the aponeurosis usually produces an excellent result. In some cases, the distal end of the aponeurosis may be found to be higher than its normal position on the lower anterior surface of the tarsus.

The *internal (transconjunctival)* approach to ptosis repair may be directed toward the Müller muscle, the tarsus, or the levator aponeurosis or muscle. *Müller muscle resections (Putterman müllerectomy)* are used in patients who have an adequate upper eyelid position following instillation of a drop of 2.5% phenylephrine hydrochloride. Müller muscle resections are typically used for repair of minimal ptosis (2 mm) and are generally considered superior to the *Fasanella-Servat procedure (tarsoconjunctival müllerectomy)* in maintaining eyelid contour and preserving the tarsus. The Fasanella-Servat ptosis repair procedure, though also directed toward small amounts of ptosis, requires removal of the superior tarsus.

When levator function is poor, the surgeon should consider utilizing the accessory elevators of the eyelid in ptosis repair. This type of surgery is most commonly required in congenital ptosis with poor levator function or in various forms of neurogenic ptosis with poor levator function.

Most patients with significant ptosis automatically elevate the forehead and brow on the affected side in an attempt to raise the eyelid and clear the visual axis; however, this maneuver is normally very inefficient because of the elasticity of the eyelid skin. In *frontalis suspension surgery* (performed when levator function is poor or absent), the eyelid is suspended directly from the frontalis muscle so that movement of the brow is efficiently transmitted to the eyelid. Thus, the patient is able to elevate the eyelid by using the frontalis muscle to lift the brow. Frontalis suspension can be performed transcutaneously or transconjunctivally (Fig 11-16).

Autogenous tensor fascia lata, banked fascia lata, and synthetic materials have been used for this purpose. *Autogenous fascia lata* has shown the best long-term results but requires harvesting and additional surgery. Generally, patients need to be at least 3 years old or weigh 35 pounds or more. *Banked fascia lata* may be obtained from a variety of sources and obviates the need for additional operative sites and harvesting. However, this material may incite immune reactions or inflammation and have poorer long-term outcomes than autogenous tissue. *Synthetic materials* such as silicone rods are commonly used; they may improve eyelid elasticity and allow easier adjustment or removal if necessary.

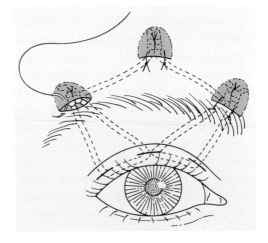

Figure 11-16 Frontalis suspension: Crawford method. *(Reprinted from Stewart WB. Surgery of the Eyelid, Orbit, and Lacrimal System. Ophthalmology Monograph 8, vol 2. San Francisco: American Academy of Ophthalmology; 1994:120.)*

There is some controversy about whether bilateral frontalis suspension should be performed in patients with unilateral ptosis. Unilateral frontalis suspension results in asymmetry in downgaze because of upper eyelid lag induced by the sling; in addition, there is less stimulus to elevate 1 brow. A bilateral procedure may improve the patient's symmetry, especially in downgaze, but it subjects the normal eyelid to surgical risks. The decision to modify a normal eyelid in an attempt to gain symmetry must be discussed by the surgeon and patient (or the parents if the patient is a child).

Carter SR, Meecham WJ, Seiff SR. Silicone frontalis slings for the correction of blepharoptosis: indications and efficacy. *Ophthalmology.* 1996;103(4):623–630.

Holds JB, McLeish WM, Anderson RL. Whitnall's sling with superior tarsectomy for the correction of severe unilateral blepharoptosis. *Arch Ophthalmol.* 1993;111(9):1285–1291.

Complications

The most common complication of blepharoptosis surgery is undercorrection. This has led some ptosis surgeons to use adjustable suture techniques or to advocate early adjustment in the office during the first 2 postoperative weeks when indicated. Judgment is required to differentiate true undercorrection from apparent undercorrection resulting from postoperative edema. Other potential complications include overcorrection, unsatisfactory or asymmetric eyelid contour, scarring, wound dehiscence, eyelid crease asymmetry, conjunctival prolapse, tarsal eversion, and lagophthalmos with exposure keratitis. Lagophthalmos following ptosis repair is most common in patients with decreased levator function. This condition is usually temporary, but it requires treatment with lubricating drops or ointments until it resolves.

Fagien S, Putterman AM, eds. *Putterman's Cosmetic Oculoplastic Surgery.* 4th ed. Philadelphia: Saunders; 2008.

Loff HJ, Wobig JL, Dailey RA. Transconjunctival frontalis suspension: a clinical evaluation. *Ophthal Plast Reconstr Surg.* 1999;15(5):349–354.

Eyelid Retraction

Eyelid retraction is present when the upper eyelid is displaced superiorly or the lower eyelid inferiorly, exposing sclera between the limbus and the eyelid margin. Lower eyelid retraction may also be a normal anatomical variant in patients with shallow orbits or certain genetic orbital or eyelid characteristics. Retraction of the eyelids often leads to lagophthalmos and exposure keratitis. The effects of these conditions can range from ocular irritation and discomfort to vision-threatening corneal decompensation.

Eyelid retraction can have local, systemic, or central nervous system causes. The most common causes of eyelid retraction are thyroid eye disease (TED), recession of the vertical rectus muscles, overly aggressive skin excision in blepharoplasty, and overcompensation for a contralateral ptosis (in accordance with Hering's law).

TED is the most common cause of both upper and lower eyelid retraction, as well as the most common cause of unilateral or bilateral proptosis (Fig 11-17). Because proptosis commonly coexists with and may mimic eyelid retraction in patients with TED, these

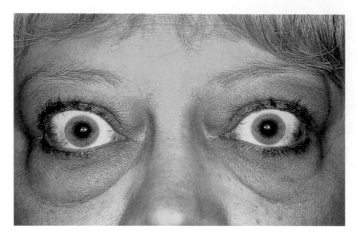

Figure 11-17 Thyroid-associated eyelid retraction. *(Courtesy of Roger A. Dailey, MD.)*

conditions must be distinguished from each other through eyelid measurements and ex-ophthalmometry. A common finding in thyroid-related eyelid retraction is *lateral flare.* In this condition, the eyelid retraction is more severe laterally than medially, resulting in an abnormal upper eyelid contour that appears to flare upward along the lateral half of the eyelid margin. The histological changes in the eyelid in TED are secondary to in-flammatory infiltration and fibrous contraction of the eyelid retractors. The sympatheti-cally innervated eyelid retractor muscles (the Müller muscle in the upper eyelid and the analogous eyelid retractor muscle in the lower eyelid) are preferentially affected by the inflammation and fibrosis of TED. See Chapter 4 for a more extensive discussion of TED.

Eyelid retraction may also be caused by recession of the vertical rectus muscles, owing to anatomical connections between the superior rectus and the levator muscles in the upper eyelid and between the inferior rectus muscle and capsulopalpebral fascia in the lower eyelid.

Another common cause of eyelid retraction, especially of the lower eyelids, is exces-sive resection of skin during cosmetic lower blepharoplasty. This surgical complication is more common in patients with preexisting lower eyelid laxity and may even manifest as frank ectropion. Midface lifting or full-thickness skin grafting may be required to correct this iatrogenic deformity. Conservative excision of skin in lower blepharoplasty, along with concomitant correction of any lower eyelid laxity, minimizes the risk of this problem.

Overcompensation for a contralateral ptosis (Hering's law) may also give the appear-ance of upper eyelid retraction. The surgeon must distinguish this condition from true eyelid retraction by observing the position of the supposedly retracted eyelid while the contralateral, presumably ptotic eyelid is either manually elevated or occluded.

Parinaud syndrome is an example of eyelid retraction caused by a central nervous system lesion. Congenital eyelid retraction occurs as a rare, isolated entity.

Lelli GJ Jr, Duong JK, Kazim M. Levator excursion as a predictor of both eyelid lag and lagoph-thalmos in thyroid eye disease. *Ophthal Plast Reconstr Surg.* 2010;26(1):7–10.

Meyer DR, Wobig JL. Detection of contralateral eyelid retraction associated with blepharopto-sis. *Ophthalmology.* 1992;99(3):366–375.

Treatment of Eyelid Retraction

The treatment of eyelid retraction is based on the underlying etiologic factors. Artificial tears, lubricants, and ointments may be sufficient to protect the cornea and minimize symptoms in cases of mild eyelid retraction. Mild eyelid retraction following lower blepharoplasty or in TED often resolves spontaneously with time. A variety of surgical techniques have been developed to correct eyelid retraction if the condition fails to resolve spontaneously or if the eyelid retraction causes an immediate threat to vision or the cornea. Various techniques involve release or recession of the eyelid retractors, with or without the use of spacers or grafts.

Eyelid retraction in TED can be managed by means of several surgical procedures. Unless there is severe exposure keratopathy, surgical intervention is indicated only after serial measurements have established stability of the disease over at least 6 months. Upper eyelid retraction can be corrected by excision or recession of the Müller muscle (anterior or posterior approach), recession of the levator aponeurosis with or without hang-back sutures or other spacer, measured myotomy of the levator muscle, or full-thickness transverse blepharotomy. Upper eyelid spacers include fascia lata, donor sclera, ear cartilage, or alloplastic materials.

If the patient has lateral flare (common in TED), a small eyelid-splitting lateral tarsorrhaphy combined with recession of the upper and lower eyelid retractors can improve the upper eyelid contour. This technique may limit the patient's lateral visual field.

As with the upper eyelids, surgical correction of lower eyelid retraction is also directed by the underlying etiologic factors. *Anterior lamellar deficiency* (eg, excess skin resection from blepharoplasty) requires recruitment of vertical skin by means of a midface lift or addition of skin with a full-thickness skin graft. *Middle lamellar deficiency* (eg, post-traumatic septal scarring) requires scar release and possible placement of a spacer graft. *Posterior lamellar deficiency* from congenital scarring or conjunctival shortage (eg, ocular cicatricial pemphigoid) may require a full-thickness mucous membrane graft.

Severe retraction of the lower eyelids, common in patients with TED, requires grafting of spacer materials between the lower eyelid retractors and the inferior tarsal border. Autogenous auricular cartilage or hard palate mucosa is a good spacer material for this type of surgery. Preserved sclera and fascia lata have also been used, as well as materials such as processed collagens (eg, Alloderm [LifeCell]; TarSys [IOP, Inc]). Some form of horizontal eyelid or lateral canthal tightening or elevation is also often necessary. However, because horizontal tightening of the lower eyelid in a patient with proptosis may exacerbate the eyelid retraction, this technique requires caution.

Bartley GB. The differential diagnosis and classification of eyelid retraction. *Ophthalmology.* 1996;103(1):168–176.

Ben Simon GJ, Mansury AM, Schwarcz RM, Modjtahedi S, McCann JD, Goldberg RA. Transconjunctival Müller muscle recession with levator disinsertion for correction of eyelid retraction associated with thyroid-related orbitopathy. *Am J Ophthalmol.* 2005;140(1):94–99 [comment in *Am J Ophthalmol.* 2006;141(1):233; author reply 233–234].

Demirci H, Hassan AS, Reck SD, Frueh BR, Elner VM. Graded full-thickness anterior blepharotomy for correction of upper eyelid retraction not associated with thyroid eye disease. *Ophthal Plast Reconstr Surg.* 2007;23(1):39–45.

Kersten RC, Kulwin DR, Levartovsky S, Tiradellis H, Tse DT. Management of lower-lid retraction with hard-palate mucosa grafting. *Arch Ophthalmol.* 1990;108(9):1339–1343.

Facial Paralysis

Paralytic Ectropion

Paralytic ectropion usually follows CN VII paralysis or palsy. Concomitant upper eyelid lagophthalmos is usually present secondary to paralytic upper eyelid orbicularis dysfunction. Poor blinking and eyelid closure lead to chronic ocular surface irritation from corneal exposure together with poor tear film replenishment and distribution. Chronically stimulated reflex tear secretion along with atonic eyelids and lacrimal pump failure account for the frequent complaint of tearing in these patients.

Neurological evaluation may be indicated to determine the cause of the CN VII paralysis. In cases resulting from stroke or intracranial surgery, clinical evaluation of corneal sensation is indicated because neurotrophic keratitis combined with paralytic lagophthalmos results in increased risk of corneal decompensation.

Lubricating drops, viscous tear supplementation, ointments, taping of the temporal half of the lower eyelid, or moisture chambers may be used alone or in combination. Such measures may be the only treatment necessary, especially for temporary paralysis. In long-term or permanent paralysis of the lower eyelid, tarsorrhaphy, medial or lateral canthoplasties, skin grafts, suspension procedures, and horizontal tightening procedures are useful in selected patients.

Tarsorrhaphies can be performed either medially or laterally. An adequate temporary tarsorrhaphy (1–3 weeks) can be achieved with nonabsorbable suture placement between the upper and lower eyelid margins. A temporary tarsorrhaphy may also be created by giving a botulinum toxin injection to the levator muscle. A permanent tarsorrhaphy involves careful de-epithelialization of the upper and lower eyelid margins, while avoiding the lash follicles. Next, absorbable or nonabsorbable sutures are placed to unite the raw surfaces of the upper and lower eyelids (Fig 11-18). In general, patients dislike the permanent tarsorrhaphy from a functional and cosmetic perspective. This procedure should be avoided, except in patients with recalcitrant corneal disease from exposure. Placement of a gold weight in the upper eyelid and repair of horizontal eyelid laxity or ectropion of the lower lid generally allow the patient to avoid permanent tarsorrhaphy.

Occasionally, a fascia lata or silicone suspension sling of the lower eyelid may be indicated. Vertical elevation of the lower eyelid is useful in reducing exposure of the inferior cornea. This elevation may be accomplished through recession of the lower lid retractors, combined with use of a spacer graft such as full-thickness hard palate mucosal or ear cartilage graft.

Paralytic Lagophthalmos

Gold weight loading of the upper eyelid is currently the most commonly performed procedure for the treatment of paralytic lagophthalmos. The patient should have some

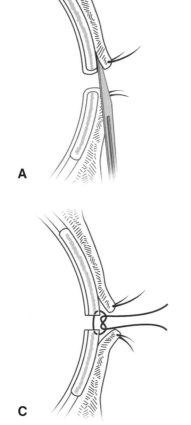

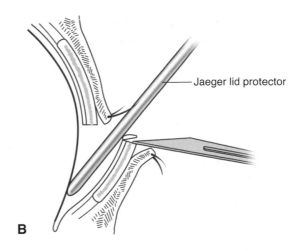

Jaeger lid protector

Figure 11-18 Tarsorrhaphy. **A,** Eyelid is split 2–3 mm deep. **B,** Epithelium is carefully removed along the upper and lower eyelid margins; the lash follicles are avoided. **C,** The raw surfaces are then united with absorbable sutures. *(Illustration by Christine Gralapp.)*

initiation of lid closure for the gold weight to work effectively. The appropriate weight can be selected through a process of preoperatively taping different sizes of gold weights to the upper eyelid skin to determine which one best achieves adequate relaxed eyelid closure with minimal eyelid ptosis in primary gaze. An upper eyelid crease incision is made through skin and orbicularis muscle. The gold weight is then sutured to the anterior surface of the tarsal plate. The gold weight implant (average weight, 0.8–1.6 g) reduces but does not usually eliminate lagophthalmos and corneal exposure. Should orbicularis function return, the weight is easily removed. A 1.2–2.2-g gold weight can also be placed behind the orbital septum, superior to the tarsus, to avoid thickening of the pretarsal area if cosmesis is a concern. Implanted eyelid springs to provide dynamic eyelid closure are infrequently used because of limited long-term success and extrusion.

Brow lift and midface suspension also can play an important role in the rehabilitation of the patient with facial nerve palsy.

Gilliland G, Wobig JL, Dailey RA. A modified surgical technique in the treatment of facial nerve palsies. *Ophthal Plast Reconstr Surg.* 1998;14(2):94–98.

Tower RN, Dailey RA. Gold weight implantation: a better way? *Ophthal Plast Reconstr Surg.* 2004;20(3):202–206.

Townsend DJ. Eyelid reanimation for the treatment of paralytic lagophthalmos: historical perspectives and current applications of the gold weight implant. *Ophthal Plast Reconstr Surg.* 1992;8(3):196–201.

Facial Dystonia

Benign Essential Blepharospasm

Benign essential blepharospasm (BEB) is a bilateral focal dystonia that affects approximately 30 of every 100,000 people. The condition is characterized by increased blinking and involuntary spasms of the eyelid protractor muscles, the orbicularis oculi, procerus, and corrugator superciliaris. The spasms generally start as mild twitches and progress over time to forceful contractures. The involuntary episodes of forced blinking or contracture may severely limit the patient's ability to drive, read, or perform activities of daily living. This condition can progress until the patient is functionally blind as a result of episodic inability to open the eyelids. Medical treatment options may include devices called *eyelid crutches,* which are attached to eyeglass frames. Women are affected more frequently than men. The age of onset is usually over 40 years. BEB is a clinical diagnosis, and neuroimaging is generally unrevealing and rarely indicated in the workup. Dry-eye syndrome and other medical conditions may result in reflex blepharospasm and must be differentiated from BEB.

Other muscles of the face may also be involved with blepharospasm. The cause of BEB is unknown; however, it is probably of central origin, in the basal ganglia. BEB can be managed by medical or surgical approaches. Oral medications have limited usefulness.

Anderson RL, Patel BC, Holds JB, Jordan DR. Blepharospasm: past, present, and future. *Ophthal Plast Reconstr Surg.* 1998;14(3):305–317.

Botulinum toxin injection

Repeated periodic injection of a botulinum toxin A—onabotulinumtoxinA (Botox, Allergan), incobotulinumtoxinA (Xeomin, Merz Pharmaceuticals), or abobotulinumtoxinA (Dysport, Tercica)—is the treatment of choice for BEB. These potent neurotoxins are derived from the bacterium *Clostridium botulinum* and alter receptor proteins in the presynaptic neuron, inhibiting the release of acetylcholine (Fig 11-19). Injection of 1 of these agents at therapeutic doses results in chemical denervation and localized muscle paralysis. Botulinum toxin injection is typically effective, but the improvement is temporary. Average onset of action is in 2–3 days, and average peak effect occurs at about 7–10 days following injection. Duration of effect also varies but is typically 3–4 months, at which point recurrence of the spasms and need for reinjection is anticipated (Fig 11-20).

RimabotulinumtoxinB (BTX-B; Myobloc, Solstice Neurosciences) is an antigenically and mechanistically distinct toxin produced by *C botulinum* that also exerts its effects at the neuromuscular junction. Compared with the type A toxins, type B, which is used in a significantly different dosage, has a quicker onset and greater diffusion in the tissues; but its duration of action is shorter. Patients treated with type B generally experience more

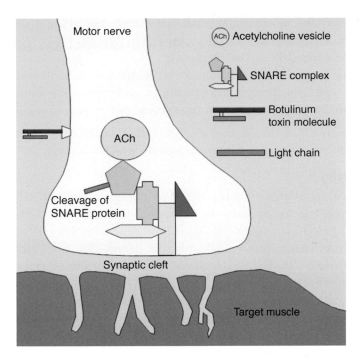

Figure 11-19 Botulinum neurotoxin binds to specific membrane acceptors, allowing internalization of the light chain. The various toxin serotypes cleave and inactivate different SNARE proteins, blocking their function. *(Reproduced from Dutton JJ, Fowler AM. Botulinum toxin in ophthalmology.* Focal Points: Clinical Modules for Ophthalmologists. *San Francisco: American Academy of Ophthalmology; 2007, module 3.)*

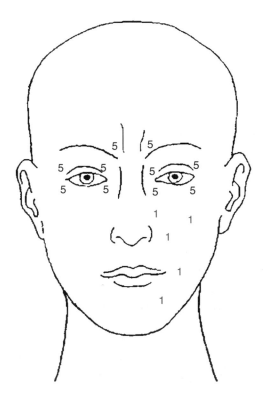

Figure 11-20 Average injection pattern of botulinum toxin type A for benign essential blepharospasm *(red)* and hemifacial spasm *(unilateral red sites plus blue). (Reproduced from Dutton JJ, Fowler AM. Botulinum toxin in ophthalmology. Focal Points: Clinical Modules for Ophthalmologists. San Francisco: American Academy of Ophthalmology; 2007, module 3.)*

discomfort at injection, and satisfaction rates are generally lower. Some patients who show a decreased clinical response or who fail to respond to treatment with type A botulinums find type B to be a safe and effective alternative.

Complications associated with botulinum toxin injection include bruising, blepharoptosis, ectropion, epiphora, diplopia, lagophthalmos, and corneal exposure. These adverse reactions are usually transient and result from spread of the toxin to adjacent muscles.

Dutton JJ, Fowler AM. Botulinum toxin in ophthalmology. *Focal Points: Clinical Modules for Ophthalmologists.* San Francisco: American Academy of Ophthalmology; 2007, module 3.

Surgical myectomy

Treatment with surgical myectomy is reserved for patients who are poorly responsive to botulinum therapy and incapacitated by the spasms. Meticulous removal of the orbital and palpebral orbicularis muscle in the upper (and sometimes lower) eyelids is an effective and permanent treatment for blepharospasm. Complications of surgical myectomy include lagophthalmos, chronic lymphedema, recurrence of spasm, and periorbital contour deformities. More limited myectomy is helpful in patients with less severe disease and may result in improved responsiveness to botulinum toxin therapy.

Many patients with blepharospasm have an associated dry-eye condition that may be aggravated by any treatment modality that decreases eyelid closure. Artificial tears, ointments, punctal plugs or occlusion, moisture chamber shields, and tinted spectacle lenses may help minimize discomfort from ocular surface problems.

Georgescu D, Vagefi MR, McMullan TF, McCann JD, Anderson RL. Upper eyelid myectomy in blepharospasm with associated apraxia of lid opening. *Am J Ophthalmol.* 2008;145(3): 541–547.

Surgical ablation of the facial nerve

Though effective in treating BEB, selective facial neurectomy has been largely abandoned. Recurrence rates as high as 30% and frequent hemifacial paralysis from facial nerve dissection limit this treatment's appeal. The results obtained with facial nerve dissection are, therefore, less satisfactory than those of direct orbicularis oculi myectomy. Some surgeons have had greater success with microsurgical ablation of selected facial nerve branches.

Fante RG, Frueh BR. Differential section of the seventh nerve as a tertiary procedure for the treatment of benign essential blepharospasm. *Ophthal Plast Reconstr Surg.* 2001;17(4): 276–280.

Muscle relaxants and sedatives

Muscle relaxants and sedatives are rarely effective in the primary treatment of BEB. Oral medications such as orphenadrine (Norflex, Graceway Pharmaceuticals), lorazepam (Ativan, Baxter Healthcare), or clonazepam (Klonopin, Teva Pharmaceuticals) are sometimes effective in suppressing mild cases of BEB, prolonging the interval between botulinum toxin injections, or helping to dampen lower facial dystonia (Meige syndrome) associated with BEB. Psychotherapy has little or no value for the patient with blepharospasm.

Hemifacial Spasm

Blepharospasm should be differentiated from hemifacial spasm (HFS). HFS is characterized by intermittent synchronous gross contractures of the entire side of the face and is rarely bilateral. HFS often begins in the periocular region and then progresses to involve the entire face. Unlike BEB, however, the spasms are present during sleep. HFS is often associated with ipsilateral facial nerve weakness. In most cases, the cause of HFS is a vascular compression of the facial nerve at the brain stem. Magnetic resonance imaging (MRI) often documents the ectatic vessel. MRI also helps rule out other cerebellopontine angle lesions that may be the cause in less than 1% of cases. Neurosurgical decompression of the facial nerve may be curative in HFS. Periodic injection of botulinum toxin is a commonly used, effective treatment option for HFS. Oral medications, including drugs with membrane-stabilizing properties, such as carbamazepine (Tegretol, Novartis) and clonazepam, are used less frequently because of their low efficacy.

Aberrant regeneration after facial nerve palsy also presents with hemifacial contracture and aberrant synkinetic facial movements. The history (eg, previous Bell palsy, trauma) and clinical examination are distinctive. Functionally troublesome synkinetic facial movements often respond well to botulinum toxin treatment at very low doses.

Involutional Periorbital Changes

Dermatochalasis

Dermatochalasis refers to redundancy of eyelid skin and is often associated with orbital fat protrusion or prolapse. Though more common in older patients, dermatochalasis also occurs in middle-aged people, particularly if there is a familial predisposition. Dermatochalasis of the upper eyelids is often associated with an indistinct or lower-than-normal eyelid crease. It also may accompany true ptosis of the upper eyelids (Fig 11-21).

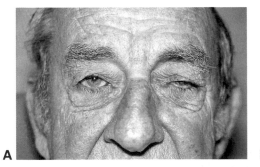 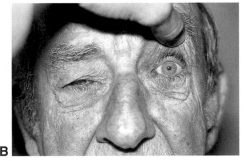

Figure 11-21 **A,** Patient with bilateral asymmetric drooping due to blepharoptosis and dermatochalasis. **B,** Elevation of more ptotic left upper eyelid reveals increased blepharoptosis on right, which had been masked by the effect of Hering's law of equal innervation to each levator muscle. *(Courtesy of Robert C. Kersten, MD.)*

Technique

Blepharoplasty begins with a thorough working knowledge of periorbital and eyelid anatomy (discussed in Chapter 9). In addition, just as the brow and glabellar areas affect the upper eyelids, the midfacial structures are influential in the position, tone, contour, and function of the lower eyelid and must be considered in the planning of lower eyelid surgery.

Surgical preparation involves marking excess skin for excision prior to the infiltration of local anesthetic. The surgeon may determine the amount of excess skin to be excised by using a pinch technique. For the upper lid, this involves placing 1 tip of the forceps in the eyelid crease. The other forceps tip is then advanced superiorly until the upper eyelid lashes begin to evert. The excess upper eyelid skin is pinched between the tips of the forceps and is marked with the surgical marking pen. The pen is then used to delineate the planned eyelid crease (often the existing upper eyelid crease) as well as the superior border of the planned area of excision. Typically, this marking process outlines a crescent or asymmetric elliptical shape on the upper eyelid. To avoid excessive skin removal, the surgeon usually leaves at least 20 mm of skin remaining between the inferior border of the brow and the upper eyelid margin. To avoid lid retraction or ectropion, the surgeon is extremely cautious with skin resection in the lower lid.

Anesthesia for blepharoplasty is typically a local infiltration of anesthetic agents with or without intravenous administration of sedatives. A rapid-onset, short-duration agent such as lidocaine 1% with epinephrine 1:100,000 may be mixed 50:50 with a slower-onset, longer-duration agent such as bupivacaine. A final epinephrine concentration of 1:200,000 is sufficient for maximizing vasoconstriction while minimizing the risk of epinephrine toxicity. Injection is best accomplished with sedation before the patient is prepared and draped and prior to surgical scrubbing. This allows enough time for the epinephrine to cause vasoconstriction and reduces perioperative bleeding. Supplemental local anesthetic and intravenous sedation is administered intraoperatively if needed.

Upper blepharoplasty

Upper blepharoplasty begins with the surgeon incising along the lines marked on the upper eyelid. The skin and underlying orbicularis oculi muscle can be excised as a single flap or in stages. The surgeon may preserve most or all of the orbicularis oculi muscle in patients with dry-eye syndrome.

In some cases, the orbital septum is incised exposing the underlying preaponeurotic fat pad. The surgeon may remove the fat by gently teasing it forward and excising it with scissors, cautery, or laser. If resection of the preaponeurotic fat pad is performed, it should go no deeper than the boundary created by the superior orbital rim. Removal of fat deeper than the rim may result in a hollow superior sulcus. The medial upper eyelid fat pad is typically prolapsed and is opened and contoured or excised in a similar manner. However, because the medial palpebral blood vessels overlie the medial upper eyelid fat pads, the surgeon must exercise caution to avoid significant bleeding in this area. The upper eyelid crease is created by the attachments of the levator aponeurosis to the orbicularis muscle and skin near the upper tarsal border. Aging often results in elevation or loss of the upper eyelid crease. The surgeon can correct a high, low, or absent eyelid crease during blepharoplasty by anchoring the eyelid skin to the levator aponeurosis with deep fixation sutures at the desired position. Alternatively, many surgeons rely on placement of the incision and excision of skin and muscle to manipulate the position of the upper eyelid crease. The upper eyelid skin can be closed with a running or subcuticular suture.

Lower blepharoplasty

Lower eyelid blepharoplasty, almost always performed for cosmetic purposes, is most often accomplished through a transconjunctival incision. At times, excess lower eyelid skin may necessitate a cutaneous incision. Skin removal during lower blepharoplasty increases the risk of lower eyelid contour abnormalities, retraction, or frank ectropion. Alternatively, excess skin can be tightened without excision through the precise application of laser skin resurfacing techniques or through chemical peeling with exfoliating solutions.

For transconjunctival surgery, preoperative evaluation defines the extent and location of lower eyelid fat prolapse and thus determines the boundaries of surgical excision. The surgery begins with retraction of the lower lid. The incision begins medially at the caruncle and then courses laterally 2–3 mm below the inferior tarsal border across the length of the eyelid. It is carried through the conjunctiva and lower eyelid retractors to gain access to the anterior face of the orbital fat pads.

Dissection then continues along the relatively avascular plane of the orbital septum toward the inferior orbital rim. Dissection along the orbital septum is also carried medially and laterally to expose the central, medial, and lateral fat compartments. The medial fat compartment is separated from the central fat compartment by the inferior oblique muscle. The surgeon must be aware of the location of the inferior oblique muscle between the nasal and central fat pads and work carefully around it to avoid damaging it during lower blepharoplasty. The medial fat pad of the lower eyelid, as in the upper eyelid, is more pale than the yellower lateral fat pads. The central fat compartment is separated from the lateral fat compartment by a fascial layer extending off the capsulopalpebral fascia; removal or incision of this fascial barrier may improve access to the lateral fat pad.

After the orbital septum overlying the fat pads is exposed and opened, the surgeon may carefully and gradually excise the fat while repeatedly checking the external contour of the lower eyelid. To improve access to and removal of the fat, the surgeon can apply pressure gently on the globe to help prolapse the fat forward. The surgeon stops the excision when the visible fat remains at or slightly behind the inferior orbital rim when gentle pressure is applied to the globe. Typically, similar volumes of fat are removed from each lower eyelid. Excessive fat removal may give the lower eyelid a hollow appearance. Alternatively, the fat can be mobilized over the inferior orbital rim and held in position to the suborbicularis oculi fat (SOOF) by sutures of the surgeon's choosing. Maintaining hemostasis throughout lower blepharoplasty is critical to the avoidance of vision-threatening complications. The conjunctival incision edges usually can be reapproximated without formal closure with sutures, although absorbable suture closure may be used.

Fagien S, Putterman AM, eds. *Putterman's Cosmetic Oculoplastic Surgery.* 4th ed. Philadelphia: Saunders; 2008.

Browpexy

Browpexy is performed through an upper eyelid blepharoplasty incision for mild to moderate brow ptosis. The sub-brow tissues are resuspended with sutures to the frontal bone periosteum above the orbital rim as part of a blepharoplasty.

McCord CD, Doxanas MT. Browplasty and browpexy: an adjunct to blepharoplasty. *Plast Reconstr Surg.* 1990;86(2):248–254.

Direct eyebrow elevation

The eyebrows can be elevated with incisions placed at the upper edge of the eyebrow. This procedure is useful for men and women with lateral eyebrow ptosis. When direct eyebrow elevation is used across the entire brow, it may result in an unacceptable arch or scar.

Booth AJ, Murray A, Tyers AG. The direct brow lift: efficacy, complications, and patient satisfaction. *Br J Ophthalmol.* 2004;88(5):688–691.

Miller TA, Rudkin G, Honig M, Elahi M, Adams J. Lateral subcutaneous brow lift and interbrow muscle resection: clinical experience and anatomic studies. *Plast Reconstr Surg.* 2000;105(3):1120–1127 [discussion, 1128].

Cosmetic Facial Surgery

Most ophthalmic plastic surgeons think that effective treatment of cosmetic and reconstructive upper eyelid problems should include consideration of eyebrow and forehead surgery. Likewise, effective lower eyelid cosmetic and reconstructive surgery should include consideration of midface and cheek surgery. Consequently, most ophthalmic plastic surgical fellowship programs in the United States include training in facial cosmetic and reconstructive surgery. Although it is important for any eyelid surgeon to understand the surgical procedures discussed here, the performance of these procedures generally requires special training, experience, and expertise.

The human face is an essential component of interpersonal communication. The aging face may communicate fatigue, depression, anger, or fear in an otherwise well-rested, well-adjusted, fully functioning person. The face is composed of smaller cosmetic units of the forehead, eyelids, cheek, nose, lips, and neck. As we age, one or more of these cosmetic units undergo changes that lead to facial imbalance, disharmony, and possibly miscommunication. If a single subunit has aged out of proportion to the rest of the face, as in dermatochalasis, an isolated repair with a bilateral upper blepharoplasty produces a nice result. On the other hand, if the patient has concomitant aging changes of the midface, lower face, and neck but undergoes only lower eyelid blepharoplasty, the result may be unsatisfactory and perpetuate further facial miscommunication, chronologic facial imbalance, and perceptual confusion.

Pathogenesis of the Aging Face

Factors that lead to involutional facial changes can be divided into 2 categories: intrinsic and extrinsic. *Intrinsic aging* refers to changes that occur as a result of chronologic aging.

Extrinsic aging results from environmental factors such as cigarette smoke, ultraviolet radiation, wind, and gravity.

The facial contours and appearance are derived from soft tissue draped over underlying bone. The soft-tissue component is composed of skin, subcutaneous fat, muscle, deeper fat pads, and fascial layers. The underlying structural element is composed of bone, cartilage, and teeth.

As the face ages, the soft-tissue component moves inferiorly and the bone component loses mass. These changes leave relatively more soft tissue to hang from its attachments to the bone. Loss of subcutaneous fat, skin atrophy, and descent of facial fat pads compound this facial sagging. Around the eyes, the lateral brow typically descends more than the medial brow, which leads to temporal hooding. The orbital septum stretches, bulges, or dehisces, allowing fat to prolapse forward. In the lower lid, midface descent produces the skeletonization of the infraorbital rim and increases the prominence of the orbital fat. This has been described as a *double convexity deformity,* and it also contributes to the increased prominence of the nasolabial fold. Sagging of the platysma muscle in the neck posterior to the mandibular ligament gives rise to jowling. The *turkey gobbler defect* in the neck is the result of redundant skin and separated medial borders of the platysma muscle at the midline.

Physical Examination of the Aging Face

Much of the surgeon's appraisal of the aging face can be obtained through close observation of the patient during the introduction and history phase of the initial meeting. From the top, the surgeon should observe the hairstyle and hair thickness, the presence of bangs, and the height of the hairline; the use of the frontalis; the position of the brow; the texture and quality of the facial skin; and the presence and location of rhytids, telangiectasias, pigmentary dyschromia, and expressive furrows.

If chemical peeling or laser skin resurfacing is being considered, the surgeon should also note the patient's Fitzpatrick skin type, which affects healing after these procedures. There are 6 skin types in the Fitzpatrick classification system, which denotes skin color and reaction of the skin to sun exposure. The higher the number, the greater the amount of skin pigment. Thus, Fitzpatrick type I refers to persons with minimal skin pigment and very fair skin. These individuals always burn with sun exposure and do not tan. Type VI represents individuals with markedly pigmented black skin, typically persons of African ancestry.

In addition, the surgeon should assess eyelid skin and fat along with eyelid margin position relative to the pupil and cornea, presence or absence of horizontal lower lid laxity, midface position, presence of jowling, accumulation of subcutaneous fat in the neck, and chin position. He or she should note any nasal deformities and tip descent and broadening, as well as thinning of the lips. The surgeon may find a side view of the neck to be particularly helpful in determining the extent of aging. Preoperative photographs should be available in the operating room.

Flynn TC. Botulinum toxin: examining duration of effect in facial aesthetic applications. *Am J Clin Dermatol.* 2010;11(3):183–199.

Lipham WJ. *Cosmetic and Clinical Applications of Botox and Dermal Fillers.* 2nd ed. Thorofare, NJ: Slack, Inc; 2008.

Forehead Rejuvenation

Many options are available for forehead rejuvenation, but the following discussion focuses on 2 methods commonly used in cosmetic surgery: the standard endoscopic brow lift and the pretrichial approach.

Endoscopic brow and forehead lift: standard approach

Endoscopic techniques allow the surgeon to raise the brow and rejuvenate the forehead (foreheadplasty) through small incisions approximately 1 cm behind the hairline (Fig 11-23). An endoscope protected by a hooded sleeve is attached through a fiberoptic light cord to a light source. A camera is also attached to the endoscope and is connected to a video monitor. Dissection is accomplished with an endoscopic periosteal elevator, sharp scissors, suction, and monopolar cautery. Key steps are the creation of an optical cavity, periosteal release at the orbital rim, and fixation of the elevated flap.

Much of the procedure is performed without the endoscope. A central subperiosteal space, or *optical pocket,* is developed posteriorly to the occiput and anteriorly to 1–2 cm above the superior orbital rim. The sheathed endoscope can then be used to complete the dissection in the area of the orbital rim where the supraorbital and supratrochlear neurovascular bundles are visualized. If indicated, the corrugator and procerus muscles are stripped or removed altogether. The central subperiosteal pocket is used to release periosteum along the superior rim, and the temporal pockets allow release of periosteum along the lateral brow. Dissection along the deep temporalis fascia spares the frontal branch of the facial nerve in the overlying temporoparietal fascia. The central and temporal pockets are joined through release of the conjoint fascia, which is firmly adherent tissue along the temporal lines.

Once elevation is completed, fixation and closure are the final steps. Fixation points are based on the preoperative brow position. The wounds are closed with surgical staples. Fixation options for the forehead flap include fixation screws, bone tunnels, fibrin sealant, bone anchors, and various soft-tissue fixation devices.

Berkowitz RL, Jacobs DI, Gorman PJ. Brow fixation with the Endotine Forehead device in endoscopic brow lift. *Plast Reconstr Surg.* 2005;116(6):1761–1770.

Jones BM, Grover R. Endoscopic brow lift: a personal review of 538 patients and comparison of fixation techniques. *Plast Reconstr Surg.* 2004;113(4):1242–1250 [discussion, 1251–1252].

Endoscopic brow lift: pretrichial approach

The pretrichial approach is used in patients who have, are or concerned about developing, a high hairline. Access is gained through a pretrichial incision instead of the small skin incisions used with the endoscopic approach. Periosteal release can be performed endoscopically through incisions in the galea, frontalis muscle, and periosteum. An appropriate amount of forehead skin is resected, and the underlying frontalis and galea are plicated with a subsequent layered closure.

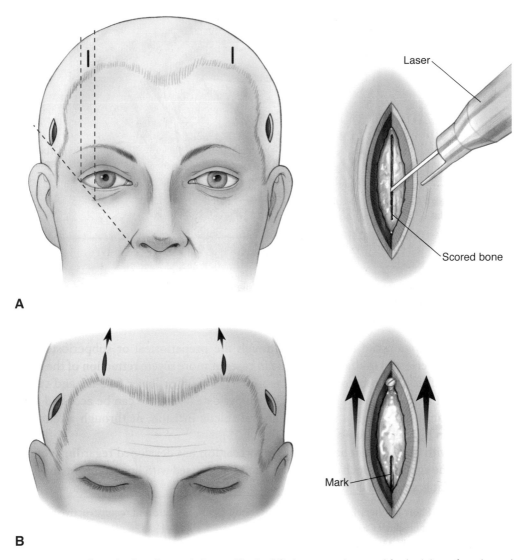

A

B

Figure 11-23 Standard endoscopic brow lift. **A,** CO_2 laser can be used for incision of scalp and scoring of bone. **B,** The scalp is retracted posteriorly, and the fixation screw is placed at the posterior aspect of the incision. *(Illustrations by Christine Gralapp.)*

Midface Rejuvenation

The entire midface should be evaluated in a patient presenting for lower eyelid blepharoplasty. With age, cheek tissue descends and orbital fat herniates, creating the double-convexity deformity. Varying degrees of elevation of the SOOF and midface, combined with conservative transconjunctival fat removal or redistribution, can restore youthful anterior projection of the midface, rendering a single smooth contour to the lower eyelid and midface region. A lower lid approach (infraciliary or transconjunctival) or a temporal endoscopic approach may be used (Fig 11-24).

musculoaponeurotic system (SMAS), and the deep-plane rhytidectomy. The classic rhytidectomy was the procedure of choice throughout most of the 1970s. The anatomical work of Mitz and Peyronie and the surgical approach of Skoog led surgeons to mobilize and secure the deeper SMAS layer, allowing better skin support and more lasting results. Rhytidectomies typically include surgical management of the neck, including liposuction with or without platysmaplasty.

The 3 rhytidectomy procedures briefly discussed in this section differ mainly in the location and extent of dissection. Although the more superficial procedures are less likely to cause facial nerve damage, they also may produce less lasting improvement. The more extensive procedures have greater risks (eg, facial nerve injury), but the likelihood that they will produce dramatic, longer-lasting improvement is also greater.

Classic (subcutaneous) rhytidectomy The standard face-lift incisions are marked. In men, a pretragal incision is generally made; a posttragal incision is generally used in women. The submental incision, if used, is placed 2 mm posterior to the submental crease.

Subcutaneous undermining of the skin is then initiated, first with a blade and then with scissors. The more medial dissection is visualized with direct illumination from a fiberoptic retractor or surgeon's headlight. After bilateral exposure, the skin is redraped in a posterosuperior manner, and skin resection is initiated. Fixation sutures are placed, but there should be essentially no traction on the flap, particularly the postauricular portion where it is the most susceptible to necrosis.

Complications of this technique are directly related to the extent of subcutaneous undermining; they include hematoma, seroma, skin necrosis, hair loss, paresthesias, motor deficits, incisional scarring, asymmetry, and contour irregularities. Hematoma is the leading surgical face-lift complication, but patient dissatisfaction may be the most common problem for the facial surgeon postoperatively.

Subcutaneous rhytidectomy with SMAS Subcutaneous rhytidectomy with SMAS plication or resection differs from the classic rhytidectomy in that the SMAS is mobilized along with subcutaneous dissection (Fig 11-26). Mobilization of the SMAS allows more skin to be repositioned with deep support for a more natural, less surgical appearance. This improves jowling and enhances the appearance of the jawline.

Deep-plane rhytidectomy The deep-plane rhytidectomy also involves mobilization of the SMAS. The extent of SMAS dissection is greater than with the combined technique, but the amount of subcutaneous dissection over the SMAS is less. Dissection is extended to the mandible for greater mobilization. The edge of the SMAS flap is attached to the firm preauricular tissues (Fig 11-27). The lateral platysma in the neck is plicated, and excess skin is resected and closed without tension. The deep-plane approach is considered the most surgically demanding.

Neck liposuction

Stab incisions, or *adits,* are made just posterior to the earlobe on each side and just anterior to the central submental crease. Microcannulas allow fat removal. A layer of fat is left on the dermis, and the liposuction cannula openings are always oriented away from the dermis to avoid injury to the vascular plexus deep to the dermis. In addition to abnormalities

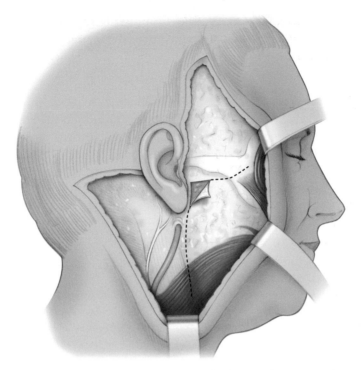

Figure 11-26 Subcutaneous rhytidectomy with superficial musculoaponeurotic system (SMAS). *(Illustration by Christine Gralapp.)*

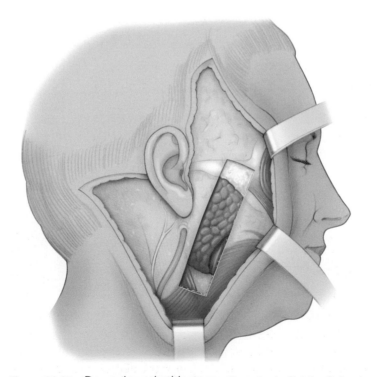

Figure 11-27 Deep-plane rhytidectomy. *(Illustration by Christine Gralapp.)*

in skin quality, damage in this area can lead to unsightly scarring of the dermis of the underlying neck musculature. The adits are left open, and a compression bandage is worn for 1 week after the procedure.

Platysmaplasty

Platysmaplasty is performed to correct platysmal bands. A subcutaneous dissection is carried out in the preplatysmal plane centrally under the chin to the level of the thyroid cartilage (Fig 11-28A). Lateral platysmal undermining and suspension may be performed as part of a rhytidectomy. Midline platysma resection and reconstruction (Fig 11-28B) are performed if midline neck support is needed. A drain and a light compression dressing are placed. Postoperatively, the cervicomental angle is more acute, yielding a more youthful look.

Baker DC. Minimal incision rhytidectomy (short scar face lift) with lateral SMASectomy: evolution and application. *Aesthet Surg J.* 2001;21(1):14–26.

Baylis HI, Goldberg RA, Shorr N. The deep plane facelift: a 20-year evolution of technique. *Ophthalmology.* 2000;107(3):490–495.

Dailey RA, Jones LT. Rejuvenation of the aging face. *Focal Points: Clinical Modules for Ophthalmologists.* San Francisco: American Academy of Ophthalmology; 2003, module 11.

Klein JA. *Tumescent Technique: Tumescent Anesthesia & Microcannular Liposuction.* St Louis: Mosby; 2000.

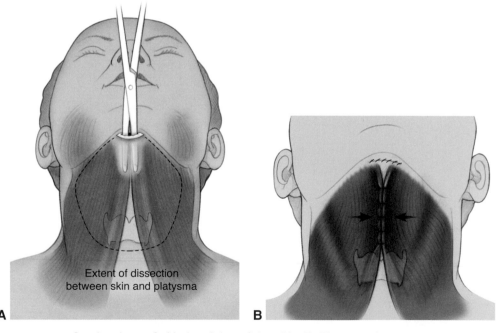

Extent of dissection between skin and platysma

A

B

Figure 11-28 Cervicoplasty. **A,** Undermining of the skin. **B,** Platysmaplasty. *(Illustrations by Christine Gralapp.)*

Conclusions

The periocular area is part of the larger anatomical superstructure of the face, whose primary function is communication. Changes produced by aging, disease, or surgery can affect the messages transmitted by this entity. If a single subunit is altered without consideration of the other subunits, facial miscommunication, chronologic facial imbalance, and perceptual confusion can result. It is therefore incumbent upon the oculofacial surgeon to understand the aging process, anatomy, and available surgical techniques before embarking on surgery that changes any portion of the face. Discussion of these issues with the patient preoperatively helps prevent patient dissatisfaction postoperatively.

PART **III**

Lacrimal System

CHAPTER 12

Development, Anatomy, and Physiology of the Lacrimal Secretory and Drainage Systems

Development

Secretory Apparatus

The lacrimal gland develops from multiple solid ectodermal buds in the anterior supero-lateral orbit. These buds branch and canalize, forming ducts and alveoli. The lacrimal glands are small and do not function fully until approximately 6 weeks after birth. This explains why newborn infants do not produce tears when crying.

Excretory Apparatus

By the end of the fifth gestational week, the nasolacrimal groove forms as a furrow lying between the nasal and maxillary prominence. In the floor of this groove, the nasolacrimal duct (NLD) develops from a linear thickening of the ectoderm. A solid cord separates from adjacent ectoderm and sinks into the mesenchyme. The cord canalizes, forming the NLD and the lacrimal sac at its cranial end. The canaliculi are thought to form similarly from invaginated ectoderm continuous with the distal cord. Caudally, the duct extends intranasally, exiting within the inferior meatus. Canalization is usually complete around the time of birth. Failure of the caudal end to completely canalize results in congenital NLD obstruction. Obstruction at the distal end (the valve of Hasner) is present in ap-proximately 50% of infants at birth. Patency usually occurs spontaneously within the first few months of life. As explained previously, lacrimation does not function normally until 6 weeks; therefore, excessive tearing may not be immediately obvious if an obstruction exists.

Normal Anatomy

Secretory Apparatus

The main lacrimal gland is an exocrine gland located in the superior lateral quadrant of the orbit within the lacrimal gland fossa. Embryologic development of the lateral horn of the levator aponeurosis indents the lacrimal gland and divides it anteriorly into orbital and palpebral lobes (see Chapter 1, Fig 1-7). The superior transverse ligament (Whitnall ligament) inserts at the division of the 2 lobes, with some fibers also projecting onto the lateral orbital tubercle.

Some 8–12 major lacrimal ducts empty into the superior cul-de-sac approximately 5 mm above the lateral tarsal border after passing posterior to the aponeurosis, through the Müller muscle and the conjunctiva. The ducts from the orbital portion run through and join the ducts of the palpebral lobe. Therefore, removal of or damage to the palpebral portion of the gland can seriously reduce secretion from the entire gland. This is the reason that biopsy of the lacrimal gland is generally performed on the orbital lobe.

Ocular surface irritation activates tear production from the lacrimal gland. The ophthalmic branch of the trigeminal nerve provides the sensory *(afferent)* pathway in this reflex tear arc. The *efferent* pathway is more complicated. Parasympathetic fibers, originating in the superior salivary nucleus of the pons, exit the brain stem with the facial nerve, cranial nerve VII (CN VII). Lacrimal fibers leave CN VII as the greater superficial petrosal nerve and pass to the sphenopalatine ganglion. From there, they are thought to enter the lacrimal gland via the superior branch of the zygomatic nerve, via an anastomosis between the zygomaticotemporal nerve and the lacrimal nerve. Whether the anastomosis between the zygomaticotemporal and lacrimal nerves is uniformly present has been debated. What role, if any, the sympathetic nervous system plays in lacrimation is not well understood.

The accessory exocrine glands of Krause and Wolfring are located deep within the superior fornix and just above the superior border of the tarsus, respectively. Aqueous lacrimal secretion has traditionally been divided into basal low-level secretion and reflex secretion. Previously, it was argued that the accessory glands provided basal tear secretion and the lacrimal gland was responsible for reflex tearing. However, recent evidence suggests that all tearing may be reflex.

The tear film composition is as follows:

- Goblet cells within the conjunctiva provide the inner layer of the tear film by secreting mucin, which allows for even distribution of the tear film over the ocular surface.
- The main and accessory lacrimal gland secretions form the intermediate aqueous layer of the tear film.
- Meibomian glands produce the oily outer layer of the tear film, which reduces the evaporation of the underlying aqueous layer.

See BCSC Section 2, *Fundamentals and Principles of Ophthalmology,* for a more detailed discussion of the tear film.

Excretory Apparatus

The entrance to the lacrimal drainage system is through puncta located medially on the margin of both the upper and the lower eyelids (Fig 12-1). The lower puncta lie slightly farther lateral than the upper puncta. Normally, the puncta are slightly inverted, lying

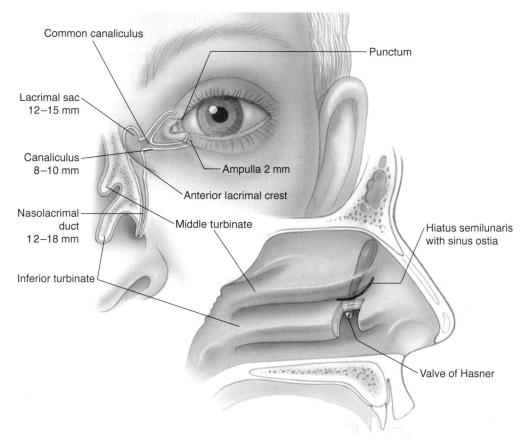

Figure 12-1 Normal anatomy of the lacrimal excretory system. Measurements are for adults. *(Illustration by Christine Gralapp.)*

against the globe within the tear lake. Each punctum is surrounded by its respective ampulla, a fleshy elevation oriented perpendicular to the eyelid margin.

Each punctum leads to its respective canaliculus. The canaliculi are lined with non-keratinized, non–mucin-producing stratified squamous epithelium. They run roughly 2 mm vertically, and then turn 90° and run 8–10 mm medially to connect with the lacrimal sac. In more than 90% of patients, the canaliculi combine to form a single common canaliculus before entering the lateral wall of the lacrimal sac.

The *valve of Rosenmüller* has traditionally been described as the structure that prevents tear reflux from the sac back into the canaliculi. The presence of a mucosal fold was detected with electron microscopy. This fold (valve of Rosenmüller) presumably functions as a 1-way valve. Additional studies suggest that the common canaliculus consistently bends from a posterior to an anterior direction behind the medial canthal tendon before entering the lacrimal sac at an acute angle. This bend, in conjunction with the fold of mucosa, may play a role in blocking reflux.

Located in the anterior medial orbit, the lacrimal sac lies within a bony fossa that is bordered by the anterior and posterior lacrimal crests, to which the medial canthal tendon attaches. The medial canthal tendon is a complex structure composed of anterior and posterior crura. The superficial head attaches to the anterior lacrimal crest; the deep head (the Horner muscle), to the posterior lacrimal crest. The medial wall of the fossa (the lamina papyracea) is composed of the lacrimal bone posteriorly and the frontal process of the maxilla anteriorly. Medial to the lamina papyracea is the middle meatus of the nose, sometimes with intervening ethmoid cells. The dome of the sac extends several millimeters above the medial canthal tendon. Superiorly, the sac is lined with fibrous tissue. This may explain why, in most cases, lacrimal sac distension extends inferior to the medial canthal tendon. Inferiorly, the lacrimal sac is continuous with the NLD. Additional structures that the surgeon should be aware of when operating in and around the lacrimal sac are the angular artery and vein, which lie 7–8 mm medial to the medial canthal angle and anastomose with the vascular systems of the face and orbit.

The NLD measures 12 mm or more in length. It travels through bone within the nasolacrimal canal, which initially curves in an inferior and slightly lateral and posterior direction. The NLD opens into the nose through an ostium under the inferior turbinate (the inferior meatus), which is usually partially covered by a mucosal fold (the valve of Hasner; see Fig 12-1). Failure of this ostium to develop is, in most cases, the cause of congenital NLD obstruction. The exact configuration of the ostium varies, but it is located fairly anteriorly in the inferior nasal meatus, approximately 2.5 cm posterior to the naris.

Physiology

Evaporation accounts for approximately 10% of tear elimination in the young and for 20% or more in the elderly. Most of the tear flow is actively pumped from the tear lake by the actions of the orbicularis muscle. Several variations in the theoretical mechanism of the tear pump have been proposed. In the mechanism described by Rosengren-Doane, the contraction of the orbicularis provides the motive power (Fig 12-2). The contraction is thought to produce positive pressure in the tear sac, forcing tears into the nose. As the eyelids open and move laterally, negative pressure is produced in the sac. This pressure is initially contained by opposition of the eyelids and therefore the puncta. When the eyelids are fully opened, the puncta pop open and the negative pressure draws tears into the canaliculi. A weakened blink interferes with the normal lacrimal pumping mechanism and explains why some patients with partial facial nerve palsies experience epiphora.

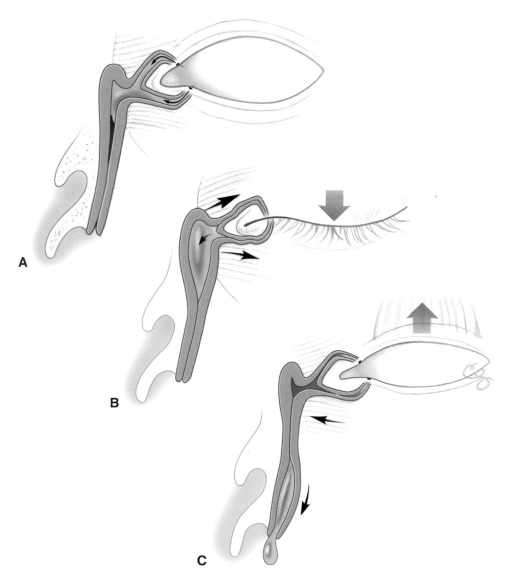

Figure 12-2 Lacrimal pump. **A,** In the relaxed state, the puncta lie in the tear lake. **B,** With eyelid closure, the orbicularis contracts. The pretarsal orbicularis squeezes and closes the canaliculi. The preseptal orbicularis, which inserts into the lacrimal sac, pulls the lacrimal sac open, creating a negative pressure that draws the tears into the sac. **C,** With eyelid opening, the orbicularis relaxes, and the elastic forces create a positive pressure in the sac that propels the tears down the duct. *(Illustration by Christine Gralapp.)*

CHAPTER 13

Abnormalities of the Lacrimal Secretory and Drainage Systems

Treatment of lacrimal drainage obstruction differs according to the cause of the obstruction and whether the obstruction involves the puncta, canaliculi, lacrimal sac, or nasolacrimal duct (NLD). Because of differing pathophysiology and management, congenital and acquired abnormalities are addressed separately.

Congenital Lacrimal Drainage Obstruction

Evaluation

The evaluation of congenital tearing is straightforward in most cases: the patient's parents give a history of tearing or mucopurulent discharge (or both) beginning shortly after birth. In rare cases, distension of the sac is present, suggesting a congenital dacrycystocele. Otherwise, distinction should be made among the following characteristics:

- constant tearing with minimal mucopurulence, which suggests an upper system block caused by punctal or canalicular dysgenesis
- constant tearing with frequent mucopurulence and matting of the lashes, which suggests complete obstruction of the NLD
- intermittent tearing with mucopurulence, which suggests intermittent obstruction of the NLD, most likely the result of impaction of a swollen inferior nasal turbinate, such as in association with an upper respiratory tract infection

Office examination includes inspection of the eyelid margins for open puncta and evaluation for extrinsic causes of reflex hypersecretion, including sources of ocular surface irritation. These causes may include infectious conjunctivitis, epiblepharon, trichiasis, and congenital glaucoma. Inspection of the medial canthal region for a distended lacrimal sac (below the tendon), inflammation, or congenital defects such as an encephalocele (above the tendon) is important. However, the single most important maneuver is digital pressure over the tear sac. A dome-shaped distension of the sac suggests congenital obstruction. If mucoid reflux is present, complete obstruction at the level of the NLD becomes the working diagnosis.

Punctal and Canalicular Agenesis and Dysgenesis

The medial eyelid margin should be carefully inspected for the presence of elevated lacrimal papillae. Close evaluation with magnification may reveal a punctum with a membranous occlusion in patients who were initially thought to have complete punctal agenesis. Such membranes can usually be opened without difficulty with a sharp probe or medium-caliber needle. Temporary intubation (discussed later in this section) or placement of a silicone plug may help prevent recurrence. If the punctum is truly absent, the surgeon may cut down through the eyelid margin in the expected area of the lateral canaliculus or perform retrograde probing through an open lacrimal sac with direct visualization of the common canalicular opening (common internal punctum). However, punctal agenesis is usually associated with the absence of underlying canalicular tissue. Occasionally, these maneuvers reveal the presence of a relatively mature canalicular system with a patent nasolacrimal sac and duct. In this case, intubation may be performed. Symptomatic patients with a single punctum frequently require surgery to relieve nasolacrimal rather than canalicular obstruction. Complete absence of the punctum and the canalicular system requires a conjunctivodacryocystorhinostomy (CDCR) when the patient is old enough to allow manipulation of, and to care for, the Jones tube. (CDCR is discussed later in this chapter under Canalicular Obstruction.)

Lyons CJ, Rosser PM, Welham RA. The management of punctal agenesis. *Ophthalmology*. 1993;100(12):1851–1855.

Congenital Nasolacrimal Duct Obstruction

Congenital obstruction of the lacrimal drainage system, which is usually caused by a membranous blockage of the valve of Hasner covering the nasal end of the NLD, may be present in roughly 50% of newborn infants. Most obstructions open spontaneously within 4–6 weeks after birth. Such an obstruction becomes clinically evident in only 2%–6% of full-term infants at 3–4 weeks of age. Of these, one-third have bilateral involvement. Approximately 90% of all symptomatic congenital NLD obstructions resolve in the first year of life.

Numerous management options are available, and they can be divided loosely into conservative (nonsurgical) and surgical. Conservative options include observation, lacrimal sac massage, and topical antibiotics. The long-term use of topical antibiotics may be needed to suppress chronic mucoid discharge with matting of the lashes.

When the obstruction fails to resolve with conservative measures, more invasive intervention may be required. Most often this consists of probing of the NLD in order to rupture a presumptive membrane occluding the NLD at the duct's exit in the nose (discussed in detail later in this chapter). In cases associated with airway obstruction or dacryocystitis, prompt treatment may be required. However, in uncomplicated cases, opinions differ regarding how long clinicians should continue with conservative management before probing.

Most cases of congenital NLD obstruction—including infants with clinical symptoms at 6 months—resolve in the first year of life. Several reports have suggested that delaying probing past 13 months of age may be associated with a decreased success rate. Most likely, the observed lower success rate of probing beyond 1 year was the result of a selection bias. If probing is delayed until after 1 year of age, a number of patients will resolve spontaneously. If probing were performed in these patients earlier than 1 year of age, these cases would be considered successfully managed with probing. Thus, the perceived success rate of later probing is lowered. Regardless, the more recent trend is for surgeons to observe these patients, with the hope of spontaneous resolution, until the patients approach 1 year of age.

Although the trend has been to perform probing with the patient under sedation if symptoms persist at 1 year of age, some advocate office probing earlier, usually at 6 months of age. In a younger child, probing in the office is more easily performed and topical anesthesia can be used, whereas children aged 1 year or older usually require general anesthesia. Probing with topical anesthetic is inexpensive and relatively safe in well-trained hands. Early office probing avoids the potential for months of mucopurulent discharge, and a visit to the operating room is not necessary. Some advocates of early office probing report that the pain associated with this procedure appears to be about the same as that of an immunization injection.

In some instances of congenital NLD obstruction, dacryocystitis may manifest as an acutely inflamed lacrimal sac with cellulitis of the overlying skin. This possibility should be discussed with the parents so that treatment with systemic antibiotics can be started promptly. Management of the pediatric patient is similar to that of the adult patient (discussed in detail later). Following resolution of the infectious process, elective probing should be performed promptly to prevent recurrence of the dacryocystitis.

Casady DR, Meyer DR, Simon JW, Stasior GO, Zobal-Ratner JL. Stepwise treatment paradigm for congenital nasolacrimal duct obstruction. *Ophthal Plast Reconstr Surg.* 2006;22(4): 243–247.

Katowitz JA, Welsh MG. Timing of initial probing and irrigation in congenital nasolacrimal duct obstruction. *Ophthalmology.* 1987;94(6):698–705.

Probing and irrigation

Probing is a delicate surgical maneuver that is facilitated by immobilization of the patient and by shrinkage of the nasal mucosa with a topical vasoconstrictor, usually oxymetazoline hydrochloride. Some clinicians avoid the use of cocaine in children because of the risk of cardiac toxicity. Others believe that cocaine can be safely administered if the concentration used is no higher than 4% and if it is not used in association with intranasal phenylephrine or epinephrine.

When probing, the physician should recall that the upper system begins at the punctum, followed first by a 2-mm vertical segment and then by a horizontal segment of 8–10 mm (canaliculus). Punctal dilation is often needed to safely introduce a size 0 or smaller Bowman probe. The surgeon initially inserts the probe into the punctum perpendicular to the eyelid margin and then advances it down the canalicular system toward the medial canthal tendon while maintaining lateral traction with the opposite hand. Manual lateral traction of the eyelid straightens the canaliculus and decreases the risk of damage to the canalicular mucosa and creation of a false passage.

Resistance to passage of the probe, along with medial movement of the eyelid soft tissue ("soft stop"), causing wrinkling of the overlying skin, may signify canalicular obstruction.

More commonly, resistance is simply due to a kink in the canaliculus created by bunching of the soft tissues in front of the probe tip. When kinking is encountered, withdrawing the probe and maintaining lateral horizontal traction while reinserting the probe should eliminate canalicular kinking (Fig 13-1). If the probe advances successfully through the common canalicular system and across the lacrimal sac, the medial wall of the lacrimal sac and adjacent lacrimal bone will be encountered, resulting in a tactile "hard stop."

The probe is then rotated superiorly against the brow until it lies adjacent to the supraorbital notch at the superior orbital rim and then directed posteriorly and slightly laterally as it is advanced down the NLD. If significant resistance is encountered at any point during the probing procedure, the probe should be withdrawn and the procedure attempted again. The distance from the punctum to the level of the inferior meatus in the infant is approximately 20 mm. Direct visualization of the probe tip is usually possible with the use of a nasal speculum and a fiberoptic headlight or endoscope along the lateral wall of the nose approximately 2.5 cm posterior to the naris. If the probe is not visualized, patency of the duct can be confirmed by irrigation with saline mixed with fluorescein. The fluorescein can be retrieved from the inferior meatus and visualized with a transparent suction catheter (Fig 13-2).

A single lacrimal probing is successful in opening a congenital NLD obstruction in 90% of patients who are 13 months old or younger. In adults, irrigation and probing are limited to the canalicular system for diagnostic purposes only. Probing of the NLD in adults is potentially traumatic and rarely effective in permanently relieving an obstruction. Merely puncturing the scar tissue within the NLD only leads to further contraction.

Intubation

Intubation is usually performed with a silicone stent and is indicated for children who have recurrent epiphora following nasolacrimal system probing or for older children when initial probing reveals significant stenosis or scarring. Intubation is also useful for upper system abnormalities such as canalicular stenosis and agenesis of the puncta. Nasolacrimal intubation after failed probing has a reported success rate of greater than 70%.

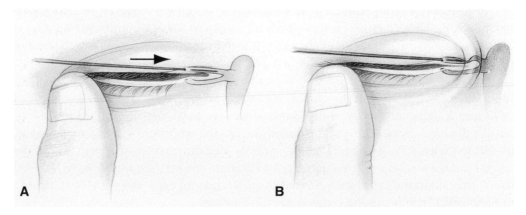

Figure 13-1 A, Bowman probe in right upper horizontal canaliculus. **B,** Attempted advancement of Bowman probe at site of canalicular atresia produces wrinkling of skin over the medial canthus. *(Illustration by Christine Gralapp.)*

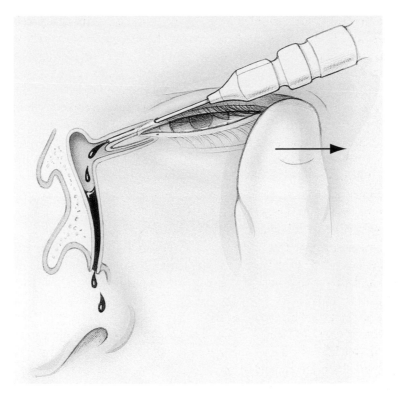

Figure 13-2 Irrigation of the nasolacrimal system. Dye is injected from the syringe, and patency of the system is confirmed by suctioning the dye from the inferior meatus of the nose. *(Illustration by Christine Gralapp.)*

Many intubation techniques and types of intubation sets have been described. Figure 13-3 illustrates one of the more commonly utilized stents (Crawford stent). Keys to successful intubation include shrinkage of the nasal mucosa with a topical vasoconstrictor and adequate lighting with a fiberoptic headlight. In more difficult cases, an endoscope can be used, and turbinate infracture is sometimes performed. The silicone tubing can be secured by a simple square knot that allows removal of the tube through the canalicular system in a retrograde fashion. Alternatively, the silicone stent may be directly sutured to the lateral wall of the nose, or the limbs of the stent can be passed through either a silicone band or a sponge in the inferior meatus of the nose. These techniques allow the stent to be retrieved through the nose. Monocanalicular stents are also available (Fig 13-4). This type of stent is passed through a single punctum to the nasal cavity, where the end of the stent is simply cut and allowed to retract loosely into the nose. The proximal end has a smooth barb and is self-secured at the punctum. The monocanalicular stent is useful when the patient has only 1 patent canaliculus.

Balloon dacryoplasty
Balloon catheter dilation of the nasolacrimal canal has been used successfully in congenital nasolacrimal obstruction. A collapsed balloon catheter is placed in a manner similar to probing and inflated inside the duct at multiple levels. The role of this modality remains

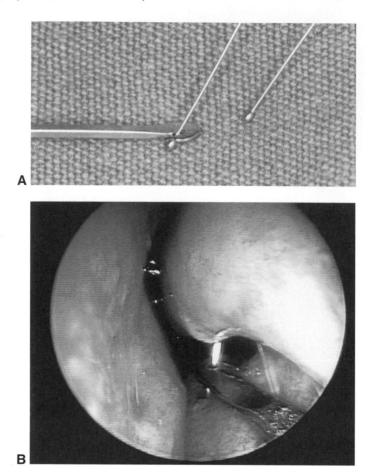

Figure 13-3 Crawford stent and hook. **A,** Hook engaging "olive tip" of stent. **B,** Intranasal view of engaged hook retrieving the stent. *(Reproduced with permission from Nerad JA.* The Requisites in Ophthalmology: Oculoplastic Surgery. *Philadelphia: Mosby; 2001:233.)*

Figure 13-4 Monocanalicular stent. At the proximal end is a soft barb and collarette, which secure the stent within the punctum. *(Courtesy of Roberta Gausas, MD.)*

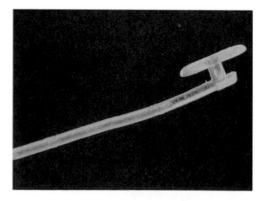

undefined in part because the necessary catheter equipment is expensive, and simple probing has a high success rate. Thus, balloon dacryoplasty is now generally limited to complicated cases or to recurrence following standard probing techniques.

Repka MX, Chandler DL, Holmes JM, et al; Pediatric Eye Disease Investigator Group. Balloon catheter dilation and nasolacrimal duct intubation for treatment of nasolacrimal duct obstruction after failed probing. *Arch Ophthalmol.* 2009;127(5):633–639.

Turbinate infracture

If the inferior turbinate seems to be impacted on the NLD at the time of probing and irrigation, medial infracturing of the inferior turbinate should be performed. This condition should be suspected in patients whose symptoms appear primarily related to upper respiratory tract infections, when swelling of the mucosa over the turbinate may cause intermittent obstruction of the inferior meatus. This procedure is most commonly performed as follows. The blunt end of a periosteal elevator is placed within the inferior meatus along the lateral surface of the inferior turbinate. The inferior turbinate is then rotated medially toward the septum. Fracturing the turbinate at its base significantly enlarges the inferior meatus and permits direct visualization of the lacrimal probe tip.

Wesley RE. Inferior turbinate fracture in the treatment of congenital nasolacrimal duct obstruction and congenital nasolacrimal duct anomaly. *Ophthalmic Surg.* 1985;16(6):368–371.

Dacryocystorhinostomy

Dacryocystorhinostomy (DCR) is usually reserved for children who have persistent epiphora following intubation and balloon dacryoplasty and for patients with extensive developmental abnormalities of the nasolacrimal drainage system that prevent probing and intubation. The details of DCR are discussed later in this chapter under Acquired Nasolacrimal Duct Obstruction.

Dolmetsch AM, Gallon MA, Holds JB. Nonlaser endoscopic endonasal dacryocystorhinostomy with adjunctive mitomycin C in children. *Ophthal Plast Reconstr Surg.* 2008;24(5):390–393.

Dacryocystocele

Mucoceles may form within the lacrimal sac or within the nasal cavity as a consequence of congenital NLD obstruction. The type of mucocele present in lacrimal sac distention has been termed a *dacryocystocele* (Fig 13-5). It occurs when the NLD is obstructed and amniotic fluid or mucus (secreted by lacrimal sac goblet cells) is trapped in the tear sac. The dacryocystocele is initially sterile and may respond to conservative management with prophylactic topical antibiotics and massage. If there is no response in 1–2 weeks or if infection develops, probing of the lacrimal drainage system may be needed. Distention of the nasal mucosa into the nasal cavity at the level of an occluded valve of Hasner may also occur. The intranasal portion often extends inferiorly under the inferior turbinate, where it can be observed during nasal examination. Excision or marsupialization of the prolapsed distended duct with nasal endoscopy is often necessary. Urgent treatment may be needed if the condition is bilateral and causes airway obstruction.

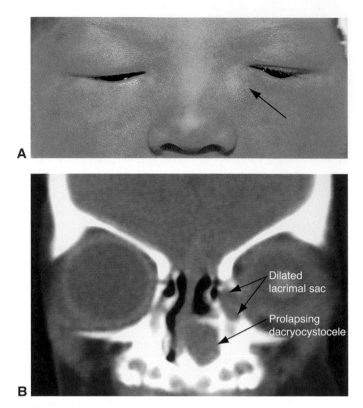

Figure 13-5 **A,** Left congenital dacryocystocele *(arrow)* 1 week postpartum. **B,** Computed tomographic scan of a congenital dacryocystocele. *(Courtesy of Pierre Arcand, MD.)*

In most cases, dacryocystoceles expand inferior to the medial canthal tendon. Congenital swelling above the medial canthal tendon, especially in the midline, should suggest alternate, often more serious, etiologies, such as a meningoencephalocele or dermoid. Proper imaging with computed tomography (CT) or magnetic resonance (MR) is mandatory to evaluate the patient for these more complex diagnoses.

Acquired Lacrimal Drainage Obstruction

Evaluation

History

Tearing patients can be loosely divided into 2 groups: those with hypersecretion of tears (lacrimation), and those with impairment of drainage (epiphora). The initial step in evaluating the tearing patient is differentiating between the 2 conditions. The following list can help guide the examiner in the assessment of the patient with tearing:

- constant versus intermittent tearing
- periods of remission versus no remission

- unilateral or bilateral condition
- subjective ocular surface discomfort
- history of allergies
- use of topical medications
- history of probing during childhood
- prior ocular surface infections
- prior sinus disease or surgery, midfacial trauma, or nasal fracture
- previous episodes of lacrimal sac inflammation
- clear tears versus tears with discharge or blood (blood in the tear meniscus may indicate malignancy)

Examination

Systematic examination helps pinpoint the cause of tearing. Similar to taking the patient's history, the initial step of the examination is to distinguish those patients with lacrimal drainage system obstruction and true epiphora from those with secondary hypersecretion.

Pseudoepiphora evaluation *Epiphora* is defined as overflow tearing. Some patients perceive their eyes as having too many tears but do not exhibit frank epiphora. These sensations are often caused by other ocular or eyelid abnormalities. For example, patients with dry eye may perceive foreign-body sensation or increased mucous production as excess tearing, but they do not exhibit true overflow of tears over the lid margin or down the cheek. In assessing pseudoepiphora, the ophthalmologist should consider the following:

- *Tear meniscus.* The size of the lacrimal lake as well as the presence of precipitated proteins and stringy mucus may indicate an abnormal tear film.
- *Tear breakup time.* The mucin layer of the tear film helps spread the other layers evenly over the corneal surface. This can be observed best after fluorescein has been placed in the conjunctival cul-de-sac. The patient is asked to open his or her eyes and refrain from blinking. The ophthalmologist then examines the tear film using a broad beam of the slit lamp. The normal time before breakup should be at least 15 seconds. Rapid tear breakup (<10 sec) may indicate poor function of the mucin layer despite a sufficient amount of tears.
- *Corneal and conjunctival epithelium evaluation.* Topical rose bengal and lissamine green can detect subtle ocular surface abnormalities by staining devitalized conjunctival and corneal epithelium. Fluorescein staining in the inferior third of the cornea indicates more severe tear film malfunction with epithelial loss.
- *Schirmer I.* This test measures tear secretion. A strip of filter paper is placed without anesthetic in the inferior cul-de-sac for 5 minutes, and the amount of wetting is recorded. The normal amount is approximately 15 mm. Hypersecretion is considered when the filter strip is rapidly inundated with tears. However, excess secretion may occur in response to the irritation from the measuring strips themselves. Serial testing should be performed to confirm this assumption. Schirmer I is one of several variations of the Schirmer test; some clinicians prefer the basic Schirmer test (measured after instillation of a topical anesthetic drop), finding it more useful in determining tear production deficiency. See also BCSC Section 8, *External Disease and Cornea,* for further discussion of tear film abnormalities.

- *Corneal irritation.* Patients should also be evaluated for mechanical irritation of the cornea. Corneal irritation from contact with eyelashes is a common cause of ocular irritation and secondary lacrimation. This can be seen in the setting of misdirected eyelashes (trichiasis) or eyelid malposition (entropion). Other ocular irritants include allergy; chronic infection, as seen, for example, with chlamydia or molluscum; and contact lens–related disease such as giant papillary conjunctivitis. Careful examination of the palpebral conjunctiva can aid in the identification of many such disorders.

Lacrimal outflow evaluation

Abnormal lacrimal outflow may result from problems in any number of structures. With eyelid malposition, tears might not have access to the puncta. Careful attention should be given to the eyelid and in particular the position of the puncta. Slit-lamp examination during the blink cycle may be needed to determine whether the punctum is properly positioned within the tear lake. Facial nerve dysfunction can result in a weakened or incomplete blink and may explain poor lacrimal pump function. Caruncular hypertrophy and conjunctival chalasis or frank prolapse can also occlude the puncta, and the patient should be evaluated for these conditions. Punctal stenosis, occlusion, or aplasia can be present.

Lacrimal sac evaluation can be invaluable. Palpation with pressure on a distended lacrimal sac may cause reflux of mucoid or mucopurulent material through the canalicular system. This reflux confirms complete NLD obstruction, and no further diagnostic tests are needed if a lacrimal sac tumor is not suspected.

Routine nasal examination may uncover an unsuspected cause of the epiphora, such as an intranasal tumor, turbinate impaction, or chronic allergic rhinitis. These conditions may occlude the nasal end of the NLD.

Diagnostic tests

The clinical evaluation of the lacrimal drainage system was originally outlined by Lester Jones. Evaluation was in the form of a dye disappearance test followed by a Jones I and Jones II test. By using this sequence (with modifications) as a guide, the physician can frequently streamline diagnostic testing.

The *dye disappearance test (DDT)* is useful for assessing the presence or absence of adequate lacrimal outflow, especially in unilateral cases. It is more heavily relied upon in children, in whom lacrimal irrigation is impossible without deep sedation. Using a drop of sterile 2% fluorescein solution or a moistened fluorescein strip, the examiner instills fluorescein into the conjunctival fornices of each eye and then observes the tear film, preferably with the cobalt blue filter of the slit lamp. Persistence of significant dye and, particularly, asymmetric clearance of the dye from the tear meniscus over a 5-minute period indicate an obstruction. Unilateral delayed dye disappearance is illustrated in Figure 13-6. If the DDT result is normal, severe lacrimal drainage dysfunction is highly unlikely. However, intermittent causes of tearing such as allergy, dacryolith, or intranasal obstruction cannot be ruled out.

Wright MM, Bersani TA, Frueh BR, Musch DC. Efficacy of the primary dye test. *Ophthalmology*. 1989;96(4):481–483.

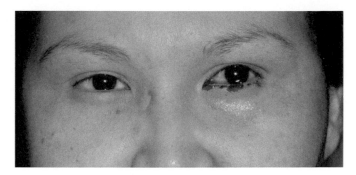

Figure 13-6 Dye disappearance test. *(Courtesy of Andrew Harrison, MD.)*

The Jones I and Jones II tests have historically been used in the evaluation of epiphora. Like the DDT, the *Jones I test,* or *primary dye test,* investigates lacrimal outflow under normal physiologic conditions. The examiner instills fluorescein into the conjunctival fornices and recovers it in the inferior nasal meatus by passing a cotton-tipped wire applicator into the region of the ostium of the NLD at 2 and 5 minutes. As this test occasionally yields abnormal results in normal patients, it is not uniformly performed.

The nonphysiologic *Jones II test* determines the presence or absence of fluorescein in the irrigating saline fluid retrieved from the nose. This test is performed as follows. The residual fluorescein is flushed from the conjunctival sac following an unsuccessful Jones I test. This is done so that the examiner can determine whether any reflux upon irrigation contains fluorescein. Irrigation of the lacrimal drainage system is performed with clear saline, which is retrieved from the inner aspect of the nose. Although some clinicians continue to use and rely on formal Jones testing, most have found retrieving the irrigating fluid from the nose to be technically difficult and have abandoned the test. Instead, they employ a simplified approach, using only the DDT and lacrimal irrigation.

Lacrimal drainage system irrigation is most frequently performed immediately after a DDT to determine the level of lacrimal drainage system occlusion (Fig 13-7). After instillation of topical anesthesia, the lower eyelid punctum is dilated, and any punctal stenosis noted. The irrigating cannula is placed in the canalicular system. To prevent canalicular kinking and difficulty in advancing the irrigating cannula, the clinician maintains lateral traction of the lower eyelid (see Fig 13-1). Canalicular stenosis or occlusion should be noted and confirmed by subsequent diagnostic probing. Once the irrigating cannula has been advanced into the horizontal canaliculus, clear saline is injected and the results noted. Careful observation and interpretation determine the area of obstruction without additional testing.

Difficulty advancing the irrigating cannula and an inability to irrigate fluid suggest *total canalicular obstruction.* If saline can be irrigated successfully but it refluxes through the upper canalicular system, and if no distension of the lacrimal sac is noted with palpation, *complete blockage of the common canaliculus* is suggested (Fig 13-8). Subsequent probing determines whether the common canalicular stenosis is total or whether it can be dilated. If mucoid material or fluorescein refluxes through the opposite punctum with

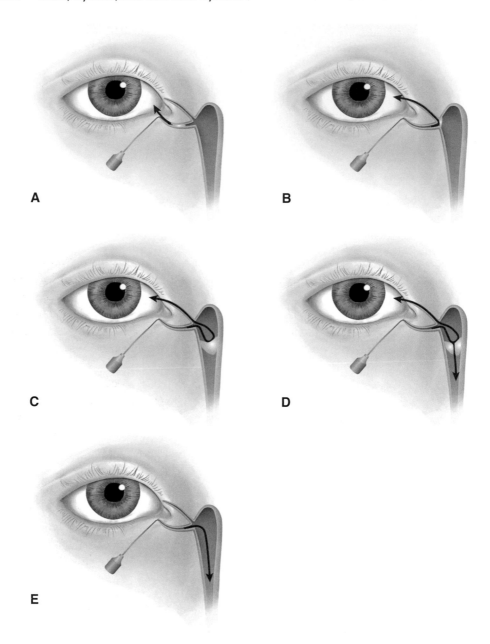

Figure 13-7 Lacrimal drainage system irrigation. **A,** Complete canalicular obstruction. The cannula is advanced with difficulty, and irrigation fluid refluxes from the same canaliculus. **B,** Complete common canalicular obstruction. A "soft stop" is encountered at the level of the lacrimal sac, and irrigated fluid refluxes through the opposite punctum. **C,** Complete nasolacrimal duct obstruction. The cannula is easily advanced to the medial wall of the lacrimal sac, then a "hard stop" is felt, and irrigation fluid refluxes through the opposite punctum. Often, the refluxed fluid contains mucus and/or pus. With an intact valve of Rosenmüller, lacrimal sac distension without reflux of irrigation fluid may be encountered. **D,** Partial nasolacrimal duct obstruction. The cannula is easily placed, and irrigation fluid passes into the nose as well as refluxing through the opposite punctum. **E,** Patent lacrimal drainage system. The cannula is placed with ease, and most of the irrigation fluid passes into the nose. *(Illustration by Cyndie C. H. Wooley.)*

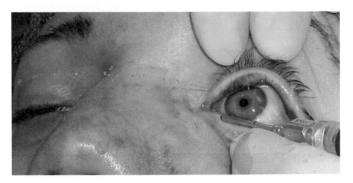

Figure 13-8 Reflux from opposite canaliculus caused by common canalicular obstruction. *(Courtesy of Morris Hartstein, MD.)*

palpable lacrimal sac distension, then the diagnosis is *complete NLD obstruction*. If saline irrigation is not associated with canalicular reflux or fluid passing down the NLD, then distension of the lacrimal sac with significant patient discomfort will occur. This result confirms a complete NLD obstruction with a functional valve of Rosenmüller preventing reflux through the canalicular system. A combination of saline reflux through the opposite canaliculus and saline irrigation through the NLD into the nose may indicate a *partial NLD stenosis*.

If saline irrigation passes freely into the nose with no reflux through the canalicular system, a *patent nasolacrimal drainage system* is present. However, it is important to note that even though this irrigation is successful under a nonphysiologic condition such as increased hydrostatic pressure on the irrigating saline, a *functional obstruction* may still be present. A dacryolith may also impair tear flow without blocking irrigation.

Diagnostic probing of the upper system (puncta, canaliculi, lacrimal sac) is useful in confirming the level of obstruction. In adults, this procedure can easily be performed with topical anesthesia. A small probe (00) should be used initially to detect any canalicular obstruction. If an obstruction is encountered, the probe is clamped at the punctum before withdrawal, thereby measuring the distance to the obstruction. A large probe may be useful to determine the extent of a partial obstruction, but the probe should not be forced through any area of resistance.

Diagnostic probing of the NLD has no place in adults because there are other means of diagnosing NLD obstruction. Also, probing in adults has limited therapeutic value, rarely producing lasting patency. In contrast, probing in infants is a useful and largely successful procedure. This reflects the differing pathophysiologies of congenital and acquired NLD obstruction, with the former often resulting from a thin membrane occluding the NLD and the latter from more extensive fibrosis of the duct itself.

Nasal endoscopy allows for direct visualization of the lacrimal passages. Diagnostic endoscopy takes only a few minutes to perform and is helpful in the evaluation of the nasal anatomy and in the identification of disease processes. Endoscopy can be performed prior to surgical correction of NLD obstruction, particularly if direct visualization is difficult.

Contrast dacryocystography and *dacryoscintigraphy* aid in the evaluation of the anatomy and function of the lacrimal drainage system. However, they are now used infrequently, primarily because alternate methods of evaluation are available such as simple irrigation and modern imaging techniques (CT and MRI). Contrast dacryocystography provides anatomical information with dye injection into the lacrimal system followed by computerized digital subtraction imaging. Dacryoscintigraphy provides physiological information using radionucleotide drops to follow tear flow using a scintigram.

Computed tomography and *magnetic resonance imaging* are useful after craniofacial injury, in congenital craniofacial deformities, or for suspected neoplasia. CT is superior in the evaluation of suspected bony abnormalities, such as fractures. It also allows assessment of the position of the cribriform plate, thereby helping to avoid injury at the time of surgery and subsequent cerebrospinal fluid leakage. MRI is superior in the evaluation of suspected soft-tissue disease, such as malignancy. Either CT or MRI may be helpful in evaluating concomitant sinus or nasal disease that may contribute to excess tearing.

Guzek JP, Ching AS, Hoang TA, et al. Clinical and radiologic lacrimal testing in patients with epiphora. *Ophthalmology.* 1997;104(11):1875–1881.

Punctal Disorders

Several punctal abnormalities can result in epiphora. Puncta may be too small (occlusion and stenosis) or too big (usually iatrogenic), or they may be malpositioned or occluded by adjacent structures.

Punctal stenosis and occlusion can occur in numerous settings, including congenital, inflammatory (Stevens-Johnson syndrome or pemphigoid), infectious (herpetic), and iatrogenic (deliberate occlusion in the treatment of dry-eye disease) conditions. Punctal stenosis is commonly associated with punctal ectropion. Punctal stenosis may be treated by dilation, punctoplasty, or stenting. Most often, the benefits of dilation are short-lived and punctoplasty is required. This is usually performed with a snip procedure, in which a small portion of the ampulla is excised. If stenosis recurs, stenting may be required during healing to prevent contraction. Treatment of complete occlusion consists of surgical canalization and, in most cases, stenting.

Abnormally large puncta can also cause epiphora, although this is somewhat counterintuitive. In this case, epiphora is thought to be the result of disruption of the lacrimal pump. The expanded opening prevents formation of an adequate seal when the eyes are closed. This in turn prevents development of negative pressure such that suctioning of the tears does not occur. Punctal enlargement is almost exclusively the result of iatrogenic injury. Stenting of the lacrimal drainage system can result in "cheese-wiring" of the puncta and adjacent canaliculi; therefore, patients with stents require periodic monitoring. Stents should be removed if punctal deformation is detected. Punctal enlargement can also result from overly aggressive punctoplasty and, occasionally, from excision of adjacent neoplasms. Damage to the puncta should be avoided because no uniformly effective treatment is available. Attempts at reconstruction usually fail, leaving a CDCR as the only reasonable alternative. Fortunately, symptoms are rarely severe enough to require this procedure.

In order to drain, tears must have access to the puncta. This access can be disrupted by a punctum that is malpositioned, such that the punctum no longer lies within the tear lake. In cases of epiphora secondary to punctal malposition, the anatomical abnormality must be corrected. Medial ectropion repair by resection of a horizontal ellipse of conjunctival and subconjunctival connective tissue below the punctum, with reapposition of the edges, rotates the punctum inward into the tear lake. This procedure may be combined with horizontal eyelid tightening if laxity is present. Frequently, punctal stenosis is also present and may require a punctoplasty.

Puncta may also become obstructed or malpositioned by adjacent structures, either a hypertrophied caruncle or conjunctiva (conjunctivochalasis). In most cases, this is easily corrected with excision of the abnormal caruncle or conjunctiva.

Canalicular Obstruction

Evaluation

Obstruction can occur within the common, upper, or lower canaliculus. Diagnostic canalicular probing may uncover a canalicular obstruction. *Partial obstruction* may be discovered during lacrimal system irrigation with partial fluid flow into the nose and partial reflux. *Total common canalicular obstruction* is characterized by flow from the lower to the upper canaliculus with no flow into the lacrimal sac during lacrimal system irrigation. After insertion, the lacrimal probe advances only about 8 mm from the punctum before encountering a tactile soft stop: the probe cannot be advanced beyond the total common canalicular obstruction. In normal conditions, a hard stop would be reached when the probe successfully passes through the open canalicular system into the lumen of the lacrimal sac and finally encounters the medial lacrimal sac and lacrimal bone. When common canalicular obstruction is present, lacrimal system irrigation results in a high-velocity reflux from the adjacent canaliculus (see Fig 13-8).

The clinician should keep in mind that what appears to be a partial obstruction may sometimes be a *total functional occlusion.* This can be seen with weakness of the lacrimal pump or inability of tears to pass through the partial obstruction under normal physiological conditions. Some functional obstructions may be overcome with irrigation by the creation of an abnormally high hydrostatic pressure.

Etiology

Lacrimal plugs Punctal and canalicular plugs, designed to obstruct the lacrimal outflow in the treatment of dry-eye disease, come in a variety of shapes and sizes. Although any type of plug can result in obstruction, this is most commonly seen with the Herrick Lacrimal Plug, which is placed deep within the canaliculus. Punctal plugs that are too small may migrate within the canaliculi and also result in obstruction. Even temporary or absorbable plugs have been known to cause a local inflammatory response and canalicular constriction. Canalicular probing is diagnostic. High-frequency ultrasound has also been used to identify silicone plugs causing obstructions within canaliculi. Once identified, the problematic plug can usually be surgically excised. Often, excision of a short segment of scarred canaliculus is required. The canaliculus is then repaired with reanastomosis over a stent. This technique is similar to reconstruction following trauma or after injury of the canaliculus during excision of a neoplasm.

White WL, Bartley GB, Hawes MJ, Linberg JV, Leventer DB. Iatrogenic complications related to the use of Herrick Lacrimal Plugs. *Ophthalmology.* 2001;108(10):1835–1837.

Medication Medications can occasionally cause canalicular obstruction. This is most often encountered with systemic chemotherapeutic agents (5-fluorouracil, docetaxel, idoxuridine). These drugs are secreted in the tears, which leads to inflammation and scarring of the canaliculi. Use of topical steroid drops and artificial tears during the chemotherapy may prevent the scarring. If this condition is identified early—before the obstruction is complete—stents can be placed to stretch constricted canaliculi and also prevent progression while the patient completes his or her course of chemotherapy. Less commonly, canalicular obstruction has also been reported to follow the use of topical medication (phospholine iodide, eserine).

Infection Numerous infections can cause canalicular obstruction. Most frequently, obstruction occurs in the setting of more diffuse conjunctival infection (vaccinia virus, herpes simplex virus). Isolated canalicular infection (canaliculitis; discussed later under Infection) can also result in obstruction.

Inflammatory disease Inflammatory conditions such as pemphigoid, Stevens-Johnson syndrome, and graft-vs-host disease often cause loss of the puncta and/or canaliculi. However, because of concurrent dry-eye disease, patients often do not suffer from epiphora.

Trauma Traumatic injury to the canaliculi can result in permanent damage if the injury is not managed in a timely, appropriate manner. This is discussed in greater detail later in this chapter in the section specifically addressing trauma.

Neoplasm When a neoplasm is present in the medial canthal area, complete resection may also include removal of the puncta and canaliculi. Complete tumor excision must be ascertained by histologic examination of excised tissue before connection of the lacrimal drainage system with the middle meatus is considered. When the distal lacrimal drainage system remains intact, the remaining portion of the canaliculi may be marsupialized to the conjunctival surface with or without intubation.

Management

Canalicular stenting *Intubation* or *stenting* of the lacrimal drainage system should be considered as first-line therapy whenever possible. Intubation of the nasolacrimal drainage system can usually be performed successfully when the patient has symptomatic canalicular constriction but not occlusion.

Reconstruction Reconstruction of an obstructed canaliculus is often successful when only a few millimeters are involved. If a limited area of total occlusion is discovered near the punctum, the occluded canaliculus can be resected, and the cut ends of the canaliculus anastomosed over a stent. When a focal obstruction is found distally or within the common canaliculus, trephining of the scarred segment establishes a patent lumen. Stenting is then required to prevent contracture and also to provide a scaffolding to direct proper epithelialization. Also, with removal of a punctal or canalicular plug, a small segment of scarred canaliculus is often excised, followed by reconstruction over a stent.

Caniculodacryocystorhinostomy If there is total obstruction at the common canaliculus, a canaliculodacryocystorhinostomy may be performed. In this procedure, the area of total common canalicular obstruction is removed, and the remaining patent canalicular system is directly anastomosed to the lacrimal sac mucosa. Use of a silicone stent for the reconstructed canalicular system is an important part of this type of reconstruction. Because the failure rate of canalicular resection surgery for total obstruction is significant, Jones tube placement is a surgical alternative.

Conjunctivodacryocystorhinostomy When 1 or both canaliculi are severely obstructed, a conjunctivodacryocystorhinostomy (CDCR) may be required. This procedure is a complete bypass of the lacrimal drainage system. A CDCR is indicated when the canalicular abnormality is so severe that the canalicular system cannot be used in the reconstruction of the tear outflow apparatus. A Pyrex glass tube (Jones tube) is placed through an opening created at the inferior half of the caruncle and then through an osteotomy site into the middle nasal meatus. A partial carunculectomy may be needed to prevent obstruction of the tube. The ocular end of the tube must be situated in the tear lake, whereas the nasal end must clear the anterior end of the middle turbinate. Subtotal resections of the anterior middle turbinate may be necessary. The surgeon should have tubes of different lengths available at the time of surgery so as to implant a tube that emerges clearly in the nose without abutting the nasal septum.

Postoperative care and complications, including obstruction of the tube with mucus and migration of the tube, can be troublesome. Forced inspiration, with the mouth and nose manually closed, creates significant airflow through the tube into the nasal airway and usually clears mucous debris and prevents obstruction. Patients should be instructed to perform this maneuver daily. They should also be informed that loss of the tube, even if only for a few days, may cause significant closure of the soft-tissue tract for the Jones tube. Periodic removal and cleaning of the Jones tube in the office, followed by immediate replacement, may be needed. Jones tubes themselves often cause chronic foreign-body sensation and mucous production and may incite pyogenic granuloma formation. Despite these drawbacks, many patients with otherwise intractable epiphora are helped by this procedure. Patients who have problems with recurrent migration or loss of the tube may benefit from placement of a frosted, angled, or modified Jones tube (Weiss Scientific Glass Blowing Company). Another alternative is the porous polyethylene-coated tube (Stryker Corporation), which allows for ingrowth of fibrous tissue into its outer covering. This ingrowth secures the tube in position.

Rosen N, Ashkenazi I, Rosner M. Patient dissatisfaction after functionally successful conjunctivodacryocystorhinostomy with Jones tube. *Am J Ophthalmol.* 1994;117(5):636–642.

Acquired Nasolacrimal Duct Obstruction

Nasolacrimal duct obstruction can usually be diagnosed with irrigation. There is a tendency for clinicians to assume that NLD obstruction is a relatively benign condition and proceed directly to a discussion of surgery. Although this is true in most cases, the alternate causes of NLD obstruction merit consideration.

Bartley GB. Acquired lacrimal drainage obstruction: an etiologic classification system, case reports, and a review of the literature. Part 1. *Ophthal Plast Reconstr Surg.* 1992;8(4):237–242. Part 3. *Ophthal Plast Reconstr Surg.* 1993;9(1):11–26.

Tucker N, Chow D, Stockl F, Codère F, Burnier M. Clinically suspected primary acquired nasolacrimal duct obstruction: clinicopathologic review of 150 patients. *Ophthalmology.* 1997;104(11):1882–1886.

Etiology

Involutional stenosis Involutional stenosis is probably the most common cause of NLD obstruction in older persons. It affects women twice as frequently as men. Although the inciting event in this process is unknown, clinicopathologic study suggests that compression of the lumen of the NLD is caused by inflammatory infiltrates and edema. This may be the result of an unidentified infection or possibly an autoimmune disease. Management almost uniformly consists of DCR.

Dacryolith Dacryoliths, or cast formation, within the lacrimal sac can also produce obstruction of the NLD. Dacryoliths consist of shed epithelial cells, lipids, and amorphous debris with or without calcium. In most cases, no inciting event or abnormality is identified. Occasionally, infection with *Actinomyces israelii* or *Candida* species or long-term administration of topical medications such as epinephrine can lead to the formation of such a cast.

Dacryoliths can form in patients with an otherwise normal lacrimal drainage system. When this occurs, patients often experience intermittent symptoms, depending on the location of the dacryolith. Dacryoliths also have a tendency to form with a preexisting obstruction; in this setting, symptoms are unremitting.

Acute impaction of a dacryolith in the NLD can produce lacrimal sac distension, which may be accompanied by substantial pain. Dacryoliths can be removed without difficulty during DCR.

Hawes MJ. The dacryolithiasis syndrome. *Ophthal Plast Reconstr Surg.* 1988;4(2):87–90.

Sinus disease Sinus disease often occurs in conjunction with, and in other instances may contribute to the development of, NLD obstruction. Patients should be asked about previous sinus surgery, as the NLD is sometimes damaged when the maxillary sinus ostium is being enlarged anteriorly.

Trauma Naso-orbital fractures may involve the NLD. Early treatment by fracture reduction with stenting of the entire lacrimal drainage system should be considered. However, such injuries are often not recognized or are initially neglected as more serious injuries are managed. In such cases, late treatment of persistent epiphora usually requires DCR.

Injuries may also occur during rhinoplasty or endoscopic sinus surgery; the management of these injuries is similar to the treatment of injuries occurring with fractures.

Inflammatory disease Granulomatous disease, including sarcoidosis, Wegener granulomatosis, and lethal midline granuloma, may also lead to NLD obstruction. When systemic disease is suspected, a biopsy of the lacrimal sac or the NLD should be performed at the time of DCR.

Lacrimal plugs As with similar cases of canalicular obstruction, dislodged punctal and canalicular plugs can migrate to and occlude the NLD. As with most forms of NLD obstruction, treatment consists of a DCR. Remaining segments of an improperly removed silicone stent have also been known to cause NLD obstruction.

Radioactive iodine Therapeutic radioactive iodine for the treatment of thyroid cancer may also lead to closure of the lacrimal apparatus. This is not seen with the lower dosages used for the treatment of the thyroid gland in patients with Graves hyperthyroidism.

Neoplasm Neoplasm should be considered in any patient presenting with NLD obstruction. In patients with an atypical presentation, including younger age and male gender, further workup is appropriate. Bloody punctal discharge or lacrimal sac distension above the medial canthal tendon is also highly suggestive of neoplasm. A history of malignancy, especially of sinus or nasopharyngeal origin, warrants further investigation. When malignancy is suspected, appropriate imaging studies (CT or MRI) should be obtained. Preoperative endoscopy is a quick and safe way to evaluate for intranasal neoplasm. In addition, if an unexpected mass or other suggestive abnormality is encountered during surgery, a biopsy should be obtained.

When a neoplasm is found to be involved with NLD obstruction, treatment should focus primarily on the neoplasm. In patients with benign tumors, a DCR or CDCR can then be performed. In patients with malignant tumors, surgical correction of the nasolacrimal drainage system should be postponed until there is certainty of clear margins or freedom from recurrence, after which a DCR or CDCR may be undertaken.

Tumors of the lacrimal sac and NLD are discussed in further detail later in this chapter in the section specifically addressing neoplasms.

Management

Intubation and stenting Some clinicians believe that partial stenosis of the NLD with symptomatic epiphora sometimes responds to surgical intubation of the entire lacrimal drainage system. This procedure should be performed only if the tubes can be passed easily. In complete NLD obstruction, intubation alone is not effective, and a DCR should be considered. Most surgeons feel that stenting has no role in the management of acquired NLD obstruction, and they routinely proceed directly to DCR.

Dacryocystorhinostomy A DCR is the treatment of choice for most patients with acquired NLD obstruction. Surgical indications include recurrent dacryocystitis, chronic mucoid reflux, painful distension of the lacrimal sac, and bothersome epiphora. For patients with dacryocystitis, active infection should be cleared, if possible, before DCR is performed.

Although there are many minor variations in surgical technique, all share the feature of creating an anastomosis between the lacrimal sac and the nasal cavity through a bony ostium. The most substantial distinction between techniques is whether the surgeon uses an internal (intranasal) approach or the more traditional external (transcutaneous) approach.

The advantages of an *internal DCR* include lack of visible scar, shorter recovery period, and less discomfort. In addition, an internal DCR can be performed in slightly less time than an external DCR. However, the success rate of an external DCR is at least equal to and probably substantially higher than that of an internal DCR. Most series report a success rate of 90% or higher for an external DCR, whereas success rates for an internal DCR have been around 70%, according to reliable accounts. When selecting a surgical technique, the surgeon should also consider that second attempts following failed DCR—no matter which approach was used—have a significantly higher failure rate. Therefore, patients should be counseled that if an internal DCR fails, the likelihood of a successful external DCR is somewhat decreased. An external DCR is also superior for management of an unexpected neoplasm or an intraoperative complication.

Thus, *external DCR* remains the preferred procedure of most ophthalmic lacrimal surgeons (Fig 13-9). Traditionally, DCR has been performed with general anesthesia, but in most adults, local anesthetic infiltration combined with anesthetic and vasoconstrictive nasal packing can be used, with the patient under monitored anesthesia care. However, monitored sedation requires both a cooperative patient and relatively deep sedation, and even in ideal circumstances, some patients report substantial discomfort.

Whether DCR is performed under general anesthesia or monitored sedation, intraoperative hemostasis can be enhanced by preoperative injection of lidocaine with epinephrine into the medial canthal soft tissues and by internal nasal packing with vasoconstrictive agents (oxymetazoline hydrochloride or cocaine 4%). The skin incision should be made so as to avoid the angular blood vessels and prevent wound contractures leading to epicanthal folds. The osteotomy adjacent to the medial wall of the lacrimal sac can be created with a rongeur, trephine, or drill. A large osteotomy site facilitates the formation of posterior and anterior mucosal flaps from both the lacrimal sac and the nasal mucosa. Suturing of the corresponding posterior flaps and anterior flaps is common, although not uniformly performed. Simultaneous stenting of the canalicular system may be needed, especially in patients who have common canalicular stenosis.

A biopsy with frozen-section examination should be considered if abnormal tissue is found. Some surgeons routinely perform a biopsy of the excised lacrimal sac. However, evidence suggests that in the absence of a grossly visible abnormality or indicative history, lacrimal sac biopsies are unlikely to reveal occult disease and should not be performed routinely.

Endonasal DCR consists of removing a nasal mucosal flap over the area corresponding to the nasolacrimal sac and duct (Fig 13-10). An osteotomy is performed to remove the frontal process of the maxilla and the lacrimal bone covering the lacrimal sac. Often, the surgeon also has to remove the uncinate process to allow proper exposure of the superior aspect of the lacrimal passage. The lacrimal sac is then opened, and the medial wall of the sac is removed, marsupializing the sac into the nose. Bicanalicular intubation is

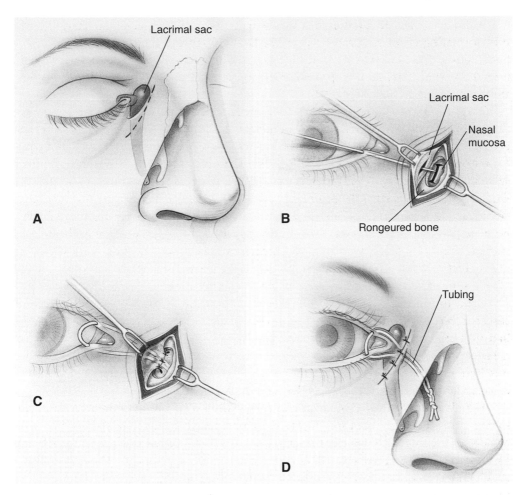

Figure 13-9 External dacryocystorhinostomy. **A,** Incision is marked 10 mm from the medial canthus, starting just above the medial canthal tendon and extending inferiorly. **B,** Bone from the lacrimal fossa and anterior lacrimal crest has been resected. Flaps have been fashioned in the nasal mucosa. A lacrimal probe extends through an incision in the lacrimal sac. **C,** Anterior lacrimal sac flap is sutured to the anterior nasal mucosal flap after a silicone tube is placed. **D,** Final position of the silicone tube following closure of the skin incision. *(Illustration by Christine Gralapp.)*

usually performed at the end of the procedure. Preserving the lacrimal and nasal mucosa may result in less scarring and a higher success rate, and techniques to preserve these structures have been proposed. Careful selection of patients with an adequate normal nasal cavity is crucial for success.

Several variations of endonasal DCR are available. Some surgeons use a fiberoptic probe passed through a canaliculus to transilluminate the lacrimal sac. This probe helps identify the thin lacrimal bone. Internal DCR can be performed endoscopically *(endoscopic DCR);* more recently, however, internal DCRs have been performed under direct visualization. Various laser systems have been used as adjuncts for bone removal. *Balloon catheters* have also been used to enlarge osteotomy sites. Many of these internal techniques

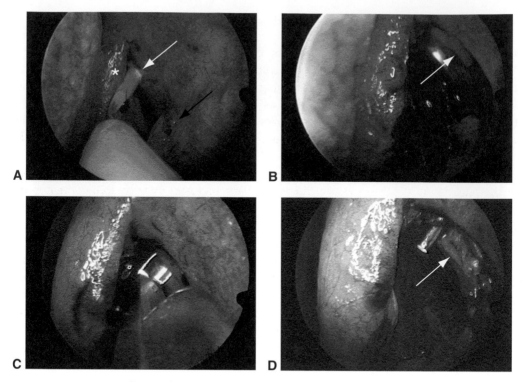

Figure 13-10 Transnasal dacryocystorhinostomy. **A,** Posterior incision behind the intracanalic-ular transilluminator *(white arrow)*, above the inferior turbinate *(black arrow)*, and just anterior to the insertion of the middle turbinate *(*)*. **B,** Frontal process of the maxilla after nasal muco-sal removal *(white arrow)*. **C,** Removal of frontal process of the maxilla with Kerrison rongeurs. **D,** Lacrimal sac has been opened *(white arrow)* and the transilluminator can be seen in the nose. *(Courtesy of François Codère, MD.)*

require expensive equipment, and most surgeons find that no matter what variation is used, the results are not comparable to the higher success rate of an external DCR.

Although DCRs are successful in most patients, failures do occur. DCR failures may be caused by fibrosis and occlusion of the osteotomy, common canalicular obstruction, or inappropriate placement or size of the bony ostium. The outcome of the DCR is also influenced by other factors, including the surgical approach used, the patient's history of trauma, the presence of active dacryocystitis, the development of postoperative infection, or hypersensitivity or foreign-body reactions to the stent. When an initial DCR fails, most surgeons attempt a second DCR before resorting to CDCR. Unfortunately, as previously noted, repeated DCR by any approach has a lower success rate. In an attempt to increase the likelihood of success, some surgeons apply mitomycin C, a potent antiproliferative alkylating agent, to the surgical site. This is thought to prevent fibrosis at the osteotomy site. The appropriate role of mitomycin C in repeat and possibly primary DCR continues to evolve.

Dolman PJ. Comparison of external dacryocystorhinostomy with nonlaser endonasal dacryo-cystorhinostomy. *Ophthalmology.* 2003;110(1):78–84.

Tarbet KJ, Custer PL. External dacryocystorhinostomy: surgical success, patient satisfaction, and economic cost. *Ophthalmology.* 1995;102(7):1065–1070.

Therapeutic Closure of the Lacrimal Drainage System

In cases of severe dry-eye disease, occlusion of the lacrimal drainage system may be helpful. Dissolvable collagen plugs may be used on a trial basis. More commonly, permanent plugs made of silicone are used. The advantages of permanent plugs are that placement is fairly straightforward and that, in most cases, they are removable. There are several varieties, and they can be divided into 2 categories: those that seat within the puncta and those that are placed within the canaliculi. Although permanent plugs are usually well tolerated, complications are occasionally encountered. Minor problems include ocular surface irritation and a foreign-body reaction. Pyogenic granulomas may develop, requiring removal of the plug. In most cases, the pyogenic granuloma regresses once the plug is removed, but surgical excision is needed on occasion. More serious complications usually relate to plug displacement.

Plug extrusion or *migration* is not uncommon. The ophthalmologist can best avoid these complications by using the appropriate size plug. There is an instrument that measures punctal diameter, and plugs are available in various sizes. When appropriately fitted, punctal plugs usually stay in place; but when they are improperly fitted, migration occurs. In most cases, a plug that is too small will simply be extruded. However, if the plug migrates within the lacrimal drainage system, obstruction of either the canaliculus or the NLD may result. Most instances of canalicular obstruction have been the result of plugs that were designed to be placed within the canaliculus. *Canaliculitis* may also result from canalicular plugs or punctal plugs that have migrated to the canaliculus.

When occlusion with plugs is not successful, the clinician may consider surgical occlusion. Surgery should be reserved for severe cases and must be performed with caution. Surgical closure is almost always permanent. If a patient suffers from subsequent epiphora, no simple solution is available, with most cases requiring a CDCR. To avoid this complication, all patients should be given a trial of temporary closure before permanent closure.

Once the decision has been made to proceed with surgical occlusion, the puncta should be closed in a stepwise fashion, 1 punctum at a time. The upper and lower puncta of the same eye should never be closed simultaneously. Complete loss of lacrimal outflow can result in epiphora even in patients with fairly severe dry-eye disease.

Numerous surgical techniques for occluding the lacrimal drainage system have been described. *Thermal obliteration* of the puncta and adjacent canaliculi can be performed with a handheld cautery unit. Although the argon laser can be used for thermal punctal occlusion, it offers no advantage over conventional techniques. *Ampullectomy* can be performed with either direct closure or placement of an overlying conjunctival graft. Often, despite fairly aggressive attempts, the puncta may persist or reform. In these recalcitrant cases, complete excision of the punctal and adjacent canalicular epithelium can be performed.

Kim BM, Osmanovic SS, Edward DP. Pyogenic granulomas after silicone punctal plugs: a clinical and histopathologic study. *Am J Ophthalmol.* 2005;139(4):678–684.

Mazow ML, McCall T, Prager TC. Lodged intracanalicular plugs as a cause of lacrimal obstruction. *Ophthal Plast Reconstr Surg.* 2007;23(2):138–142.

Trauma

Canaliculus

Most traumatic injuries to the canaliculi occur in 1 of 2 ways: by direct laceration, such as a stab wound or dog bite; or by traction, which occurs when sudden lateral displacement of the eyelid tears the medial canthal tendon and associated canaliculus. Being without tarsal support, the canaliculus lies within the weakest part of the eyelid and is often the first structure to yield. Whenever blunt trauma, such as from a fist or an air bag, results in a full-thickness eyelid laceration, the clinician should suspect and evaluate for an associated medial injury. The avulsion injury often appears trivial on superficial inspection, with its full extent revealed only on detailed examination of the area. When possible, diagnostic canalicular probing and irrigation may be helpful.

Because some patients who have only 1 functioning canaliculus may be asymptomatic, some clinicians consider the repair of an isolated single canalicular laceration to be optional. However, it is estimated that among patients with only 1 functioning canaliculus, 10% suffer from constant or nearly constant epiphora and 40% have symptomatic epiphora with ocular irritation, leaving only 50% fairly asymptomatic. Moreover, the success rate of a primary repair is much higher than that of a secondary reconstruction. Therefore, given the common occurrence of epiphora and the difficulties associated with delayed reconstruction, most surgeons recommend repair of all canalicular lacerations.

Repair of injured canaliculi should be performed as soon as possible, preferably within 48 hours of injury. The first step of the repair is locating the severed ends of the canalicular system. This can often be frustrating, but the controlled conditions of an operating room, including the use of general anesthesia and magnification with optimal illumination, facilitate the search. A thorough understanding of the medial canthal anatomy guides the surgeon to the appropriate area to begin exploration for the medial end of the severed canaliculus. Laterally, the canaliculus is located near the eyelid margin, but for lacerations close to the lacrimal sac, the canaliculus is deep to the anterior limb of the medial canthal tendon. Irrigation using air, fluorescein, or yellow viscoelastic through an intact adjacent canaliculus may be helpful. Methylene blue should be avoided, as it tends to stain the entire operative field. In difficult cases, the careful use of a smooth-tipped pigtail probe may be helpful for identification of the medial cut end. The probe is introduced through the opposite, uninvolved punctum, passed through the common canaliculus, and finally passed through the medial cut end.

Stenting of the injured canaliculus is usually performed to help prevent postoperative canalicular strictures. By putting the stent on traction, the surgeon draws together the severed canalicular ends and other soft-tissue structures, replacing them in their normal anatomical positions. Direct anastomosis of the cut canaliculus over the silicone tube can be accomplished with closure of the pericanalicular tissues. Direct suturing of the canalicular ends is probably not necessary. Lacrimal intubation also facilitates the soft-tissue reconstruction of the medial canthal tendon and eyelid margin.

Traditionally, bicanalicular stents have been used, but monocanalicular stents are gaining popularity (see Fig 13-4). One type of monocanalicular stent is attached distally to a metal guiding probe. This probe is retrieved intranasally. Thus, the monocanalicular stent can be used in soft-tissue approximation similar to the way a bicanalicular system is used. Another monocanalicular stent is inserted into the punctum and directly into the lacerated canaliculus to bridge the laceration. Other advantages of monocanalicular stents are the greatly reduced risk of punctal injury, or cheese-wiring, and their easier retrieval.

Stents are usually left in place for 3 months or longer. However, cheese-wiring, ocular irritation, infection, local inflammation, or pyogenic granuloma formation may necessitate early removal. Bicanalicular stents are usually cut at the medial canthus and retrieved from the nose. Monocanalicular stents are simply pulled through the punctum.

Jordan DR, Nerad JA, Tse DT. The pigtail probe, revisited. *Ophthalmology.* 1990;97(4):512–519.

Jordan DR, Ziai S, Gilberg SM, Mawn LA. Pathogenesis of canalicular lacerations. *Ophthal Plast Reconstr Surg.* 2008;24(5):394–398.

Kersten RC, Kulwin DR. "One-stitch" canalicular repair. A simplified approach for repair of canalicular laceration. *Ophthalmology.* 1996;103(5):785–789.

Reifler D. Management of canalicular laceration. *Surv Ophthalmol.* 1991;36(2):113–132.

Lacrimal Sac and Nasolacrimal Duct

The lacrimal sac and NLD may be injured by direct laceration or by fracture of surrounding bones. Injuries of the lacrimal sac or NLD may also occur during rhinoplasty or endoscopic sinus surgery when the physiologic maxillary sinus ostium is being enlarged anteriorly. Early treatment of the lacrimal sac and NLD is appropriate and consists of fracture reduction and soft-tissue repair, with silicone intubation of the entire lacrimal drainage system. Late treatment of persistent epiphora may require DCR.

Neuhaus RW. Orbital complications secondary to endoscopic sinus surgery. *Ophthalmology.* 1990;97(11):1512–1518.

Infection

Lacrimal Gland (Dacryoadenitis)

Acute inflammation of the lacrimal gland *(dacryoadenitis)* is most often seen in sterile inflammatory disease and occasionally is the consequence of malignancy, such as lymphoproliferative disease. Noninfectious disease of the lacrimal gland is covered in Chapter 4. Dacryoadenitis is extremely rare, and occurrence of gross purulence and abscess formation are even more uncommon. Most cases are the result of bacterial infection, which may develop secondary to an adjacent infection, after trauma, or hematogenously. Infections have also been reported to originate within a ductal cyst. Given the rare occurrence of these infections, large case series are lacking, as well as a precise breakdown of causative organisms and suggestions on management. Moreover, many nonsuppurative cases are treated empirically without isolation of the alleged pathogen. Presumably, most cases are due to gram-positive bacteria, although cases due to gram-negative bacteria have been documented. There are numerous reports of dacryoadenitis related to tuberculosis, with the formation of discrete tuberculomas in several cases. Epstein-Barr virus is the most frequently reported viral pathogen. There have also been numerous isolated reports of uncommon pathogens, including methicillin-resistant *Staphylococcus aureus*.

Canaliculus (Canaliculitis)

Canaliculitis, though usually of limited consequence, can be a challenge for patients and clinicians. Infection within the canaliculus is caused by a variety of bacteria, viruses, and mycotic organisms. The most common pathogen is a filamentous gram-positive rod, *Actinomyces israelii*.

The patient presents with persistent weeping, sometimes accompanied by a follicular conjunctivitis centered in the medial canthus. The punctum is often erythematous and dilated, or "pouting." A cotton tip applicator can be used to apply pressure to the canaliculus (ie, milking). The expression of purulent discharge confirms the diagnosis (Fig 13-11).

Canaliculitis can be somewhat difficult to eradicate, and the clinician should warn the patient that treatment may consist of several stages. A culture should be obtained when the patient presents. Conservative management then consists of warm compresses, digital massage, and topical antibiotic therapy. Initially, a broad-spectrum antibiotic is selected and then refined when culture sensitivities become available. Many patients require more aggressive treatment, particularly those with *Actinomyces* infection, which has a tendency to form concretions, or "stones." Within these stones, organisms are protected from lethal antibiotic concentrations. Occasionally, curettage through the punctum is successful. However, in most cases a canaliculotomy is required to completely remove all particulate matter.

The canaliculotomy should be limited to the horizontal canaliculus and approached from the conjunctival surface. The incision is left open to heal by second intention and does not require stenting. Some surgeons irrigate or paint the canaliculus with povidone-iodine or use specially formulated penicillin-fortified drops perioperatively. If the infection is the consequence of an obstruction, such as iatrogenic plug placement, the surgeon may need to correct the obstruction in order to prevent recurrence.

Lacrimal Sac (Dacryocystitis)

Inflammation of the lacrimal sac *(acute dacryocystitis)* has various causes. However, in most cases the common factor is complete NLD obstruction that prevents normal drainage

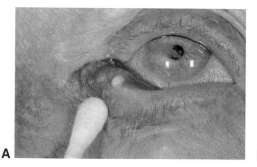
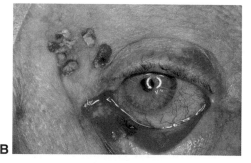

Figure 13-11 Canaliculitis. **A,** Pouting punctum expressing purulent material. **B,** Several small stones curetted from canaliculitis. *(Courtesy of Jeffrey A. Nerad, MD.)*

from the lacrimal sac into the nose. Chronic tear retention and stasis lead to secondary infection. Clinical findings include edema and erythema with distension of the lacrimal sac below the medial canthal tendon (Fig 13-12). The degree of discomfort ranges none to severe pain. Complications include dacryocystocele formation, chronic conjunctivitis, and spread to adjacent structures (orbital or facial cellulitis).

The following are guidelines for treating acute dacryocystitis:

- Irrigation or probing of the canalicular system should be avoided until the infection subsides. In most cases, irrigation is not needed to establish the diagnosis and is extremely painful in the setting of active infection.
- Similarly, diagnostic or therapeutic probing of the NLD is not indicated in adults with acute dacryocystitis.
- Topical antibiotics are of limited value. They do not reach the site of the infection because of stasis within the lacrimal drainage system. They also do not penetrate sufficiently within the adjacent soft tissue.
- Oral antibiotics are effective in most infections. Gram-positive bacteria are the most common cause of acute dacryocystitis. However, the clinician should suspect gram-negative organisms in patients who are diabetic or immunocompromised or in those who have been exposed to atypical pathogens (eg, individuals residing in nursing homes).
- Parenteral antibiotics are necessary for the treatment of severe cases, especially if cellulitis or orbital extension is present.
- Aspiration of the lacrimal sac may be performed if a pyocele–mucocele is localized and approaching the skin. Information regarding appropriate systemic antibiotic therapy may be obtained from smears and cultures of the aspirate material.
- A localized abscess involving the lacrimal sac and adjacent soft tissues requires incision and drainage. The incised abscess is packed open and allowed to heal by second intention. This treatment should be reserved for severe cases and those that do not respond to more conservative measures, because a chronically draining epithelialized fistula that communicates with the lacrimal sac can form.

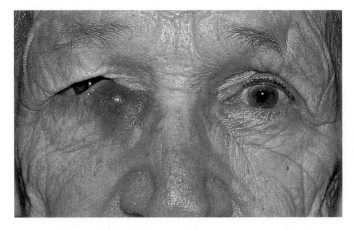

Figure 13-12 Acute dacryocystitis with cellulitis.

Dacryocystitis indicating total NLD obstruction requires a DCR in most cases because of inevitable persistent epiphora and recurrent infection. In general, such surgery is deferred until resolution of the acute inflammation. Some patients, however, continue to have a subacute infection until definitive drainage surgery is performed.

Chronic dacryocystitis, a smoldering low-grade infection, may develop in some individuals. This usually results in distension of the lacrimal sac. Massage may reflux mucoid material through the canalicular system onto the surface of the eye. Diagnostic probing and irrigation should be confined to the upper system in adults, because probing of the NLD does not achieve permanent patency in adults. If a tumor is not suspected, no further diagnostic evaluation is indicated to confirm the diagnosis of a total NLD obstruction. Chronic dacryocystitis needs to be surgically resolved before elective intraocular surgery.

Neoplasm

Lacrimal Gland

Neoplasms of the lacrimal gland are discussed in Chapter 5.

Lacrimal Drainage System

Neoplastic causes of acquired obstruction of the lacrimal drainage system may be classified into the following groups:

- primary lacrimal drainage system tumors (most commonly papilloma and squamous cell carcinoma)
- primary tumors of tissues surrounding the lacrimal drainage system that secondarily invade or compromise lacrimal system structures (most commonly eyelid skin basal and squamous cell carcinoma; also included are adenoid cystic carcinoma, capillary hemangioma, inverted papilloma, epidermoid carcinoma, osteoma, and lymphoma)
- tumors metastatic to the nasolacrimal region

Primary lacrimal sac tumors are rare and may present clinically as a mass located above the medial canthal tendon. They are often associated with epiphora or chronic dacryocystitis. Dacryocystitis associated with tumor may differ from simple NLD obstruction in that the irrigation fluid may pass into the nose. Also, with irrigation, blood may reflux from the punctum; and, more ominously, some patients may report spontaneous bleeding. Tumors that invade the skin may produce ulceration with telangiectasia over the lacrimal sac. Metastasis to regional lymph nodes may also occur. Dacryocystography is useful to outline uneven, mottled densities in the dilated lacrimal sac. However, CT or MRI is far superior in identifying neoplasms and determining disease extent. CT also has the advantage of clearly revealing bone erosion.

Histologically, approximately 45% of lacrimal sac tumors are benign and 55% are malignant. Squamous cell papillomas and carcinomas are the most common tumors of the sac. Many papillomas initially grow in an inverted pattern and into the lacrimal sac wall and, consequently, their excision is often incomplete. With recurrence, malignant degeneration may occur.

Treatment of benign lacrimal sac tumors commonly requires a *dacryocystectomy.* Malignancies may require a dacryocystectomy combined with a lateral rhinotomy, performed by an otolaryngologist. *Exenteration,* including bone removal in the medial canthal area, is necessary if a malignant epithelial tumor has involved bone and the soft tissues of the orbit (see Chapter 8). *Radiation* is useful in treating lymphomatous lesions or as a palliative measure in extensive epithelial lesions. The recurrence rate for invasive squamous and transitional cell carcinoma of the lacrimal sac is approximately 50%, with 50% of these being fatal. See Chapter 5 for further discussion.

Parmar DN, Rose GE. Management of lacrimal sac tumours. *Eye (Lond).* 2003;17(5):599–606.

Developmental Abnormalities

Lacrimal Secretory System

Congenital abnormalities of the lacrimal gland are relatively uncommon. Abnormalities include hypoplasia and agenesis of the lacrimal gland. Either can occur in isolation or, in some cases, in conjunction with congenital abnormalities of the salivary glands. Though usually occurring sporadically, both aplasia and hypoplasia have been reported to occur with an apparent autosomal dominant pattern. Lacrimal gland prolapse has been reported in association with craniosynostosis syndromes. Ectopic lacrimal gland tissue has also been found within the orbit.

Occasionally, children are born with an aberrant ductule, previously referred to as a *lacrimal gland fistula,* which exits externally through the eyelid overlying the lacrimal gland. These aberrant ductules exit laterally several millimeters above the eyelash line and are usually accompanied by an adjacent cluster of eyelashes. Tears produced from the aberrant ductules can mimic epiphora. These ductules can be successfully managed with simple excision.

Lacrimal Drainage System

Most developmental abnormalities of the lacrimal drainage system relate to (1) failure of the epithelial core to completely separate from the surface ectoderm from which it originated (multiple puncta or lacrimal–cutaneous fistula) or (2) incomplete patency, either at the eyelid (punctal/canalicular hypoplasia or aplasia) or intranasally (NLD obstruction).

Duplication

Uncommonly, multiple puncta and additional canaliculi develop. When the extra opening is on the eyelid margin, it is usually inconsequential and requires no treatment. The term *lacrimal–cutaneous fistula* has been used to describe those fistulas exiting through the skin infranasal to the medial canthus; this abnormality is discussed next.

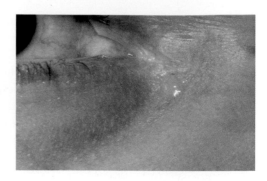

Figure 13-13 Congenital lacrimal–cutaneous fistula draining to the skin surface. *(Courtesy of Andrew Harrison, MD.)*

Congenital lacrimal–cutaneous fistulas

A congenital lacrimal–cutaneous fistula from an otherwise normal canalicular system or lacrimal sac is occasionally encountered infranasal to the medial canthal area (Fig 13-13). These fistulas are frequently asymptomatic or associated with a minimal amount of tears. Approximately one-third of patients have an underlying NLD obstruction, wherein chronic mucoid discharge from the affected nasolacrimal sac may be present.

In symptomatic patients, direct surgical excision of the epithelium-lined fistulous tract with direct suture closure is indicated. In patients with underlying NLD obstruction and chronic dacryocystitis, silicone intubation of the NLD may also be required.

> Birchansky LD, Nerad JA, Kersten RC, Kulwin DR. Management of congenital lacrimal sac fistula. *Arch Ophthalmol.* 1990;108(3):388–390.

Aplasia and hypoplasia

Punctal hypoplasia or stenosis is encountered more frequently than true aplasia. Moreover, in many cases of presumed aplasia, close evaluation with magnification reveals an intact punctum with a thin overlying membrane. Management of punctal stenosis, membranes, and aplasia is covered in the section addressing lacrimal drainage obstruction.

Nasolacrimal duct obstruction

In most cases, congenital NLD obstruction is due to failure of the duct to fully canalize; however, associations with more severe abnormalities have been described. For example, major facial cleft deformities can pass through or be adjacent to the nasolacrimal drainage pathways and produce outflow disorders.

> Sevel D. Development and congenital abnormalities of the nasolacrimal apparatus. *J Pediatr Ophthalmol Strabismus.* 1981;18(5):13–19.

Basic Texts

Orbit, Eyelids, and Lacrimal System

Albert DM, Lucarelli MJ, eds. *Clinical Atlas of Procedures in Ophthalmic Surgery*. Chicago: AMA Press; 2004.

Baker SR. *Local Flaps in Facial Reconstruction*. 2nd ed. St Louis: Mosby; 2007.

Bron AJ, Tripathi RC, Tripathi BJ. *Wolff's Anatomy of the Eye and Orbit*. 8th ed. Philadelphia: A Hodder Arnold Publication; 1997.

Chen WP. *Asian Blepharoplasty and the Eyelid Crease*. 2nd ed. Philadelphia: Butterworth-Heinemann; 2006.

Dutton JJ. *Atlas of Clinical and Surgical Orbital Anatomy*. Philadelphia: WB Saunders; 1994.

Dutton JJ, Byrne SF, Proia AD. *Diagnostic Atlas of Orbital Diseases*. Philadelphia: WB Saunders; 2000.

Fagien S. *Putterman's Cosmetic Oculoplastic Surgery*. 4th ed. Philadelphia: Saunders; 2007.

Holck D. *Evaluation and Treatment of Orbital Fractures: A Multidisciplinary Approach*. Philadelphia: Saunders; 2005.

Hurwitz JJ, ed. *The Lacrimal System*. Philadelphia: Lippincott-Raven; 1996.

Lemke BN, Della Rocca RC, eds. *Surgery of the Eyelids and Orbit: An Anatomical Approach*. East Norwalk, CT: Appleton & Lange; 1992.

Levine M. *Manual of Oculoplastic Surgery*. 4th ed. Thorofare, NJ: SLACK Incorporated; 2010.

McCord CD, Tanenbaum M, Nunery WR, eds. *Oculoplastic Surgery*. 3rd ed. New York: Raven Press; 1995.

Nerad J. *Techniques in Ophthalmic Plastic Surgery: A Personal Tutorial*. Philadelphia: Saunders; 2009.

Nesi FA, Lisman RD, Levine RM, eds. *Smith's Ophthalmic Plastic and Reconstructive Surgery*. 2nd ed. St Louis: Mosby; 1998.

Rootman J, ed. *Diseases of the Orbit: A Multidisciplinary Approach*. 2nd ed. Philadelphia: Lippincott Williams & Wilkins; 2002.

Shields JA, Shields CL. *Eyelid, Conjunctival, and Orbital Tumors: An Atlas and Textbook*. 2nd ed. Philadelphia: Lippincott Williams & Wilkins; 2007.

Spencer WH, ed. *Ophthalmic Pathology: An Atlas and Textbook*. 4th ed. Philadelphia: WB Saunders; 1996.

Tyers AG, Collin JRO. *Colour Atlas of Ophthalmic Plastic Surgery*. 3rd ed. Oxford: Butterworth-Heinemann; 2007.

Zide BM. *Surgical Anatomy Around the Orbit: The System of Zones*. Philadelphia: Lippincott Williams & Wilkins; 2005.

Related Academy Materials

Focal Points: Clinical Modules for Ophthalmologists

Alford MA. Management of trichiasis (Module 4, 2001).

Biesman BS. Lasers in periorbital surgery (Module 7, 2000).

Cockerham KP, Cockerham GC, Zwick OM. Orbital inflammation (Module 9, 2007).

Cockerham KP, Kennerdel JS. Thyroid-associated orbitopathy (Module 1, 1997).

Dailey RA. Rejuvenation of the aging face (Module 2, 2004).

Dailey RA. Upper eyelid blepharoplasty (Module 8, 1995).

de Imus GC, Arpey CJ. Periorbital skin cancers: the dermatologist's perspective (Module 1, 2006).

de la Garza AG, Carter KD, Kersten RC, Purdy EP. Evaluation and treatment of benign eyelid lesions (Module 5, 2010).

Dresner SC. Ophthalmic management of facial nerve paralysis (Module 4, 2000).

Dutton JJ, Fowler AM. Botulinum toxin in ophthalmology (Module 3, 2007).

Gossman MD. Management of eyelid trauma (Module 10, 1996).

Howard GR. Management of acquired ptosis (Module 8, 1999).

Khan JA, Steinsapir KD, McCracken M. Facial fillers (Module 4, 2011).

Laquis SJ, Haik BG. Orbital imaging (Module 12, 2004).

Lauer SA. Ectropion and entropion (Module 10, 1994).

Lucarelli JM, Kaltreider SA. Advances in evisceration and enucleation (Module 6, 2004).

Lyon DB. Evaluation of the tearing adult patient (Module 9, 2002).

Meyer DR. Congenital ptosis (Module 2, 2001).

Patel BCK, Anderson RL. Essential blepharospasm and related diseases (Module 5, 2000).

Rubin PAD, Bilyk JR, Shore JW. Management of orbital trauma: fractures, hemorrhage, and traumatic optic neuropathy (Module 7, 1994).

Spinelli HM, Riou J-P. Aesthetic surgery of the lower eyelid (Module 7, 1995).

Wiggs EO, Popham JK. Evaluation and surgery of the lacrimal drainage system in adults (Module 12, 1995).

Print Publications

Arnold AC, ed. *Basic Principles of Ophthalmic Surgery* (2006).

Dunn JP, Langer PD, eds. *Basic Techniques of Ophthalmic Surgery* (2009).

Rockwood EJ, ed. *ProVision: Preferred Responses in Ophthalmology, Series 4.* Self-Assessment Program, 2-vol set (2007).

Wilson FM II, Blomquist PH, eds. *Practical Ophthalmology: A Manual for Beginning Residents.* 6th ed. (2009).

Academy Maintenance of Certification (MOC)

MOC Exam Review Course (2011).

Preferred Practice Patterns

Preferred Practice Patterns are available at http://one.aao.org/CE/PracticeGuidelines/PPP.aspx.

Preferred Practice Patterns Committee, Cornea/External Disease Panel. *Conjunctivitis* (2008).

Ophthalmic Technology Assessments

Ophthalmic Technology Assessments are available at http://one.aao.org/CE/PracticeGuidelines/Ophthalmic.aspx and are published in the Academy's journal, *Ophthalmology*. Individual reprints may be ordered at http://www.aao.org/store.

Ophthalmic Technology Assessment Committee. *Cosmetic Oculofacial Applications of Botulinum Toxin* (2005).
Ophthalmic Technology Assessment Committee. *Endonasal Dacryocystorhinostomy* (2002; reviewed for currency 2006).
Ophthalmic Technology Assessment Committee. *Functional Indications for Upper and Lower Eyelid Blepharoplasty* (1999; reviewed for currency 2003).
Ophthalmic Technology Assessment Committee. *Laser Blepharoplasty and Skin Resurfacing* (1998; reviewed for currency 2008).
Ophthalmic Technology Assessment Committee. *Orbital Implants in Enucleation Surgery* (2003; reviewed for currency 2008).
Ophthalmic Technology Assessment Committee. *Orbital Radiation for Graves Ophthalmopathy* (2008).

CDs/DVDs

Clinical Skills DVD series. *Plastic Surgery of the Eyelids* (DVD-ROM; reviewed for currency 2010).
Johns KJ, ed. *Eye Care Skills: Presentations for Physicians and Other Health Care Professionals* (CD-ROM; 2009).

Online Materials

Focal Points modules; http://one.aao.org/CE/EducationalProducts/FocalPoints.aspx
Hatton MP, ed. Cosmetic Facial Surgery (January 2009). ONE Network online course; http://one.aao.org/CE/EducationalContent/Courses.aspx

Lin LK, ed. Oculoplastic Trauma (August 2009). ONE Network online course; http://one
.aao.org/CE/EducationalContent/Courses.aspx

Ophthalmic Technology Assessments; http://one.aao.org/CE/PracticeGuidelines/
Ophthalmic.aspx

Practicing Ophthalmologists Learning System (2011); http://one.aao.org/CE/POLS/
Default.aspx

Preferred Practice Patterns; http://one.aao.org/CE/PracticeGuidelines/PPP.aspx

Rockwood EJ, ed. *ProVision: Preferred Responses in Ophthalmology, Series 4.* Self-
Assessment Program, 2-vol set (2007); http://one.aao.org/CE/EducationalProducts/
Provision.aspx

**To order any of these materials, please order online at www.aao.org/store or call
the Academy's Customer Service toll-free number 866-561-8558 in the U.S. If
outside the U.S., call 415-561-8540 between 8:00 AM and 5:00 PM PST.**

Requesting Continuing Medical Education Credit

The American Academy of Ophthalmology is accredited by the Accreditation Council for Continuing Medical Education to provide continuing medical education for physicians.

The American Academy of Ophthalmology designates this enduring material for a maximum of 10 *AMA PRA Category 1 Credits™*. Physicians should claim only the credit commensurate with the extent of their participation in the activity.

The American Medical Association requires that all learners participating in activities involving enduring materials complete a formal assessment before claiming continuing medical education (CME) credit. To assess your achievement in this activity and ensure that a specified level of knowledge has been reached, a posttest for this Section of the Basic and Clinical Science Course is provided. A minimum score of 80% must be obtained to pass the test and claim CME credit.

To take the posttest and request CME credit online:

1. Go to www.aao.org/cme and log in.
2. Select the appropriate Academy activity. You will be directed to the posttest.
3. Once you have passed the test with a score of 80% or higher, you will be directed to your transcript. *If you are not an Academy member, you will be able to print out a certificate of participation once you have passed the test.*

To take the posttest and request CME credit using a paper form:

1. Complete the CME Posttest Request Form on the following page and return it to the address provided. *Please note that there is a $20.00 processing fee for all paper requests.* The posttest will be mailed to you.
2. Return the completed test as directed. Once you have passed the test with a score of 80% or higher, your transcript will be updated automatically. To receive verification of your CME credits, be sure to check the appropriate box on the posttest.

   Please note that test results will not be provided. If you do not achieve a minimum score of 80%, another test will be sent to you automatically, at no charge. If you do not reach the specified level of knowledge (80%) on your second attempt, you will need to pay an additional processing fee to receive the third test.

Note: Submission of the CME Posttest Request Form does not represent claiming CME credit.

• **Credit must be claimed by June 1, 2014** •

For assistance, contact the Academy's Customer Service department at 866-561-8558 (US only) or 415-561-8540 between 8:00 AM and 5:00 PM (PST), Monday through Friday, or send an e-mail to customer_service@aao.org.

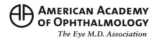
AMERICAN ACADEMY
OF OPHTHALMOLOGY
The Eye M.D. Association

CME Posttest Request Form
Basic and Clinical Science Course, 2012–2013
Section 7

Please note that requesting CME credit with this form will incur a fee of $20.00. (Prepayment required.)

☐ Yes, please send me the posttest for BCSC Section 7. I choose not to report my CME credit online for free. I have enclosed a payment of **$20.00** for processing.

Academy Member ID Number (if known): _____

Name: _____
      First   Last

Address: _____

_____
    City   State/Province   ZIP/Postal Code   Country

Phone Number: _____ Fax Number: _____

E-mail Address: _____

Method of Payment: ☐ Check   ☐ Credit Card   Make checks payable to AAO.

Credit Card Type: ☐ Visa   ☐ MasterCard   ☐ American Express   ☐ Discover

Card Number: _____ Expiration Date: _____

Credit must be claimed by June 1, 2014. Please note that submission of this form does not represent claiming CME credits.

Test results will not be sent. If a participant does not achieve an 80% pass rate, one new posttest will be sent at no charge. Additional processing fees are incurred thereafter.

Please mail completed form to:
American Academy of Ophthalmology, CME Posttest
Dept. 34051
PO Box 39000
San Francisco, CA 94139

Please allow 3 weeks for delivery of the posttest.

Academy use only:

PN: _____   MC: _____

Study Questions

Please note that these questions are *not* part of your CME reporting process. They are provided here for self-assessment and identification of personal professional practice gaps. The required CME posttest is available online or by request (see "Requesting CME Credit").

Following the questions are a blank answer sheet and answers with discussions. Although a concerted effort has been made to avoid ambiguity and redundancy in these questions, the authors recognize that differences of opinion may occur regarding the "best" answer. The discussions are provided to demonstrate the rationale used to derive the answer. They may also be helpful in confirming that your approach to the problem was correct or, if necessary, in fixing the principle in your memory. The Section 7 faculty would like to thank the Self-Assessment Committee for working with them to provide these study questions and discussions.

1. When removing bone from the medial wall of the orbit in an orbital decompression, the surgeon can locate the ethmoidal arteries along the
   a. sphenoethmoidal recess
   b. superior orbital fissure
   c. frontoethmoidal suture
   d. infraorbital canal

2. Orbital computed tomography (CT) scanning of a patient with a dural cavernous sinus fistula is likely to show enlargement of which one of the following blood vessels?
   a. central retinal vein
   b. pterygopalatine venous plexus
   c. superior ophthalmic vein
   d. inferior ophthalmic vein

3. What disease might be indicated by a salmon- or pink-colored mass in the conjunctival cul-de-sac?
   a. orbital lymphoma
   b. systemic lupus erythematosus
   c. lymphangioma
   d. xanthogranuloma

4. What condition typically presents with proptosis and axial displacement of the globe?
   a. maxillary sinus tumors invading the orbital floor
   b. lacrimal gland tumors
   c. frontoethmoidal mucoceles
   d. intraconal cavernous hemangioma

5. What is the best technique for visualizing the orbitocranial junction?

   a. magnetic resonance imaging (MRI)

   b. CT scanning

   c. ultrasonography

   d. plain films

6. A 61-year-old man presents with a 1-week history of redness and pain of the right eye. He wonders if this is related to his chronic sinus problems. On examination, his visual acuity is 20/20. His right upper eyelid is swollen. The right conjunctiva is injected with dilated episcleral vessels inferiorly. The underlying sclera appears inflamed. His ocular motility is limited, and there is 2 mm of proptosis in the right eye. A CT scan shows a diffuse infiltrate in the right inferior orbit. There is also thickening of the left nasal mucosa. Which of the following tests would be most beneficial in diagnosing this patient's condition?

   a. serum rheumatoid factor

   b. conjunctival culture for bacterial and viral pathogens

   c. serum erythrocyte sedimentation rate (ESR) and C-reactive protein

   d. serum antineutrophil cytoplasmic antibodies (ANCAs)

7. A previously healthy 6-year-old child presents with proptosis of the left eye. Family photographs reveal some prominence of the eye for the past year. One week prior to presentation, the child had a seizure of undetermined cause. Fundus examination reveals choroidal folds in the left eye. Which one of the following diagnostic tests is least useful in this case?

   a. fluorescein angiography

   b. orbital ultrasound

   c. MRI

   d. CT scan

8. What advantages does CT scanning of the orbit offer over MRI?

   a. better view of bone

   b. better soft tissue detail

   c. better image of the orbital apex

   d. more motion artifact

9. Which of the following lesions is most likely to be found in the superonasal quadrant of the orbit?

   a. Wegener granulomatosis

   b. mucocele

   c. benign mixed tumor

   d. meningioma

10. Perineural invasion and pain are associated with which of the following orbital tumors?
    a. esthesioneuroblastoma
    b. adenocarcinoma of the lacrimal gland
    c. adenoid cystic carcinoma of the lacrimal gland
    d. rhabdomyosarcoma

11. All of the following orbital diseases may improve with corticosteroids *except*
    a. thyroid eye disease
    b. orbital mucocele
    c. nonspecific orbital inflammation
    d. orbital lymphoma

12. A patient presents with a lacrimal fossa lesion. CT scanning shows a poorly circumscribed lesion with bone destruction. The most likely diagnosis is
    a. lymphoma
    b. adenoid cystic carcinoma of the lacrimal gland
    c. benign mixed tumor
    d. nonspecific orbital inflammation

13. A patient with declining visual acuity has an optic nerve sheath meningioma that does not extend outside the orbit. Which of the following is the best treatment?
    a. systemic corticosteroid therapy
    b. fractionated stereotactic radiation therapy
    c. proton beam radiation
    d. exenteration

14. The most common cause of unilateral proptosis in adults is
    a. lymphoma
    b. cavernous hemangioma
    c. thyroid eye disease
    d. meningioma

15. What is the study of choice for the evaluation of fractures in acute orbital trauma?
    a. MRI
    b. CT scanning
    c. nerve conduction
    d. orbital ultrasound

16. A 30-year-old man is evaluated in the emergency room for trauma to the right orbit. The patient has marked proptosis and an intraocular pressure of 40 mm Hg on the affected side. A CT scan shows intraorbital hemorrhage. Which of the following actions would be the least effective in acutely reducing intraocular pressure?
    a. lateral canthotomy and cantholysis
    b. administration of topical aqueous suppressants
    c. administration of intravenous mannitol
    d. administration of high-dose oral corticosteroids

17. Naso-orbital-ethmoidal fractures are most commonly associated with which one of the following findings?
    a. epiphora
    b. infraorbital nerve hypesthesia
    c. facial nerve palsy
    d. trismus

18. The best approach to an intraconal orbital tumor located between the optic nerve and the lateral rectus is
    a. transcaruncular orbitotomy
    b. vertical eyelid-splitting orbitotomy
    c. medial orbitotomy
    d. lateral orbitotomy

19. Dermoid and epidermoid cysts of the orbit are typically located
    a. deep in the orbit when seen in young children
    b. within the lacrimal gland
    c. along the inferior orbital rim
    d. in the superior temporal or superior nasal orbital quadrant

20. A biopsy is obtained for a presumed lymphoproliferative disorder. The appropriate way to submit the tissue is
    a. alcohol-fixed
    b. fresh
    c. formalin-fixed
    d. frozen

21. During decompression of the orbital floor, diplopia and dystopia can be minimized by preserving
    a. the palatine bone
    b. the orbital strut between the medial wall and floor
    c. the zygomatic bone
    d. the ethmoid bone

22. Which of the following is most important in the management of dermoid cysts of the orbit?
    a. deferring surgery until age 8 to avoid causing bony deformity
    b. filling in any bony defects with bone substitute (eg, hydroxyapatite)
    c. early removal to avoid malignant transformation
    d. removal of all cyst walls and cyst content

23. The primary advantage of nonporous compared to porous orbital implants is
    a. better orbital volume replacement
    b. lower exposure rates
    c. increased implant stability
    d. better prosthesis motility

24. The principle drawback to using a dermis-fat graft for acquired anophthalmos in adults is
    a. donor site morbidity
    b. unpredictable resorption of volume
    c. high extrusion rate
    d. high infection rate

25. What is the treatment of choice for keratocanthoma?
    a. observation
    b. corticosteroid injection
    c. incisional biopsy followed by complete surgical excision
    d. cryotherapy

26. When planning reconstruction of an eyelid defect, the surgeon should
    a. replace both anterior and posterior lamella with grafts
    b. avoid undermining adjacent tissue
    c. minimize vertical tension
    d. allow wounds to granulate prior to reconstruction

27. Appropriate management of multiple or recurrent chalazia includes
    a. needle biopsy
    b. shave biopsy
    c. local injection with triamcinolone
    d. full-thickness biopsy

28. The following measurements are obtained bilaterally in a patient with congenital ptosis: margin–reflex distance (MRD), +1 mm; eyelid fissure, 5 mm; and eyelid excursion, 4 mm. Which of the following bilateral surgical procedures is the most appropriate?

    a. frontalis suspension

    b. maximal external levator resection

    c. Fasanella-Servat

    d. müllerectomy

29. In a tarsal strip lateral canthoplasty, the strip is sutured to the

    a. opposite eyelid margin tarsus

    b. opposite limb of the lateral canthal ligament

    c. periosteum inside the lateral orbital rim

    d. periosteum external to the lateral orbital rim

30. The lacrimal sac is located

    a. between the anterior and posterior crura of the medial canthal tendon

    b. in the lacrimal gland fossa

    c. under the inferior turbinate

    d. anterior to the orbicularis muscle

31. A 45-year-old man has a mass medial to the inferior punctum and a yellow discharge from the punctum. Which of the following is the most appropriate management option?

    a. curettage with possible incision of the punctum

    b. aspiration of the mass with a large-bore needle

    c. oral steroids

    d. dacryocystorhinostomy (DCR)

32. The cause of congenital nasolacrimal obstruction is

    a. maldevelopment of the valve of Rosenmüller

    b. membranous block of the valve of Hasner

    c. retention of amniotic fluid in the nasolacrimal sac

    d. trauma during delivery

Answer Sheet for Section 7 Study Questions

Question	Answer	Question	Answer
1	a b c d	17	a b c d
2	a b c d	18	a b c d
3	a b c d	19	a b c d
4	a b c d	20	a b c d
5	a b c d	21	a b c d
6	a b c d	22	a b c d
7	a b c d	23	a b c d
8	a b c d	24	a b c d
9	a b c d	25	a b c d
10	a b c d	26	a b c d
11	a b c d	27	a b c d
12	a b c d	28	a b c d
13	a b c d	29	a b c d
14	a b c d	30	a b c d
15	a b c d	31	a b c d
16	a b c d	32	a b c d

Answers

1. **c.** The frontoethmoidal suture line defines the junction between the orbit and sinuses (below) and the anterior cranial fossa (above). This suture line is the superior-most level reached along the medial orbital wall in orbital decompression surgery. The anterior and posterior ethmoidal arteries pass through their respective foramina in this suture line, providing further anatomic clues to define the location within the orbit.

2. **c.** The superior ophthalmic vein drains into the cavernous sinus and is typically seen on neuroimaging studies coursing across the superior orbit. This vein enlarges in conditions such as dural cavernous sinus fistula that increase venous pressure within the cavernous sinus, with the superior ophthalmic vein transmitting this pressure into the orbit.

3. **a.** Orbital lymphoma primarily affects the anterior orbit and may be seen protruding beneath the conjunctiva in the cul-de-sac. Systemic lupus erythematosus may cause telangiectasia and edema of the eyelids. Lymphangioma has a vascular appearance and may affect the conjunctiva. Necrobiotic xanthogranuloma is associated with skin lesions with a propensity to ulcerate and fibrose.

4. **d.** An enlarging mass in the intraconal space such as a cavernous hemangioma would mechanically push the globe forward, resulting in axial proptosis. Maxillary sinus tumors are more likely to cause the globe to move superiorly (hyperglobus), and frontoethmoidal mucoceles will push the globe inferolaterally. An enlarging lesion in the lacrimal gland fossa will cause inferomedial displacement and proptosis.

5. **a.** MRI provides excellent tissue contrast of structures in the orbital apex, intracanalicular portion of the optic nerve, and orbitocranial processes. CT provides poor definition of the orbital apex. Ultrasonography is of limited value in assessing lesions of the posterior orbit because of sound attenuation. Plain films do not provide the level of definition obtained with CT or MRI.

6. **d.** The patient has a diffuse orbital inflammatory process with possibly related sinus disease on the opposite side. Inflammation associated with rheumatoid disease or an infectious process is unlikely to cause this. Giant cell arteritis associated with an elevated ESR and C-reactive protein rarely causes an orbital ischemic syndrome, but the patient is unlikely to retain good vision at that point. Wegener granulomatosis is associated with elevated serum cytoplasmic ANCAs and may cause a diffuse orbital inflammation with sinus involvement and small-vessel vasculitis affecting any organ system.

7. **a.** Although fluorescein angiography may highlight the choroidal folds, the pathology most likely to be the primary cause of problems in this patient will occur in the orbit and brain. CT, MRI, or ultrasound would be useful in the diagnostic evaluation of an orbital mass or an orbital mass with a possible intracranial lesion.

8. **a.** CT scanning offers exquisite detail of bone, which has little or no signal on MRI. The newest CT scanners have very short image acquisition times, whereas the physics of MRI demand a longer image acquisition time that makes motion artifact a potential problem. MRI generally outdoes CT in soft tissue contrast and imaging of the orbital apex, where surrounding bone may obscure soft tissue changes on CT.

9. **b.** Mucoceles, resulting from obstruction of the sinus excretory ducts, most commonly arise from the frontal or ethmoidal sinuses, thereby producing a superonasal mass when they expand into the orbit.

10. **c.** Although also malignant, rhabdomyosarcoma, lacrimal gland adenocarcinoma, and esthesioneuroblastoma are not associated with the rate of perineural invasion that is seen in adenoid cystic carcinoma of the lacrimal gland, the most common malignant tumor of the lacrimal gland.

11. **b.** Orbital inflammatory processes would be expected to respond to anti-inflammatory agents such as steroids. Orbital lymphoma initially improves with steroids, although it would not be expected to resolve completely and would generally recur. An orbital mucocele is not an inflammatory process and should not respond to steroids.

12. **b.** Orbital bone destruction is most commonly seen in the highly malignant adenoid cystic carcinoma of the lacrimal gland; however, even aggressive histologic variants of orbital lymphoproliferative disease have been associated with bone destruction as well.

13. **b.** Treatment of optic nerve sheath meningiomas is tailored to the individual patient based on the amount of visual loss and presence or absence of intracranial extension. Progressive visual loss with a tumor confined within the orbit is best treated with stereotactic radiotherapy. Attempts at surgical resection mostly result in visual loss or spread of tumor.

14. **c.** Thyroid eye disease is the most common cause of both unilateral and bilateral proptosis in adults. Proptosis is seen in up to 60% of patients with thyroid eye disease.

15. **b.** Excellent bony detail with simultaneous resolution of soft tissues makes CT scanning the study of choice in the evaluation for fractures with acute orbital trauma. MRI and orbital ultrasound studies may provide better detail of certain soft tissues and have greater utility in the evaluation of certain foreign bodies, but do not provide the bony detail seen in CT.

16. **d.** The trauma with proptosis suggests extrinsic compression of the globe, which raises intraocular pressure. A lateral canthotomy and cantholysis will typically lower intraocular pressure in this situation. Mannitol and topical aqueous suppressants will lower intraocular pressure arising from intrinsic or extrinsic factors. High-dose corticosteroids are postulated to have neuroprotective effects, but also carry numerous risks. They have no direct immediate effect on intraocular pressure.

17. **a.** Naso-orbital-ethmoidal fractures frequently involve the bones and soft tissues around the canthal tendons and lacrimal apparatus, including the nasolacrimal duct. Tearing due to damage at any of these levels is a frequent accompaniment to these fractures.

18. **d.** Lateral orbitotomy provides the most direct route to this lesion located between the nerve and the lateral rectus muscle. Medial incisions such as the transcaruncular and medial orbitotomy would lead to the medial orbital space on the opposite side of orbit compared to the lesion. The eyelid-splitting incision would also take the surgeon through a less-direct route to the lateral wall.

19. **d.** These lesions are thought to occur at lines of fetal suture closure. They are commonly (70%) located around the frontozygomatic suture line. They also occur at other fetal tissue suture lines, especially in the head and neck.

20. **b.** An essential step in pathologic examination for lymphoproliferative disease is the use of flow cytometry or other examinations for cell surface markers, to determine whether there is a monoclonal proliferation suggesting lymphoma. The specimen may be divided, with a portion submitted in formalin, but studies of fresh tissue are the most definitive.

21. **b.** Complete removal of the orbital floor with release of the periosteum may result in downward displacement of the globe following orbital decompression. Risks for this are diminished if the anterior portion of the medial orbital strut is left intact.

22. **d.** The surgical goal is to remove the entire lesion with the cyst wall intact. Leaving behind any of the wall of a dermoid cyst will result in recurrence of the lesion. Leaving any keratin contents behind will result in an acute inflammatory reaction. Dermoid cysts are often removed when they become clinically apparent to prevent rupture and an inflammatory reaction. Bone remodeling rarely requires intervention, and malignant transformation is rare.

23. **b.** Nonporous implants are an excellent, cost-effective choice for patients not requiring implant integration and have a lower rate of extrusion when compared to porous implants. They transfer motility to the ocular prosthesis only though passive movement.

24. **b.** Although dermis-fat grafts tend to grow with surrounding orbit in children, in adults resorption is unpredictable. They are valuable when there is limited conjunctiva in the socket and can be used as patch grafts in cases of implant exposure.

25. **c.** Although gradual involution over months has been observed with keratoacanthoma, this is regarded as a low-grade squamous cell carcinoma. Thus complete surgical excision is recommended.

26. **c.** Vertical tension on the eyelids can cause eyelid retraction or ectropion. When planning reconstruction of an eyelid defect, the tension of closure should be directed horizontally.

27. **d.** Recurrent chalazion may represent an underlying malignancy. Sebaceous adenocarcinoma may originate in the tarsal plate or the lash margin. A superficial shave biopsy may reveal chronic inflammation, but miss an underlying tumor. Thus a full-thickness diagnostic biopsy of the eyelid is recommended.

28. **a.** Frontalis suspension is correct, because this is a severe, bilateral ptosis with poor levator function. Müllerectomy and the Fasanella-Servat procedure generally work better in patients with mild cases of ptosis with better levator function. Large levator resections can work with in patients with poor levator function but in a unilateral, not bilateral, case.

29. **c.** The lateral tarsal strip needs to be attached to the periosteum inside the orbital rim so that the eyelid will be well-apposed to the globe. Suturing the strip to the external periosteum would leave the eyelid too distracted from the globe. Attachment to the opposite eyelid margin and canthal limb would not provide adequate support or place the eyelid in the proper position with respect to the globe.

30. **a.** The lacrimal sac is located in the anterior medial orbit within a bony fossa that is bordered by the anterior and posterior lacrimal crests, to which the anterior and posterior crura of the medial canthal tendon attach.

31. **a.** The initial treatment of canaliculitis is curettage, which may require snip incision of the puncta to allow access. Some surgeons advocate initial conservative treatment with warm soaks, digital massage, and topical antibiotic therapy.

32. **b.** The most common cause of congenital nasolacrimal obstruction is a membranous block of the valve of Hasner at the distal end of the duct. Congenital dacryocystoceles (amniotoceles) are caused by retained amniotic fluid in the nasolacrimal sac due to proximal and distal obstruction.

Index

(*f* = figure; *t* = table)